Pediatric Eye Care

edited by

SIMON BARNARD AND DAVID EDGAR

b

**Blackwell
Science**

© 1996 by
Blackwell Science Ltd
Editorial Offices:
Osney Mead, Oxford OX2 0EL
25 John Street, London WC1N 2BL
23 Ainslie Place, Edinburgh EH3 6AJ
238 Main Street, Cambridge
  Massachusetts 02142, USA
54 University Street, Carlton
  Victoria 3053, Australia

Other Editorial Offices:
  Arnette Blackwell SA
    1, rue de Lille, 75007 Paris
    France

  Blackwell Wissenschafts-Verlag GmbH
    Kurfürstendamm 57
    10707 Berlin, Germany

  Feldgasse 13, A-1238 Wien
  Austria

First published 1996

Set in $10\frac{1}{2}$ on 13 Plantin
by Best-set Typesetter Ltd., Hong Kong
Printed and bound in Great Britain
by The University Press, Cambridge
The colour plates in Chapter 12 have also appeared in *The Child's Eye: Diagnosis of Ophthalmic Disorders in Children* by B. Dhillon and G.T. Millar, published by Oxford Medical Publications in 1994.

DISTRIBUTORS
Marston Book Services Ltd
PO Box 87
Oxford OX2 0DT
(*Orders*: Tel: 01865 791155
        Fax: 01865 791927
        Telex: 837515)

North America
  Blackwell Science, Inc.
  238 Main Street
  Cambridge, MA 02142
  (*Orders*: Tel: 800 215-1000
          617 876-7000
          Fax: 617 492-5263)

Australia
  Blackwell Science Pty Ltd
  54 University Street
  Carlton, Victoria 3053
  (*Orders*: Tel: 03 347-0300
          Fax: 03 349-3016)

A catalogue record for this title
is available from the British Library

ISBN 0 632 03979 5

Library of Congress
Cataloging-in-Publication Data
is available.

This book is dedicated to the memory of Tere Simons

Contents

Section 3   Abnormal Neurological, Ocular and Orbital Conditions, 241

Section 4   Management and Treatment of the Child Patient, 281

Foreword

E.G. Woodward

*Head of Department and Professor of Optometry & Visual
Science, City University, London*

The stated intention of this book is to be a comprehensive guide to primary care in pediatric optometric practice. Primary care is defined as that sector of health care to which a patient has direct access without the need for referral from another health-care professional. The fact that an optometrist will usually be the first professional to see a child with actual, or potential, visual problems, only serves to emphasize the importance of this text.

Section 1 deals with basic science without which no profound understanding of the subject can exist. This is particularly so in an area where there has been so much new knowledge and development in the last few years. The remaining sections of the book cover the examination of children, disorders of the eye and the neurodevelopmental system, followed by a final section dealing with the management and treatment of the child patient. Perhaps of equal clinical importance, the relationship between practitioner and parent is also explored here.

The editors are to be complimented on assembling such a distinguished panel of experts to contribute to this text. Their disciplines include optometry, medicine, psychology and the basic science. It is an index of the regard in which the editors are held, that such a group of authors agreed to participate, and the result is a text which is both comprehensive in the academic sense, yet of immediate value to any clinician dealing with children.

It is with some pride that I note that so many of the authors have at some point in their career been connected with City University. The editors are both members of the academic staff of the Department of Optometry & Visual Science, both are parents, and their acquired expertise is evident from the scope and style of the text. There is no doubt that this book has achieved its stated objective and that it will become the pre-eminent textbook in this area for many years to come.

Preface

In the last decade there have been enormous and exciting advances in the understanding of visual development in children which have been matched by the development of new clinical tests. There has also been an increase in interest from optometrists wishing to develop their skills to enable them to provide optimum care for this most precious section of our community, children.

This book was written with the aim of providing a comprehensive guide to primary pediatric eye care both for the student of optometry and orthoptics, and also for the practising clinician – optometrist, orthoptist, ophthalmologist and pediatrician.

We are very fortunate to have so many experts in the field who have contributed chapters. Our only sadness is the loss to us, and to the optometric profession, of Tere Simons, who died during the writing of this book, which we dedicate to her. Tere's chapter on embryology, for which she personally drew all the figures, will always remind us of her.

Apart from teaching and practising within a university clinic environment, both of us have experience in private and hospital practice and one of us is a partner in a practice specializing almost entirely in children. Accordingly, we have tried to balance the academic content of this text with a practising clinician's view. We hope to offer some of our and the contributing authors' experience and thereby help the reader to develop her or his examination routine, and patient and parent management skills.

We hope that the book will encourage further interest in pediatric eye care, and be of assistance to students not only of the optometry and orthoptics degree courses, and to practising optometrists studying for the British College of Optometrists Fellowship, but also to the practitioner – optometric, orthoptic or medical – who is simply interested in reading more.

Finally, since we started on this project, both of us have become proud (and exhausted) fathers, and we now know a little of the story from the other side.

David Edgar, Simon Barnard

List of Contributors

Editors

N.A. Simon Barnard BSc (Hons), FBCO, FAAO, DCLP,
Lecturer in Clinical Optometry & Head of Pediatric Clinics, Department of Optometry & Visual Science, City University, London.

David F. Edgar BSc (Hons), FBCO, FAAO,
Senior Lecturer in Optometry & Director of Clinics, Department of Optometry & Visual Science, City University, London.

Authors

Jennifer Birch BSc (Hons), MPhil, DIC, FBA, SMSA,
Senior Lecturer, Department of Optometry & Visual Science, City University, London.

Baljean Dhillon B.Med.Sc, BM BS (Notts), FRCS (Glasg.), FRCOphth., MD,
Consultant Ophthalmologist, Princess Alexandra Eye Pavillion, The Royal Infirmary of Edinburgh, Edinburgh.

Bruce J. W. Evans BSc (Hons), PhD, MBCO, DCLP, FAAO,
Senior Lecturer, Institute of Optometry, London.

Brian Fleck BSc (Hons), MBCh.B., FRCS (Ed.), FRCOphth., MD,
Consultant Ophthalmologist, Princess Alexandra Eye Pavillion, The Royal Infirmary of Edinburgh, Edinburgh.

Elizabeth Gould FBCO,
Senior Optometrist, Moorfields Eye Hospital, London.

Elizabeth Green MD, BA (Hons), DCH,
Consultant Neurodevelopmental Pediatrician, MacKeith Centre, Royal Alexandra Hospital for Sick Children, Brighton, East Sussex.

Annette Grounds BSc (Hons), PhD, DIC, ARCS, FBCO,
Senior Optometrist, Clinical Coordinator and Research Director, Colchester Primary Ophthalmic Clinic, Essex County Hospital, Colchester, Essex.

Marcelle Jay PhD,
Senior Lecturer in Genetics, Institute of Ophthalmology and Moorfields Eye Hospital, Department of Clinical Ophthalmology, London.

Adrian Jennings PhD, MSc, FBCO,
Senior Lecturer and Clinical Director, Department of Optometry & Vision Sciences, University of Manchester Institute of Science and Technology, Manchester.

Stanley D. Klein, PhD,
Professor of Psychology and Director of Counselling Service, The New England College of Optometry, Boston, USA & Editor-in-Chief; *Exceptional Parent Magazine*.

Judith Morris BSc (Hons), MSc, FBCO, FAAO,
Director, The Institute of Optometry, London.

Henri Obstfeld MPhil, FBOAHD, FBCO, DCLP,
Senior Lecturer, Department of Optometry & Visual Science, City University, London.

Janet Silver MPhil, FBCO,
Principal Optometrist, Moorfields Eye Hospital, London.

Teresa Simons BSc (Hons), PhD, FBCO,
The late Teresa Simons was formerly lecturer in Ocular Anatomy, Department of Optometry & Visual Science, City University, London.

David Thomson BSc (Hons), PhD, MBCO,
Senior Lecturer in Optometry, Department of Optometry & Visual Science, City University, London.

Ivan Wood PhD, MSc, FBCO, FAAO,
Senior Lecturer, Department of Optometry & Vision Sciences, University of Manchester Institute of Science and Technology, Manchester.

SECTION 1
DEVELOPMENT

CHAPTER 1

Genetics

Marcelle Jay

1.1   Introduction

The unit of inheritance is the gene and the molecular basis of the gene is DNA – the molecule of life. The structure of DNA is such that it replicates at every cell division, and it provides a template for the formation of the gene products which determine the function of a cell. DNA is carried by chromosomes, and the number of chromosomes varies among different species. In man, there are 46 chromosomes disposed in pairs, 22 pairs being called autosomes and one pair called sex chromosomes, which together form the karyotype, the name given to an individual's complement of chromosomes. The sex chromosomes are identical in the female who has two X chromosomes, but in the male the sex chromosomes consist of one X chromosome and one Y chromosome. The karyotype of the normal male is 46,XY and of the normal female, 46,XX. In the same way as the word karyotype is used to describe the chromosome complement of an individual, the genotype is the term used to describe a person's genetic constitution, usually with reference to one specific gene, or else more generally. Externally observable characteristics are known as the phenotype, a descriptive term also often used in connection with the clinical appearance. For example, a male with Down's syndrome (or trisomy 21) would be described as having the karyotype 47,XY,21+, and his phenotype would include mental subnormality and the characteristic facial appearance of individuals with Down's syndrome.

In normal somatic cell division, each chromosome is replicated and daughter cells have the same number of chromosomes as the parent cell. The formation of gametes, sperm and ova, differs however, as each gamete carries half the total chromosome number made up from one chromosome from each pair. Each ovum carries 22 autosomes and an X chromosome, while each sperm carries 22 autosomes and either an X or a Y chromosome. The father determines the sex of his child, depending on whether the ovum has been fertilized by an X or a Y chromosome-bearing sperm. The fertilized ovum is called a zygote and will have inherited its genes from its parents.

Errors in the process of cell division or in the formation of gametes can give rise to abnormalities of chromosome number or chromosome structure. The presence of three chromosomes instead of two is termed trisomy, and a common such abnormality is trisomy 21 or Down's syndrome which occurs in about one in 600 live births. Absence of one chromosome of a pair is called monosomy, and absence of part of a chromosome is termed partial monosomy or more commonly deletion.

A chromosome spread normally shows chromosomes disposed in random fashion. However, a photograph of the spread can be cut and each individual chromosome pair may be arranged in descending order of size, and the pairs numbered from 1 to 22. Each chromosome is further described in terms of a short arm called 'p' and a long arm called 'q'. When chromosomes are stained, they show a pattern of alternating dark and light bands. This pattern is reproducible whatever the stain used, and has led to a numbering system which defines any given region in terms of long or short arm and a band and sub-band number. For example, 13 q 14 refers to chromosome 13, long arm, band 1, sub-band 4.

The position or site of a gene on a chromosome is called the locus, and since genes act in pairs (one on each chromosome of a pair), a locus refers to a pair of genes. Genes of a pair are not necessarily identical; for example, one may have undergone a mutation; or there may be alternative forms which occur in nature. These alternative forms are called alleles. Individuals may be homozygous, which means that both alleles for a gene are identical, or heterozygous, which is the term used to describe individuals who possess different alleles for a given gene. Males have only one X chromosome, half the number females have, so that a male with an X-linked disorder is termed hemizygous.

1.2   Autosomal dominant transmission

A disorder is autosomal dominant when it is expressed by the presence of one abnormal gene on one of the autosomes, so that affected individuals are heterozygous. Males and females are equally affected, and there is direct transmission from an affected parent to an affected child. Affected individuals with an unaffected spouse have a 50% risk of having an affected child depending on which chromosome of the relevant pair has been transmitted. This risk is the same for every pregnancy, and does not depend on whether a child born previously is affected or not.

There is a tendency for like to marry like, and this is termed assortative mating. In terms of visual impairments, there are many opportunities for the visually handicapped to meet during their school years or during vocational and guide-dog training. It is, however, very rare to find a marriage between two people with the same autosomal dominant disorder, though not uncommon to find a marriage between two people with different autosomal dominant disorders.

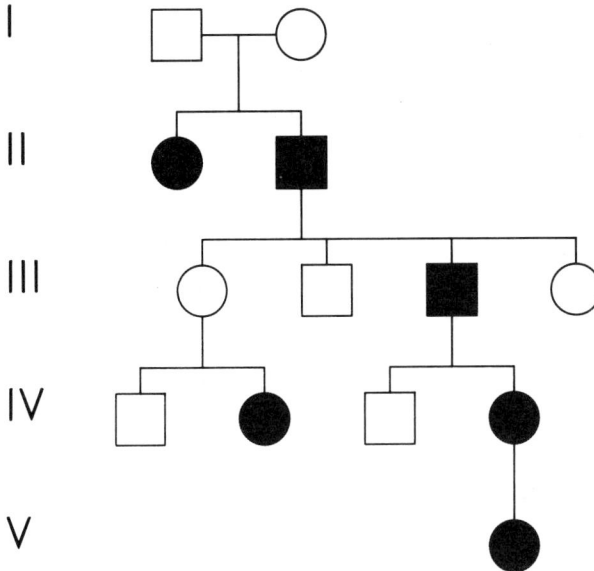

Fig. 1.1 Autosomal dominant inheritance showing transmission over four generations and reduced penetrance in one individual.

In each case of assortative mating, the risk of having an affected child can be calculated from the risk inherent to each parent: the risk for a child being affected with either of the parents' disorders is one in two, and the risk of that child being affected with both disorders is one in four. It is fortunately unusual to find children who have inherited both disorders, and it is possible that one of the reasons for this is that prospective parents are deterred by the risks involved.

Unaffected individuals with a family history of autosomal dominant disease usually have unaffected children. The exception may arise through incomplete penetrance, which is the occurrence of individuals who carry the gene because they have an affected parent and an affected child, but who appear unaffected themselves. Incomplete penetrance occurs in a number of autosomal dominant disorders which include retinoblastoma and autosomal dominant forms of retinitis pigmentosa. This incomplete gene expression may appear to occur because there is no means of detecting an underlying biochemical defect.

Autosomal dominant traits are characterized by variable expressivity, that is the degree to which individuals are affected. This degree can apply to the degree of severity, and also to the spectrum of clinical signs present. There is, for example, wide intrafamilial variation in the manifestation of autosomal dominant retinitis pigmentosa with some individuals more severely affected than others of the same age and therefore presumably at the same stage in the evolution of the disorder. Another example of variable expressivity is Marfan syndrome, a disorder of connective tissue, where affected individuals are tall and thin, and may or may not have myopia, dislocated lens, skeletal abnormalities and heart defects. Incomplete penetrance may be an example of the extreme case of variable expressivity, that is, a case where the expressivity is nil.

A pedigree illustrating autosomal dominant transmission has been shown in Fig. 1.1 (see above). Pedigrees are drawn using squares to represent males and circles to represent females. Solid symbols indicate affected males or females. Any individual on a pedigree may be described by means of a conventional system of numbering whereby generations are numbered from the top with roman numerals, and individuals within a given generation are numbered from left to right using arabic numerals. For example, in the pedigree shown in Fig. 1.1, individual III.1 shows reduced penetrance; individuals I.1 and I.2 are shown as unaffected as it is not known from the family history whether the mutation originated in one or the other.

1.3   Autosomal recessive transmission

A disorder is autosomal recessive when it is expressed by the presence of two abnormal genes, one on each chromosome of a pair of autosomes, so that affected individuals are homozygous. Males and females are equally affected, and have received one abnormal gene from each parent. The parents are hetero-zygous and clinically unaffected. A pedigree illustrating autosomal recessive inheritance is shown in Fig. 1.2. There are two instances of first cousin marriages since the fathers of II.1 and II.2 are brothers, and the mothers of III.4 and III.5 are sisters. Inspection of the pedigree will show that I.1 and I.3 must have been heterozygous for the abnormal gene and the origin of the mutation may have been many generations away.

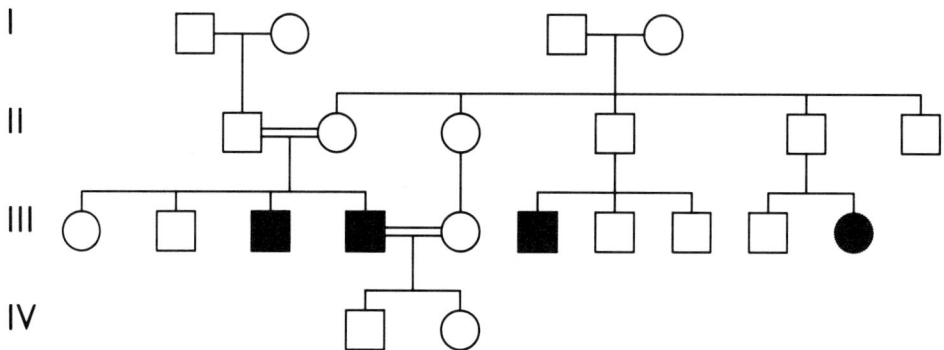

Fig. 1.2 Autosomal recessive inheritance and multiple consanguineous (first-cousin) marriage.

The consequences of autosomal recessive inheritance are different in the case of the heterozygous and the homozygous individual. In the case of two hetero-zygous parents, the risk of an affected child is 25% with each pregnancy. This risk is derived from the fact that each parent, being heterozygous, has a 50% chance of transmitting the abnormal gene; the probability that both parents have transmitted their abnormal gene is therefore the product of both probabilities, namely 50% × 50% = 25%. The probability that two carrier parents have an unaffected child is 75%, but of these, two out of three will be carriers like their parents. All carriers are clinically unaffected, but they contribute to the fre-quency of carriers in the population. Until recently, the detection of the carrier state in many autosomal recessive disorders was not possible. However, recent advances in molecular biology have made carrier detection possible in an in-creasing number of conditions, even though the underlying cause of the defect may not be known – and, at the time of writing, this is true of most ophthalmic disorders.

Affected individuals with an unaffected and unrelated partner have a small risk of transmitting their disorder, but all their children will be carriers. In conditions which are fairly rare with a prevalence of between 1:20000 and 1:2000, the carrier frequency in the population at large is between 1.4% and 4.3%; the risk of an affected child is half the carrier frequency, i.e. between 0.7% and 2.1%. This risk is smaller than that of having a child with any congenital abnormality. If the partner of an affected individual is unaffected but related, for example a cousin, then the likelihood of this partner being a carrier is very much increased, and the union of an affected and a carrier individual has a 50% risk of producing an affected child.

Parental consanguinity, that is the union of parents who are blood relatives, has some influence in autosomal recessive inheritance. Some very rare autosomal recessive disorders are associated with an increase in parental consanguinity, which is of the order of 50% in some parts of the Middle East, and of 0.5% in the UK. A result of a high rate of consanguinous marriage is the existence of pedigrees of autosomal recessive disorders which show pseudo-dominance, that is transmission from one generation to another due to the union of affected and carrier individuals (homozygote and heterozygote).

Finally, as with autosomal dominant disorders, the situation may arise where two individuals affected with an autosomal recessive disorder have a child. The risk to such a child is 100% provided both parents are affected with the same disorder. However, some disorders have different allelic forms, or may appear similar but have a different genetic basis for each autosomal recessive disorder. In this case, all the children will be heterozygous for both disorders and they are termed compound heterozygotes.

1.4　　X-linked transmission

This form of transmission is fairly simple to recognize from the family history, since affected individuals are usually male and have affected male maternal relatives, for example an affected maternal grandfather or maternal uncles. As X-linked disorders usually affect only one sex, this mode of transmission is also described as sex-linked, but the term X-linked is preferable.

Affected males are called hemizygotes and have an abnormal allele on their X chromosome. As a result of the mechanism of sex determination, affected males never transmit this allele to their sons who receive their Y chromosome from their fathers. The daughters of affected males receive an X chromosome from each parent, and obligatorily the X chromosome with the abnormal allele from their fathers, so that they are termed obligate heterozygotes.

X-linked disorders are transmitted by heterozygotes to their sons who have a 50% risk of being affected depending on which X chromosome they have received from their mothers. Similarly, the daughters of heterozygotes have a 50% risk of being themselves heterozygotes. Pedigrees of X-linked disorders (as in Fig. 1.3) show a step-wise transmission as affected males always receive the abnormal gene through one or more generations of heterozygous females.

While X-linked disorders usually affect males, it is possible for females to be affected. This situation arises particularly in the more common X-linked

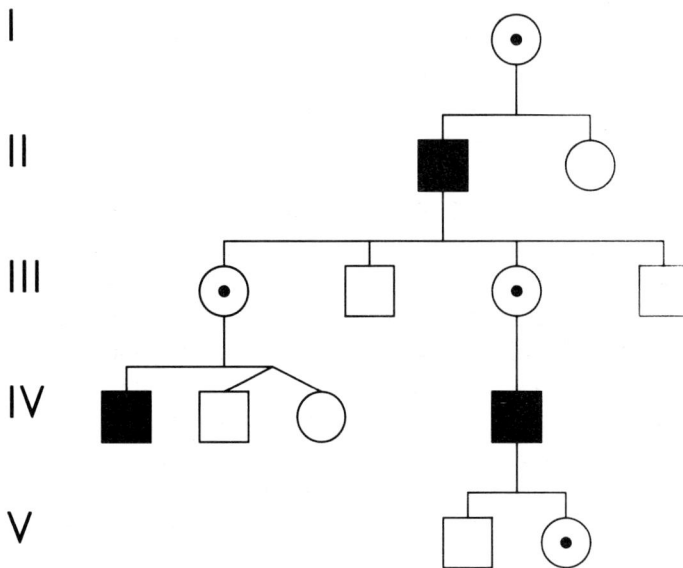

Fig. 1.3 X-linked transmission over five generations. Obligate heterozygotes are indicated by a dot within a circle.

disorders such as colour deficiency where 8% of males are affected, and the frequency of heterozygotes is such that marriages of hemizygotes and heterozygotes are not uncommon. Such unions produce females who are either heterozygous or homozygous, that is, carriers or affected, and males who have a 50% risk of being affected.

There are many X-linked disorders with ocular manifestations, which vary in the degree of severity; similarly, the expression of the carrier state varies from one disorder to another. For example, the carriers of X-linked retinoschisis and Norrie disease have no clinically detectable abnormalities, although identification of heterozygotes by other means, using molecular biology, is likely to be possible in the near future. The carriers for choroideremia, X-linked retinitis pigmentosa (RP) and X-linked ocular albinism can be identified by fundus appearance. It is apparent that there is a wide variation in the expression of carrier abnormalities among and within families.

This variable expressivity in heterozygotes of X-linked disorders is a consequence of the features underlying the Lyon hypothesis. This was formulated by Mary Lyon following her work on coat colour in mice. Mouse and human genes show considerable homology, and in particular, the determination of sex in mice is the same as in man. In both species, males are distinguished from females at the chromosome level by the possession of an X and a Y chromosome, while the female has two X chromosomes. Given that the majority of genes on the Y chromosome determine male sexual characteristics, a dosage compensation effect must exist to allow for two X chromosomes in the female and one X chromosome in the male. The Lyon hypothesis states that early in embryogenesis, one of the two X chromosomes in each cell in the female is inactivated at random. The inactivated X chromosome is either maternal or paternal in origin. Once inactivation has occurred, the descendants of each cell will carry the same inactivated X chromosome which then forms the Barr body (i.e. inactivated X chromosome).

As a result of the Lyon hypothesis, females effectively have two cell lines in terms of their X chromosome, each cell line having either an active paternally-derived or an active maternally-derived X chromosome. Heterozygotes for X-linked disorders would therefore be expected to show one population of cells with the characteristics of the disorder, while the other population of cells would be normal. X-linked ocular albinism is the only condition which is the perfect illustration of this principle as the fundus appearance in heterozygotes looks like a mosaic of depigmented and normally pigmented areas.

The relationship between clinical appearance in the heterozygote and in the hemizygote is not clear as in other conditions such as X-linked RP and choroideremia, however the variability of expression does exist. Manifesting heterozygotes have been described in choroideremia and in X-linked ocular albinism. These are heterozygotes in whom the clinical picture resembles that of the affected males, and they can be regarded as examples of the extreme of inactivation with a preponderance of paternally derived X-chromosomes. The whole spectrum of inactivation of the 'normal' X chromosome is illustrated by the fundus changes found in heterozygotes for X-linked RP. These changes range from the most subtle and discrete to changes which may resemble those found in the affected males. The signs are also progressive and age-related, and their extent reflects the proportion of active X chromosomes bearing the mutated gene.

1.5   Genetic heterogeneity

Retinitis pigmentosa (RP) is the name given to a group of disorders which have a similar appearance (phenotype) but which have different genetic bases. RP is an example of genetic heterogeneity, which may be allelic or non-allelic, the different genes being at the same locus if the heterogeneity is allelic, or at different loci if non-allelic. In the case of RP, there are several non-allelic forms since RP may be autosomal dominant, autosomal recessive or X-linked. In addition, autosomal dominant RP may be further subdivided on the basis of electrophysiological and psychophysical tests, but it is not yet possible to state whether these two subdivisions are allelic. At the time of writing, there are seven different chromosomal loci for autosomal dominant RP, and over 60 mutations associated with one of these loci, that of the gene coding for rhodopsin.

RP is often diagnosed in sporadic cases, such as in patients who have no family history of the disorder. In a few instances the disorder may be an example of a 'phenocopy', or non-genetic mimic of a genetic disorder, which is due to environmental factors. Phenocopies of RP are often called pseudo-retinitis pigmentosa and occur as a result of trauma, inflammation, or they may be viral in origin. Chloroquine or some phenothiazines in large doses cause an RP-like appearance of the fundus, as may measles and congenital syphilis.

1.6   Non-mendelian inheritance

Leber's optic atrophy is a disorder where the pattern of inheritance cannot be explained in classical Mendelian terms. It is a disorder which affects males predominantly, and there is no transmission in the male line, so that affected males do not have affected descendants. Females are either affected or carriers and descent takes place through the female who will have a high proportion of affected or carrier offspring.

This pattern of inheritance is thought to be an example of mitochondrial inheritance. Mitochondrial chromosomes are present in the cytoplasm as opposed to the nucleus of the cell. Sperm have no mitochondrial chromosome as they have no cytoplasm, but mitochondrial chromosomes are found in ova and hence transmitted by females to their children of either sex. In Leber's optic atrophy, carrier females have a high proportion of affected sons, and a high proportion of daughters who are either carriers or affected. The departure from an expected 100% of affected or carrier children is probably due to incomplete penetrance of the abnormal gene.

Not to be confused with Leber's optic atrophy, with its sudden onset of visual loss in the second and third decades, is congenital optic atrophy. The majority of cases of congenital optic atrophy are non-hereditary, and those which are genetically determined are usually autosomal dominant, but there are rare forms which are autosomal recessive. The inheritance patterns of optic atrophy and of some classical ophthalmological disorders is given in Table 1.1.

Table 1.1   Some classical ophthalmological conditions and their inheritance patterns.

Condition	Inheritance
Aniridia	AD
Best's vitelliform macular dystrophy	AD
Colour defects protan and deutan	XL
tritan	AD
Choroideremia	XL
Congenital cataract	AD, AR, (XL – rare)
Congenital glaucoma	Multifactorial
Congenital optic atrophy	Non-hereditary
	AD, (AR – rare)
Corneal dystrophies	AD, AR
Galactokinase deficiency	AR
Galactosaemia	AR
Glaucoma, open-angle	Multifactorial
Gyrate atrophy	AR
Leber's amaurosis	AR
Leber's optic atrophy	Mitochondrial
Ocular albinism	XL, AR
Oculocutaneous albinism (OCA)	AR
Retinitis pigmentosa (RP)	AD, AR, XL
Retinoblastoma (when bilateral)	AD
Stargardt disease	AR
Strabismus	Multifactorial

AD = autosomal dominant
AR = autosomal recessive
XL = X-linked

1.7   Multifactorial inheritance

Some other conditions, such as strabismus, also do not follow a clear pattern of Mendelian inheritance, but seem to show a familial tendency in that the incidence among close relatives is greater than the incidence in the general population; the familial incidence is, however, much smaller than in Mendelian inheritance. These conditions are thought to be multifactorial, that is they are due to genetic and environmental factors. The genetic factors usually consist of several genes rather than one gene, and are termed polygenic.

The risk of recurrence (i.e. another child being born with the same defect to the same parents) is usually derived from an analysis of the various risk factors involved. For example, the relationship to the patient is a risk factor, with the risk highest for the first-degree relatives (brothers and sisters) and then decreasing for second- and third-degree relatives (nephews, nieces, and first cousins). Other risk factors are related to the incidence of the disorder in the general population, to the severity of the disease in the patient, and to the number of relatives affected. It is from all these considerations, and also from the result of twin studies, that a general empirical risk figure is calculated.

Multifactorial inheritance is the basis of several common systemic disorders, the classical example being pyloric stenosis. Among common ophthalmic disorders are strabismus, refractive errors and glaucoma. All of these are heterogeneous groups of disorders, of which only some are multifactorial.

Strabismus is sometimes given as an example of a multifactorial disorder. It is important to distinguish isolated strabismus from strabismus occuring as part of a disorder which may have a Mendelian form of inheritance. Isolated strabismus is not a single disease, but several and can be thought of as a group of conditions, and the evidence for multifactorial inheritance is that there is a raised familial incidence. In particular, studies of twins have shown that identical twins are concordant, that is, they both manifest the trait. The genetic component of concomitant strabismus may be related to anatomical factors such as the shape of the eye, the alignment of the eyes in the orbit, the interpupillary distance, and these anatomical features are genetically determined and polygenic.

Disorders of ocular motility have different modes of inheritance, for example hereditary congenital ophthalmoplegia is autosomal dominant, while Duane syndrome is probably autosomal dominant with incomplete penetrance, although most cases are sporadic and probably non-hereditary.

Similarly, the inheritance of refractive errors depends on the type of refractive error. As a general rule, low refractive errors are multifactorial, while high refractive errors are usually autosomal recessive or occasionally autosomal dominant. Since refractive errors are common, there are many myopic and astigmatic parents who are curious to know whether their children will have the same conditions. The answer depends very much on the family history and it is not always simple to derive.

1.8   Inborn errors of metabolism

Some disorders are the result of a biochemical defect, or inborn error of metabolism. Enzymes which control one or more steps of a chemical pathway may be absent or defective, and enzymes are produced by genes. An example of an inborn error of metabolism is the congenital cataract due to galactokinase deficiency. This condition is rare, and autosomal recessive, with affected (homozygous) persons having no galactokinase activity. The heterozygotes have values of galactokinase which are intermediate between normal and affected.

Oculocutaneous albinism (OCA) which affects skin, hair and eyes is another example of an enzyme defect, in this case the enzyme is tyrosinase which controls the formation of the melanin pigments. OCA can be subdivided into several forms which include tyrosinase positive and tyrosinase negative (ty-pos and ty-neg) forms. Ty-neg albinos have an absence of tyrosinase so that no melanin pigments are formed. The exact defect in ty-pos albinos is not known, but it is possibly a block to tyrosinase in the metabolic pathway concerned with the synthesis of melanin. Both ty-pos and ty-neg OCA are autosomal recessive, but non-allelic. The two forms are due to different genes and therefore the children of a marriage between a ty-pos and a ty-neg albino will be unaffected although they will be compound heterozygotes. There are also less common forms of oculocutaneous albinism which are distinguished from the ty-pos and ty-neg forms by the degree of pigmentation of hair, skin and eyes. The molecular basis of the different forms of albinism is being worked out at the present time. Strabismus, nystagmus and reduced visual acuity are usually found in all forms of albinism. Albinism restricted to the eye is termed ocular albinism and may be autosomal recessive or X-linked.

Recent and exciting advances in the field of molecular biology are revolutionizing our concept of human genetics. It is now possible to study DNA in a way undreamt of twenty years ago. It is already possible to undertake prenatal diagnosis in a number of conditions, and the treatment of genetic disorders should be possible in the foreseeable future. This, however, is a subject on its own, and the reader is urged towards the recommended texts for a fuller understanding of how genetic factors affect ocular development and visual conditions.

1.9   Further reading

Fraser-Roberts, J.A. and Pembrey, M.E. (1985) *An Introduction to Medical Genetics.* Oxford University Press, Oxford.

Harper, P.S. (1981) *Practical Genetic Counselling.* John Wright and Sons Ltd, Bristol.

Weatherall, D.J. (1985) *The New Genetics and Clinical Practice.* Oxford University Press, Oxford.

CHAPTER 2

Embryology of the Eye and Adnexa

Teresa Simons

2.1 Introduction

The study of embryological development requires constant reference to either the time for which development has been proceeding, or the size to which the organism has grown. Both of these factors present problems. Time of fertilization is rarely known with certainty, and rate of development varies and therefore the 'age' of the embryo or fetus is questionable. For descriptions of the fetal period, the GL (greatest length in millimetres), i.e. the greatest length of the body with the exclusion of the lower limbs is now used (O'Rahilly & Müller, 1984), as size and the state of development are more consistent.

However, when referring to the embryonic period, it is standard to use the approximate age in days (time of fertilization being day 1), as very small differences in size occur until the fetal period.

This author has found that reference to the size of the fetus conveys little information without constant resource to a table of age–length relationships, whereas the approximate time of development is immediately comprehensible.

The text of this chapter therefore refers mainly to days or weeks of development rather than the greatest length, although this is included occasionally for reference, as is Table 2.1 which gives the approximate age–length relationships for the human embryo (day 1 to 8 weeks) and fetus (8 weeks to term). The figures are taken from O'Rahilly & Müller (1987), and Ozanics & Jakobiec (1982), and are approximations only, as measurements in the literature vary greatly.

For the purposes of this chapter, in which the author has set out to review the normal development of the human eye, a fundamental knowledge of the events leading up to the first indication of a developing eye in the embryo will be assumed (for revision see Sadler, 1985; O'Rahilly & Müller, 1987).

2.2 Origins of ocular tissues

Four types of embryological tissues participate in the formation of the human eye. These are neural ectoderm, surface ectoderm, mesoderm and neural crest cells.

Table 2.1 Age–length relationship in the human embryo and fetus.

Age	Size (mm)	Dia. of eye cup or globe (mm)	
1 day–4 weeks	0.1–6 ⎫	<1	Embryonic period
1 month–2 months	6–40 ⎭		
2 " 3 "	40–70	1–2	
3 " 4 "	70–120 ⎫	3–6	
4 " 5 "	120–170 ⎭		
5 " 6 "	170–220 ⎫	6–10	Fetal period
6 " 7 "	220–260 ⎭		
7 " 8 "	260–300 ⎫	10–15	
8 " 9 "	300–500 or more ⎭		
Full term	550 crown to heel	17	

(1) *Neural ectoderm*

This forms the walls of the optic vesicle, and subsequently the optic cup which eventually differentiate into the retina and its pigment epithelium, the iris epithelium and muscles, the ciliary epithelium and the glia of the optic nerve.

(2) *Surface ectoderm*

From this tissue are derived the lens, corneal epithelium, conjunctiva, eyelid epithelium and glands, and the lacrimal gland.

(3) *Mesoderm*

A large part of the body's connective tissue is derived from mesoderm which begins to condense into the paired somites at approximately 20 days. It was once believed that the ocular and adnexal connective tissues were derived in a similar way, from mesoderm, but it is now known that mesoderm actually contributes very little to the eye, due in part to the fact that there are no paired somites in the head and neck region. The extraocular muscles and vascular endothelia are thought to be the only ocular structures derived from mesodermal tissue (Ozanics & Jakobiec, 1982).

(4) *Neural crest cells*

These are neuroectodermal cells that proliferate from the crest of the neural folds when the folds fuse to form the neural tube at approximately 24 days. They migrate to many body sites and are known either as secondary mesenchyme, mesectoderm or ectomesenchyme.

In the eye, they develop into the keratocytes, corneal endothelium, trabecular meshwork (Tripathi & Tripathi, 1989), iris and choroidal stroma, ciliary muscle, sclera, fibroblasts and the meninges of the optic nerve.

In the following description, the word mesenchyme will be used to refer to those cells derived from the neural crest.

2.3 Development of the optic vesicle and lens

The development of the nervous system and the eye are closely linked in the embryo. Müller and O'Rahilly (1985), observed the initial formation of the neural tube at 22 days, together with the optic sulcus, a bilateral groove in the anterior neural crest (destined to become the forebrain or prosencephalon). By 24 days (fetal length approximately 4 mm) the neural tube has closed completely and the optic sulcus has become the optic vesicle, completely enclosed within the caudal surface ectoderm and laterally positioned (Fig. 2.1).

The lateral wall of the optic vesicle is at first in direct contact with the surface ectoderm (Bartelmez & Blount, 1954), surface and neural ectoderm elsewhere being separated by mesoderm. This surface ectoderm gives rise eventually to the lens, corneal epithelium, conjunctiva and lids, and epithelia-derived lid structures, e.g. hairs and glands.

At 28 days, the surface ectoderm in contact with the optic vesicle appears thickened, and shows a slight indentation against the lower part of the optic vesicle (Fig. 2.2). This is the lens plate, or disc. A similar thickening of tissue is occurring on the optic vesicle and is termed the retinal disc (O'Rahilly, 1966).

The formation of the secondary optic vesicle or optic cup by the indentation of the retinal disc occurs by 32 days (5–7 mm). The indentation is anterior and also inferior, so forming a shallow groove at the 6 o'clock position from the optic cup margin almost to the wall of the forebrain. This groove is termed the retinal, choroidal or fetal fissure, and allows the hyaloid artery to reach the developing lens (see section on vasculature, Fig. 2.21). The choroidal fissure disappears during the seventh week, as its walls fuse together. Failure of the fissure to close results in a residual cleft or coloboma in the 6 o'clock position, most commonly in the iris (coloboma iridis), but occasionally also involving the ciliary body, retina, choroid and optic nerve.

The invagination forming the secondary optic vesicle progresses rapidly, the two original walls of the optic vesicle soon becoming apposed.

The lens plate or disc meanwhile has also become indented, producing a lens pit (Fig. 2.3). By 33 days, the lens pit has closed, forming a hollow ball of ectodermal cells called the lens vesicle (Streeter, 1945). It separates from the surface ectoderm a short while later, and almost immediately after separation the cells of the posterior wall elongate towards the anterior aspect, so producing a D-shaped cavity (Fig. 2.4) (O'Rahilly, 1966).

At 44 days (13–17 mm), the cavity of the lens vesicle is almost completely filled with the elongating cells of the posterior wall, termed the primary lens fibres (Fig. 2.5) (Streeter, 1945). The cells of the anterior wall remain basically

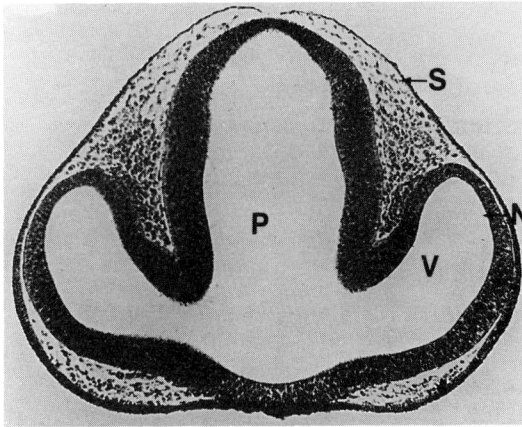

Fig. 2.1 Transverse section through the anterior part of the prosencephalon (P) and primary optic vesicles (V) of a three- to four-week-old embryo. (S = surface ectoderm. N = neural ectoderm.) Original magnification ×100 (from O'Rahilly, 1966).

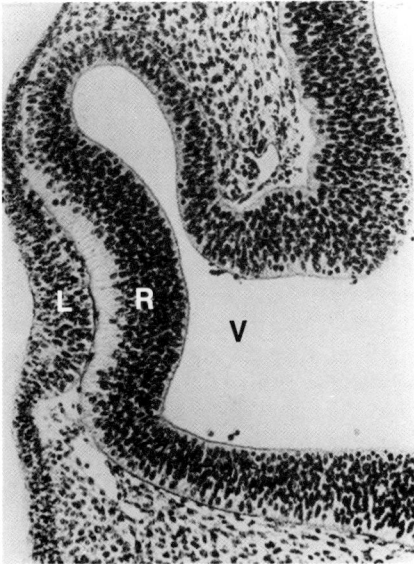

2.2

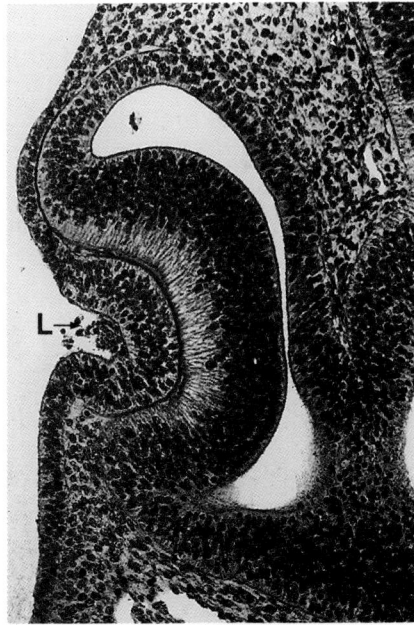

2.3

Fig. 2.2 Sagittal section through the lens plate (L) and primary optic vesicle (V) of a four week-old embryo. R = retinal disc. Original magnification ×200 (from O'Rahilly, 1966).

Fig. 2.3 Sagittal section showing the indentation of the surface ectoderm into the secondary optic vesicle, or optic up, resulting in the formation of the lens pit (L) in a four to five week-old embryo. Original magnification ×200 (from O'Rahilly, 1966).

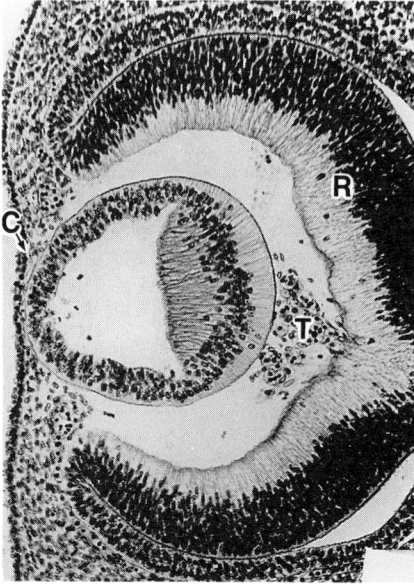
2.4

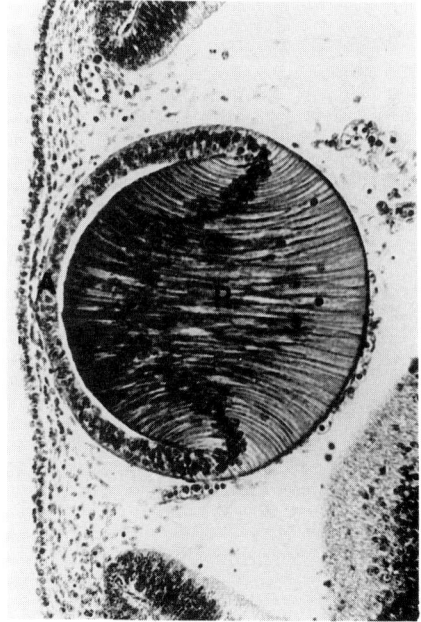
2.5

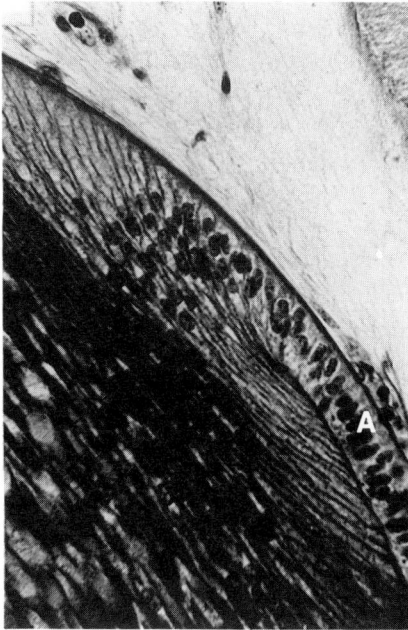
2.6

Fig. 2.4 Horizontal section through an embryonic eye at six weeks. Note the elongating cells of the posterior part of the lens, gradually filling the D-shaped lens cavity. Part of the hyaloid vascular system is visible (T); R = developing neuroretina; C = surface ectoderm forming the future corneal epithelium. Original magnification ×200 (from O'Rahilly, 1966).

Fig. 2.5 Horizontal section through the lens of a six- to seven-week-old embryo. The lens cavity has almost been obliterated by the primary lens fibres (P); A = anterior epithelium. Original magnification ×200 (from O'Rahilly, 1966).

Fig. 2.6 Part of the lens of an eight week-old fetus, showing the formation of the nuclear bow from developing secondary lens fibres at the equator of the lens. A = anterior epithelium. Original magnification ×300 (from O'Rahilly, 1966).

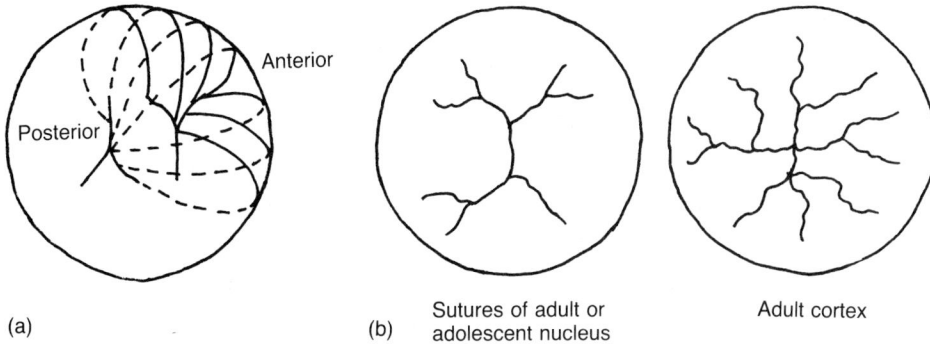

Sutures of adult or
adolescent nucleus

Adult cortex

(a)

(b)

Fig. 2.7 (a) Diagrammatic representation of the formation of the Y-sutures of the fetal lens (towards the end of the third month of gestation). (b) Diagram of the appearance of the lens sutures at various ages (after Mann, 1964).

unchanged, forming the simple cuboidal anterior epithelium of the adult lens. The hyaline capsule can also be identified at this time, believed to be secreted by the cells of the lens vesicle (Mann, 1964).

Apart from an overall enlargement, the lens remains in this state until 50 days (26–30 mm) when secondary lens fibres begin to develop from anterior epithelial cells which have migrated towards the equator. These elongate and grow forward beneath the anterior capsule, and also backwards towards the posterior pole, a shift in their nuclear distribution giving rise to the lens bow (Fig. 2.6).

By the end of the third month the innermost cells have lost their nuclei and other cell organelles, leaving a finely filamentous cytoplasm. All the new fibres formed are of exactly equal length, being just too short to reach from the anterior to posterior poles. The fibres therefore do not meet at a point, but produce a linear pattern (first seen at 35 mm) on and within the lens, both anteriorly and posteriorly. The two patterns thus formed are termed the Y-sutures, which continue to change in appearance as the lens ages throughout life and further secondary fibres are produced (Figs 2.7(a) and (b)).

2.3.1   Lens maturation

The shape of the lens and its orientation with respect to the optical axis continually adjust within the developing eye. Up to 30 mm (< two months), the antero–posterior diameter is greater than the equatorial. The continued production of secondary fibres causes the equatorial diameter to increase rapidly, making the lens increasingly more ellipsoid.

At birth the lens is still more spherical than in the adult, the comparative measurements are shown in Table 2.2.

Table 2.2   **Comparative lengths of the lens in newborns and adults.**

	Newborn	*Adult*
Equatorial diameter	6.7 mm	9.1 mm
Antero–posterior diameter	3.76 mm	3.6 mm
Eyeball length	17 mm (approx.)	24 mm (approx.)

(Mann, 1964)

2.4   Development of the retina

At 26 days (4 mm) the retinal disc is in contact with the surface ectoderm and consists of three or four compact rows of cells (Rhodes, 1979). At 29–30 days, the optic cup has formed, inner and outer layers now being identifiable. The outer wall of the cup is a non-thickened cellular layer (Fig. 2.2), formed of simple pseudostratified columnar epithelium (Mann, 1964).

By 32–33 days (7 mm), a very narrow space is left between the inner and outer walls of the optic cup (Fig. 2.3). The inner wall or retinal disc is a primitive neuroepithelium with five or six layers of oval nuclei in its outer two thirds and an inner, cell-free marginal zone (Rhodes, 1979). The outermost layer of cells (the germinating or proliferating layer) at this time projects cilia to the surface of the adjacent layer of cells, which is the outer wall of the optic cup. These cilia disappear during the seventh week to be replaced by the precursors of the photoreceptor outer segments (Ozanics & Jakobiec, 1982).

The pigment epithelium has two to three layers of pseudostratified columnar cells that enclose pigment granules at three weeks (6–7 mm), this layer producing the earliest pigment in the body (Ozanics & Jakobiec, 1982).

A thin basal lamina covers the inner surface of the marginal layer at five weeks and this, together with a contribution of basal lamina-like material from the developing Müller cell processes at a later stage, becomes the primitive internal limiting membrane (Ozanics & Jakobiec, 1982). During the fifth week, the external limiting membrane is also visible, being formed of zonula adherens between the outer plasma membranes of adjacent neuroblasts.

Cell division occurs in the proliferative layer of the inner wall of the cup, increasing the thickness and surface area of the primitive retina, so that by seven weeks adult thickness (0.2 mm) is reached (Mann, 1964).

Two distinct layers of cells can now be seen, the inner and outer neuroblastic layers, which are separated by a narrow, relatively cell-free region called the transient nerve fibre layer of Chievitz (Fig. 2.8). Although several authors claim that this layer does not represent any particular layer of the adult retina, being purely transient (Mann, 1964; Spira & Hollenberg, 1973; Ozanics & Jakobiec, 1982), Rhodes (1979), states that remnants of Chievitz become the definitive inner plexiform layer which develops during the ninth to twelfth week (40 mm to 83 mm).

Retinal development proceeds more rapidly at the posterior pole, so that by seven weeks the inner neuroblastic layer has given rise to Müller cells and ganglion cells, the axons of the latter growing out into the marginal layer to form the nerve fibre layer (Rhodes, 1979). The inner limiting membrane covering the nerve fibre layer, is seen by electron microscopy at seven weeks to consist of processes of cells with ovoid nuclei, located in the inner neuroblastic layers, and a thin uninterrupted basal lamina (Spira & Hollenberg, 1973).

The ganglion cell layer of the whole retina is established between nine and twelve weeks, the transient fibre layer of Chievitz having disappeared and the inner plexiform layer now being apparent (Fig. 2.9). The photoreceptors, amacrine cells, horizontal and bipolar cells develop from the outer neuroblastic layer according to Rhodes (1979), though Mann (1964) states that amacrine cells develop from the inner neuroblastic layer. Cones differentiate from the outer row of the outer neuroblastic layer by about 10 weeks or 51 mm (Rhodes, 1979). Rods are slower to develop, a few appearing in the primitive outer nuclear layer at 12–13 weeks (Fig. 2.10).

Bipolar cells differentiate mostly from the middle portion of the outer neuroblastic layer, with horizontal cells and photoreceptors arising from the outermost region. By 10–12 weeks (Fig. 2.10) the outer plexiform layer separates the immature horizontal and bipolar cell nuclei from those of the receptors (Ozanics & Jakobiec, 1982).

The primitive outer segments of the photoreceptors seem to exist at 10 weeks, the cells nearest the pigment epithelium possessing a pair of centrioles, one of which extends into a short ciliary process towards the pigment epithelium (Yamada & Ishikawa, 1965). These processes begin to differentiate into photoreceptors at six months.

By 15 weeks (Fig. 2.11), most of the cells and layers of the retina are present, although differentiation continues with the further development of the bipolar and horizontal cells. Rhodes (1979), could identify bipolar and horizontal cell nuclei in the inner nuclear layer by mid-term (159–200 mm, 16–20 weeks). Also at mid-term, the two photoreceptor types are easily distinguishable, cones having pale round nuclei and rods having darker elongated nuclei (Spira & Hollenberg, 1973). According to these same authors, proliferation of cells in the outermost row of outer neuroblasts ceases in the human posterior retina between 13 and 15 weeks of gestation. Mann (1964), previously suggested that mitosis ceased at seven to nine weeks.

Differentiation of the photoreceptors continues into the second half of pregnancy. Primitive inner and outer segments appear by 23 weeks, and by 27 weeks, tubular structures appear in the distal portion of the outer segment. By 36 weeks the structural features of the outer segment are similar to those of the

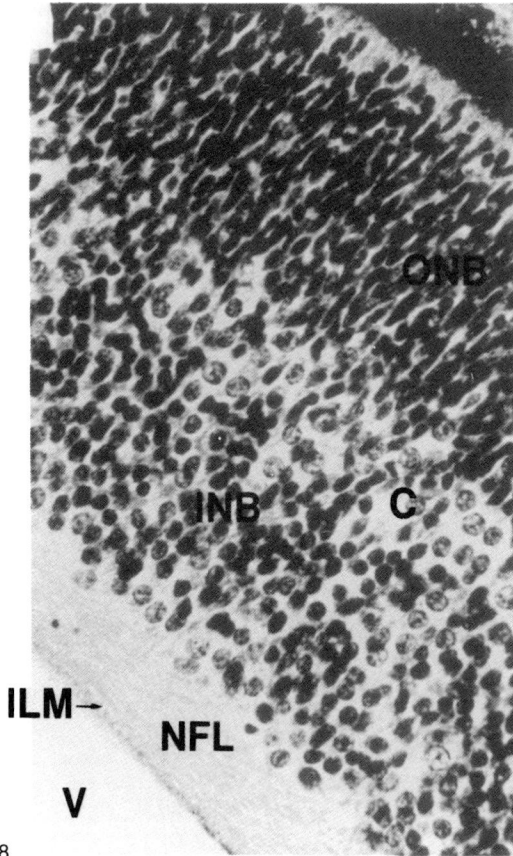

2.8

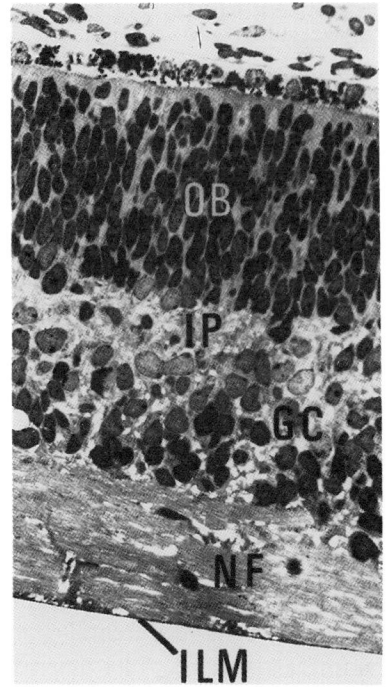

2.9

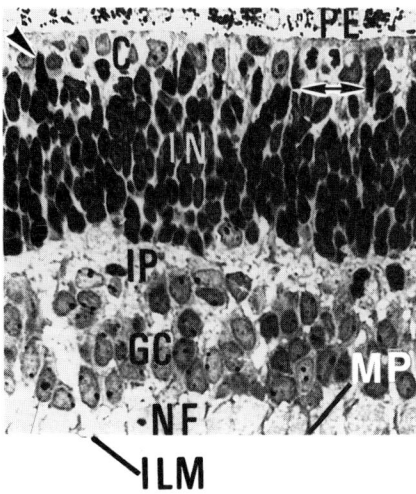

2.10

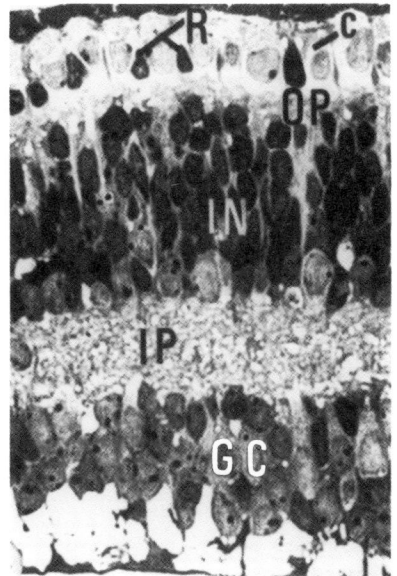

2.11

adult retina, stacked lamellar sacs filling most of the outer segment (Yamada & Ishikawa, 1965).

2.4.1   Development of the fovea

The earliest evidence of maculogenesis in the human retina is a localized increase in the number of superimposed nuclei in the ganglion cell layer at the posterior pole temporal to the disc at 22 weeks (Fig. 2.12), beneath which lies a prominent zone of cone photoreceptors (Hendricksson & Yuodelis, 1984). Between 24 and 26 weeks a depression appears (Fig. 2.13), as the ganglion and inner nuclear layer cells move laterally, the photoreceptor layer at this time being only one cone thick. At 34–36 weeks, the cones at the centre of the foveolar pit are short and appear less mature than the surrounding cones on the slope which are very elongated.

Just after birth (five to eight days) the ganglion cell layer is no more than one cell thick and the inner nuclear layer has thinned to less than 3 cells thick in the centre of the foveal pit (Fig. 2.14). The transient layer of Chievitz is still very prominent in the inner nuclear layer of the slope.

According to Hendricksson and Yuodelis (1984), the human fovea does not complete its development until well after birth, possibly as late as 45 months postpartum, the cone outer segment growth occurring almost entirely after birth (Figs 2.15 and 2.16).

←——

Fig. 2.8 Section through the retina of an embryo at seven to eight weeks showing ONB, INB, outer and inner neuroblastic layers; C = nerve fibre layer of Chievitz; ILM = internal limiting membrane; V = vitreous. Original magnification ×400 (from O'Rahilly, 1966).

Fig. 2.9 Section through the retina at approximately ten weeks. PE = pigment epithelium; OB = outer neuroblastic layer; IP = inner plexiform layer; GC = presumptive ganglion cell layer; NF = nerve fibre layer; ILM = internal limiting membrane. Magnification ×1068 (from Spira and Hollenberg, 1973).

Fig. 2.10 Section through the retina at 12 weeks. PE = pigment epithelium; C = cones. Double-headed arrow = outer plexiform layer; IN = inner nuclear layer; IP = inner plexiform layer; GC = ganglion cell layer; NF = nerve fibre layer; MF = radial fibres of Müller; ILM = inner limiting membrane. Original magnification ×1225 (from Spira and Hollenberg, 1973).

Fig. 2.11 Section through the retina at 15 weeks. Most of the layers of the retina are now identifiable, although the outer segments of the photoreceptors do not appear until the second half of gestation. R = rods; C = cones. OP and IP = outer and inner plexiform layers; IN = inner nuclear layer; GC = ganglion cell layer. Original magnification ×1725 (from Spira & Hollenberg, 1973).

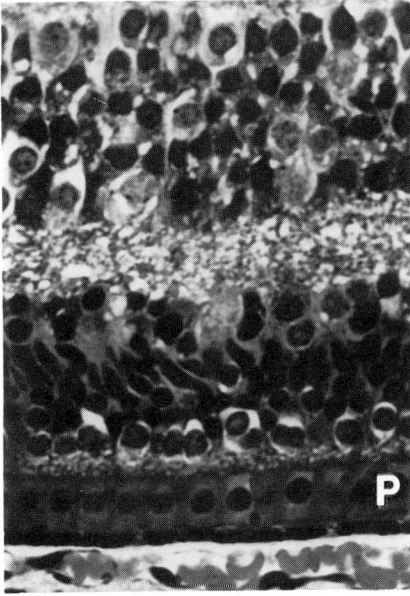

2.12

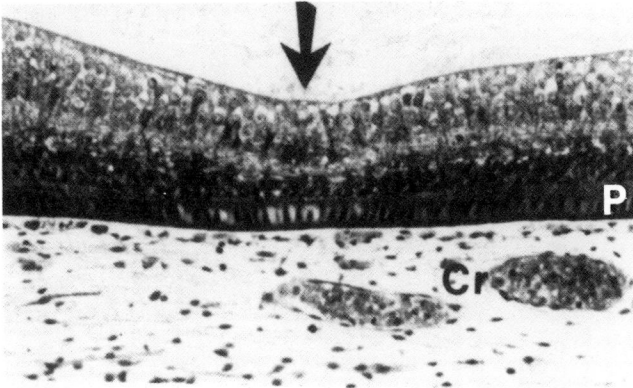

2.13

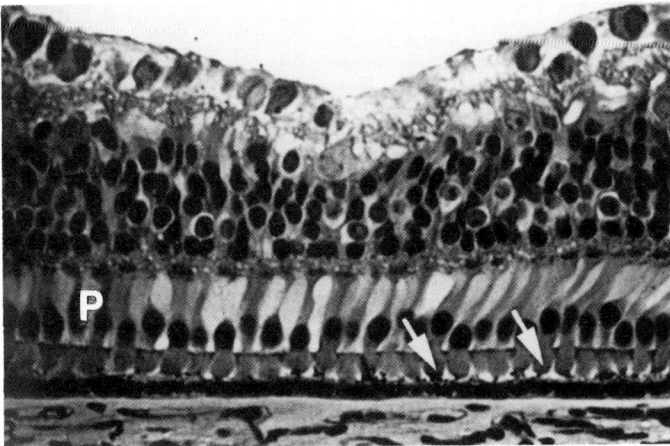

2.14

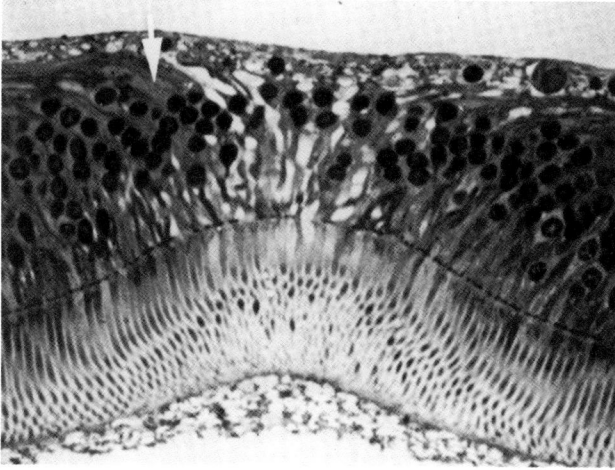

Fig. 2.15 Foveola from 45 month-old child in which the entire thickness of the retina is formed from dark-staining cones and pale-staining glial processes. The cone inner and outer segments are thin and elongated. The arrow indicates the fibres of Henle. Original magnification ×173 (from Hendrickson and Yuodelis, 1984).

2.5 Development of the optic nerve

The choroidal fissure begins to close during the fifth week (8–10 mm), the central part of the optic cup fusing first, followed by its inner and outer margins. Closure of the cup is complete at the end of five weeks (see Fig. 2.21 in the section on vasculature), that of the optic stalk occurring slightly later at six to seven weeks (Ozanics & Jakobiec, 1982).

Initially, the wall of the optic stalk is composed of undifferentiated neuro-

---

Fig. 2.12 Section through the foveal region of the retina of a 24–26 week fetus showing the beginning of the foveal depression which involves the thinning of inner nuclear and retinal ganglion cell layers (arrow). P = outer nuclear layer, Cr = choroid. Original magnification ×162 (from Hendrickson & Yuodelis, 1984).

Fig. 2.13 Centre of future fovea from a 22 week fetus. The photoreceptor layer (P) consists entirely of cones which lack both inner and outer segments at this time. All of the characteristic neurons and glia are present in inner and ganglion cell layers. Both plexiform layers are present. Original magnification ×1971 (from Hendrickson & Yuodelis, 1984).

Fig. 2.14 Centre of foveal depression from five day-old infant. The photoreceptor layer (P) contains pale glial processes and darker staining cones marked by their promonent nuclei. The cones have a large round inner segment which bulges above the outer limiting membrane (arrow). Tiny dark-staining outer segments can be seen just below the pigment epithelium. Original magnification ×173 (from Hendrickson & Yuodelis, 1984).

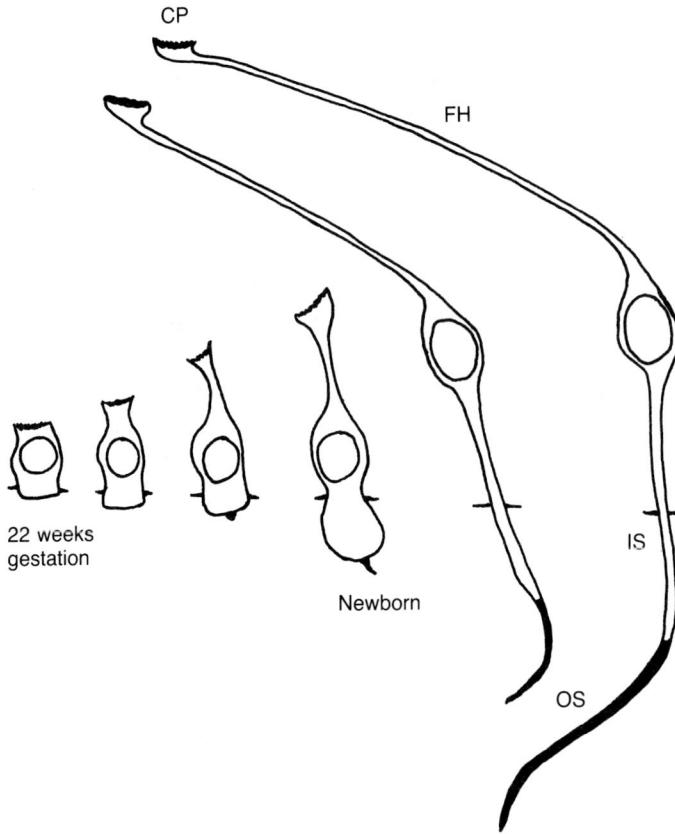

Fig. 2.16 Schematic drawing indicating the stage of development of the foveal cones at (left to right) 22, 24–26, and 34–36 weeks of gestation; newborn; and 15 and 45 months postpartum. The inner segment (IS) develops before birth, while most of the outer segment (OS) develops after. Both the fibre of Henle (FH) and cone pedicle (CP) are present before birth. All four of these structures show a striking thinning and elongation over this developmental span especially at postnatal ages (drawn to comparative scale). (Redrawn with permission from Hendrickson & Yuodelis, 1984.)

epithelium. With the appearance of nerve fibres from the ganglion cells in the retina, cells at the centre of the optic stalk become vacuolated. Axons from the retina grow in among the vacuolated cells which gradually disappear. The stalk is almost completely filled with retinal nerve fibres by seven weeks (Mann, 1964) although the number of axons in the optic nerve does not remain constant during development. Provis *et al.* (1985), and Sturrock (1987b), found that the number of axons in the human optic nerve reaches a peak of approximately 5 million at 14 weeks, and then drops by 2.5 million between 14 and 30 weeks.

The glial cells of the optic nerve begin to develop from stalk cells at about seven weeks, (Ozanics & Jakobiec, 1982). After two months, the nerve is composed of bundles of fibres, separated by parallel rows of longitudinally aligned glial cells and their processes (Rhodes, 1978), and the thin-walled hyaloid artery occupies almost a third of the diameter of the nerve.

By eight to fourteen weeks, the optic nerve is surrounded by loosely packed layers of connective tissue, but by 18 weeks the meninges are well-differentiated (Sturrock, 1987a).

Myelination of the nerve fibres proceeds from the optic tract toward the optic nerve head (Sattler, 1915), and first appears in the tract and intracranial optic nerve at 32 weeks (Magoon & Robb, 1981). Classical literature states that myelination of the optic nerve is virtually complete at birth (Duke-Elder & Cooke, 1963; Mann, 1964) but more recent observations on human material (Magoon & Robb, 1981) indicate that by full-term, some fibres in the optic nerve near the globe begin to become myelinated but the amount of myelin around individual nerves increases dramatically during the ensuing months, up to two years of age and less rapidly thereafter.

2.5.1 Optic disc

By the ninth week, a conical group of glial cells have developed in the disc along the distal wall of the hyaloid canal, and this is termed Bergmeister's papilla (Rhodes, 1978). The cells of the papilla proliferate so that at four-and-a-half months there is a mantle around the regressing artery (Ozanics & Jakobiec, 1982). Excavation of the disc in the fully developed eye depends on the extent of degeneration of the glia late in gestation, these cells occasionally remaining as a postnatal remnant on the optic disc in man with no detrimental effect on vision (Yanoff & Fine, 1975).

2.6 Development of the anterior eye

2.6.1 Cornea

Following the separation of the lens vesicle from the surface ectoderm at 33 days (7–9 mm), the ectoderm is restored (Fig. 2.4) and constitutes the anterior epithelium of the future cornea, being composed of two cell layers and having its own basement membrane (Wulle & Richter, 1978).

By seven weeks (19 mm) a wave of mesenchymal cells has moved from the periphery into the space between ectoderm and lens epithelium and has formed the future corneal endothelium. This is at first a double row of flattened cells (Wulle, 1972). At this stage the space between the epithelium and endothelium, the primary stroma, contains collagen fibrils, the synthesis of which is thought to be contributed to by the epithelial cells (Wulle & Richter, 1978). The ability of corneal epithelium to synthesize collagen has been demonstrated in other animals (Hay & Revel, 1969; Trelstad & Coulombe, 1971; Gradinger & Leuenberger, 1973).

A second wave of mesenchymal cells grows inward from the tissue at the margin of the optic cup, and these differentiate into cells of a fibroblastic nature (Duke-Elder & Cooke, 1963) so that by eight weeks (Fig. 2.17), the stroma is composed of approximately 15 layers of cells and developing collagen fibrils. The epithelium at this stage consists of surface squamous cells and basal columnar cells resting on a basal lamina. The wing cells appear later at four or five months. Ozanics and Jakobiec (1982) reported that Bowman's layer is visible by electron microscopy at three to four months. It is acellular, and possibly formed by the anterior fibroblasts of the stroma.

In the fourth month the endothelium consists of a single layer of cells, and Descemet's membrane is recognizable as a fine layered basal lamella (Wulle, 1972). By the eighth month, Descemet's membrane has increased in thickness, and its structure appears more condensed.

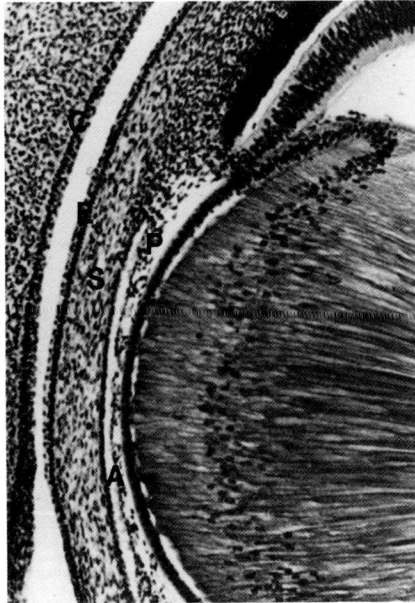

Fig. 2.17 Section through the anterior eye of a fetus at seven to eight weeks. C = palpebral conjunctiva; E = corneal epithelium; S = corneal stroma; P = pupillary membrane; A = anterior chamber. Original magnification ×400 (from O'Rahilly, 1966).

2.6.2   Sclera

The sclera develops from periocular mesenchyme, and by six to seven weeks, differentiation of this tissue into fibroblasts is in progress (Sellheyer & Spitznas, 1988a). These authors agreed with previous reports (Duke-Elder & Cooke, 1963; Weale, 1982) that differentiation begins anteriorly, in the region of the future limbus, and progresses to the posterior cup. Mann (1964), observed that by five months the sclera is well-differentiated around the whole globe.

2.6.3   Anterior chamber

The mechanisms involved in the formation of the anterior chamber and filtration angle have given rise to much speculation over the years, and several theories have been postulated.

One of the earliest of these theories suggested that atrophy of the mesenchymal tissue occurs in the filtration angle (Seefelder, 1910; Anderson, 1939; Mann, 1960). Alternatively, it was suggested that the chamber angle is opened by splitting or cleavage of the mesenchymal tissue (Rytkola, 1952; Burian & Braley, 1956; Maumenee, 1959).

Smelser & Ozanics (1971), and Remé & Lalive d'Epinay (1981), favoured the theory of rarefaction of the reticular mesenchyme with a rearrangement of the cells, this theory being a slight variation on that of cleavage. More recently, Sevel *et al.* (1985), reappraised the situation, and were able to divide the development of the anterior chamber into three stages:

(1)   Passive (lenticular) phase: 44–54 days;
(2)   Active (expanding) phase: 2–5 months;
(3)   Maturation of filtration angle: 5 months–1 year.

They suggest that a cavity, lined with flattened mesenchymal cells is first created by the lens receding from the cornea. With time, the anterior chamber expands both in depth and peripherally, the depth being achieved by the cornea growing faster than the region of the limbus and thus bowing anteriorly, and the lens receding further. At the same time a cleft develops in the mesenchymal tissue at the periphery, increasing in depth and length so that the mesenchymal cells lining the anterior chamber become attenuated peripherally. This results in the peripheral expansion of the chamber. Figure 2.18 shows the chamber angle at 15 weeks.

By the end of the fifth month the trabecular meshwork has begun to develop, and the canal of Schlemm begins to take form. After the fifth month, the phase of maturation is noted, the corneal endothelium merging with the cells of the trabecular meshwork as the mesenchymal cells in the acutely shaped filtration

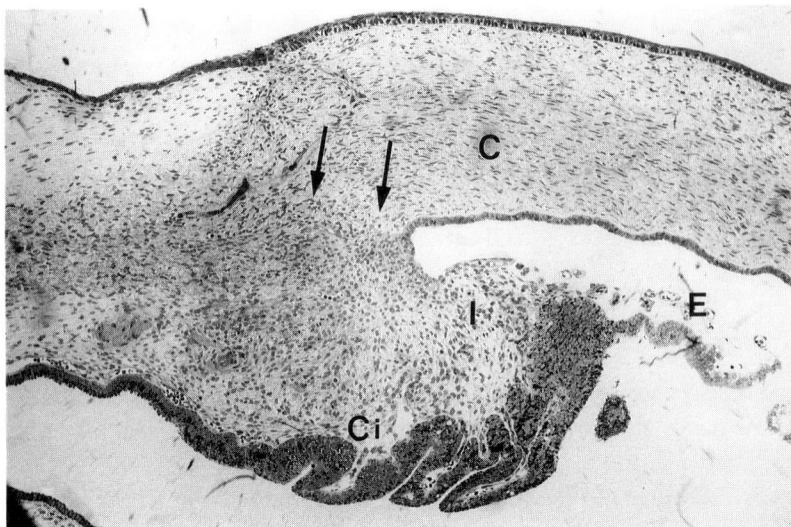

Fig. 2.18 Section through the chamber angle at the fifteenth week. Primitive corneal (C) and iris (I) tissue forms the angle recessus. The arrows indicate the demarcation between the corneo–scleral and ciliary–iris regions. E = pupillary membrane; Ci = ciliary body. Original magnification ×75 (photomicrograph kindly donated by Professor Charlotte Remé).

angle degenerate. This fissuring of the angle occurs beyond term, and probably continues for the first year of life according to these authors.

2.6.4 Ciliary body

Mesenchyme and neuroectoderm both contribute to the formation of the ciliary body; the stroma and muscle are derived from mesenchyme and the ciliary epithelium from the neuroectoderm forming the walls of the optic cup.

The first ciliary folds were identified 100–150 μm from the growing anterior rim of the optic cup at 10 weeks by light microscopy (Wulle, 1972) and more recently by scanning electron microscopy (Fig. 2.19) (Sellheyer & Spitznas, 1988b). Both sets of autors agree that the first folding occurs in the pigmented epithelium, followed in week 11 by that of the non-pigmented epithelium. Zonule fibres have been identified in week 12 by light microscopy (Ozanics & Jakobiec, 1982).

According to Sellheyer & Spitznas (1988b), the principle structure of the ciliary body, judging from its topography, is established during week 24 (Fig. 2.20) when the pars plana has just become discernible. Approximately 70–80 ciliary processes could be recognized (Streeten, 1982; Sellheyer & Spitznas, 1988b). However, the ciliary processes at this time appear smooth, unlike those at birth which exhibit numerous secondary surface infoldings (Streeten, 1982).

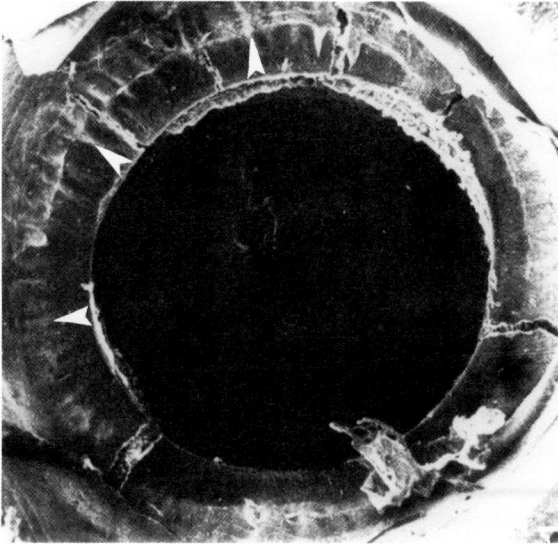

Fig. 2.19 Scanning electron micrograph of the anterior eye segment from a 10-week-old fetus. The lens and cornea have been removed. The arrowheads indicate the beginnings of the ciliary folds. Original magnification ×160 (from Sellheyer & Spitznas, 1988).

Meanwhile, the growing tip of the optic cup has extended beyond the developing ciliary body, and forms the iris (see below).

2.6.5 Ciliary muscle

This begins to develop from mesenchyme, external to the growing ciliary processes, during the third month (Mann, 1964; Duke-Elder & Cooke, 1963). The meridional (longitudinal) bundles of ciliary muscle cells are the first to complete their development, which happens during the fifth month. Oblique and circular muscle fibres develop more slowly and appear during the sixth month (Duke-Elder & Cooke, 1963). According to Mann (1964), the circular fibres are well formed by the end of the seventh month, but continue to develop for a variable time after birth.

The ciliary region is supplied with recurrent vessels from the major iridic circle after the sixth month.

2.6.6 Iris

With the continued growth of both walls of the optic cup forward from the area of developing ciliary processes at the end of the third month, the vascular iris stroma begins to form. This is closely linked with changes in the anterior tunica

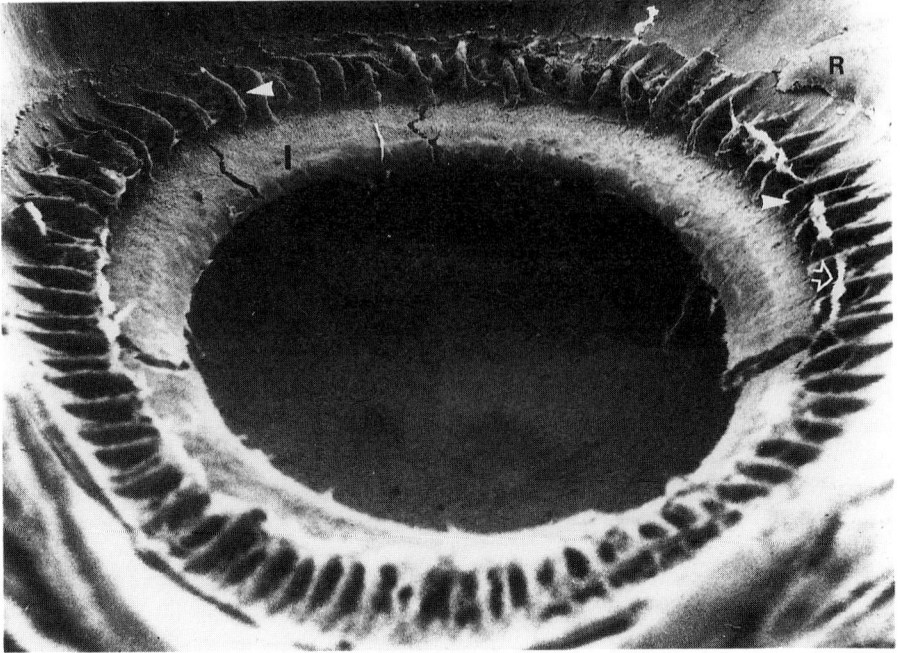

Fig. 2.20 Scanning electron micrograph of the anterior eye segment at week 24. The lens and cornea have been removed. The retina (R) in most parts of the anterior eye cup is artificially removed. Arrowheads = ciliary processes; hollow arrowhead = condensed fibrillar material; I = iris. Original magnification ×27 (from Sellheyer and Spitznas, 1988).

vasculosa lentis, or lamina iridopupillaris (see the section on vasculature). The peripheral part of this structure is composed of blood vessels and mesenchyme, and becomes incorporated into the iris stroma, while the central, pupillary region eventually disappears leaving the pupil.

While the iris stroma is developing, the nasal and temporal long ciliary arteries bifurcate in the ciliary body and the branches unite with peripheral vessels of the lamina iridopupillaris to form the major iridic circle (Ozanics & Jakobiec, 1982).

Anterior ciliary arteries penetrating the sclera during the fourth month send tributaries to join the major iridic circle, and during the fifth month loop vessels supply the iris stroma from branches of the long ciliary arteries.

At first, like the future ciliary epithelium, the iris epithelium consists of an anterior layer of pigmented cells and a posterior layer of non-pigmented cells. The posterior layer gradually becomes pigmented, the pigmentation extending from the tip of the iris towards the root, the whole process occupying the period of between three and seven months (Mann, 1964). Figure 2.18 shows the beginnings of the iris at 15 weeks.

The sphincter and dilator muscles of the iris, unlike most muscles of the body including the ciliary muscle, are not derived from mesenchyme but from the neural ectoderm, which forms the iris epithelial cells. This was first noted by Nassbaum (1893), and confirmed by Szilli (1901). According to Mund *et al.* (1972), and Ruprecht & Wulle (1973), the earliest sign of muscle development in the human iris is at 11 to 12 weeks, when fibrillar material appears in the basal part of the anterior epithelial layer near the tip of the iris. Definite myofibrils can be recognized in the fifth month when the developing muscle cells are still closely apposed to the iris epithelium. Not until the eighth month is the sphincter pupillae seen to lie free within the iris stroma, attached only at the pupil margin.

The dilator muscle is slower to develop than the sphincter both in the human (Mund *et al.*, 1972) and in the rat (Imaizumi & Kuwabara, 1971; Lai, 1972). In man it appears during the sixth month, the anterior epithelial cells peripheral to the developing sphincter muscle cells differentiating to form a sheet of myoepithelial cells, extending to the root of the iris. This unusual muscle never separates from the epithelial layer.

2.7   Development of the choroid and vascular system

Endothelial blood spaces in the mesenchyme around the outer wall of the optic cup appear very early in development. The primitive choriocapillaris is seen at seven weeks as an incomplete chain of capillaries outside the retinal pigment epithelium (Mund *et al.*, 1972), these same authors observing Bruch's membrane by light microscopy at 11 weeks. Following the completion of the choriocapillaris at 35 days, the vessels at the anterior rim of the cup coalesce to form the *annular vessel* (Fig. 2.21), a circular vessel around the margin. The suprachoroid is found during the third month (Duke-Elder & Cooke, 1963), and during the third and fourth month, and the fourth and fifth month respectively the large external (Haller's) and medium sized internal vessels (Sattler's) become visible (Heimann, 1972).

Pigment is present in the choroid at 27 weeks only in the peripapillary region, but progresses anteriorly with age so that it is widespread in this part of the eye at term (Mund *et al.*, 1972).

At the end of the third month, six to eight short posterior ciliary arteries penetrate the sclera around the optic nerve head. There are also two long posterior ciliary arteries which pass over the choriocapillaris to fork out in its distal third, the terminal branches forming a circle peripheral to the region destined to become the ciliary body (Heimann, 1972). Vortex veins develop from the merging of some capillaries in the anterior part of the choroid (Fig. 2.21).

At the end of the fourth month, the anterior ciliary arteries have formed and

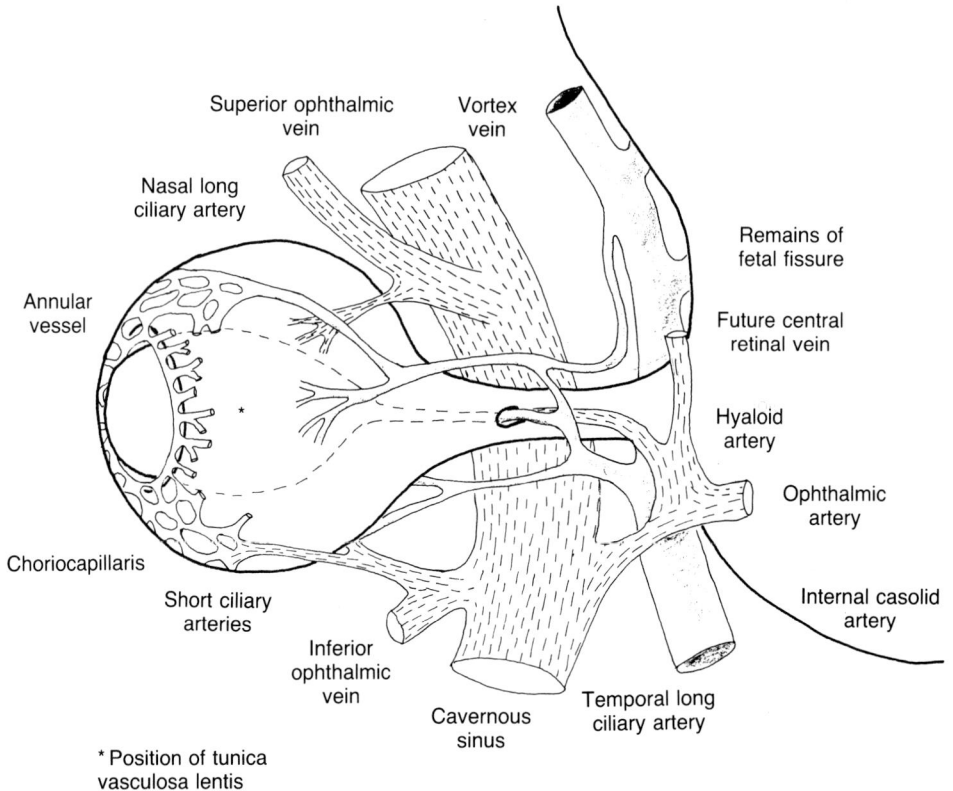

Fig. 2.21 Schematic diagram of the primitive embryonic ocular vasculature at approximately six weeks (adapted from the film 'Embryology of the Eye', American Academy of Ophthalmology).

contribute to the major iridic circle, together with branches of the long posterior ciliary arteries (Heimann, 1972).

The sixth to ninth month sees the formation of recurrent arterial branches arising from the major iridic circle, supplying the developing iris and ciliary body.

2.7.1 Hyaloid system and vitreous

The vitreous space at 29 and 30 days is narrow, but contains cells originating from the mesenchyme surrounding the outer surface of the optic cup (Balazs *et al.*, 1980). These undifferentiated cells enter the vitreal space through the annular opening between the lens vesicle and the rim of the optic cup, and through the open embryonic fissure.

Classic textbooks state that at about 5 mm the primitive internal carotid artery gives rise to a vessel, the hyaloid artery, which penetrates the fetal fissure and enters the primary optic vesicle. Inside the vesicle the artery branches into the primary vitreous forming a network of vessels, the *vasa hyaloidea propria* (Fig. 2.22).

At five weeks (8–9 mm) the hyaloid artery reaches the posterior pole of the lens, and a second network of blood vessels spreads over the posterior surface of the lens, so forming the *posterior tunica vasculosa lentis*. Branches also distribute over the equator, and anastomose with the annular vessel at the optic cup margin.

Balazs *et al.* (1980) reexamined the development of the hyaloid system, and concluded that the whole structure develops *in situ*, from the differentiation of mesenchymal cells already present in the vitreous, rather than from the inward migration and branching from the hyaloid artery.

The posterior part of the hyaloid system appears to be fully developed by nine to ten weeks (Mann, 1964; Balazs *et al.*, 1980), although Sellheyer & Spitznas (1987) recently reported that it is complete as early as seven weeks.

Anteriorly, the lens becomes covered by several tiers of looped vessels derived from the annular vessel. This is the *anterior tunica vasculosa lentis* (Fig. 2.22),

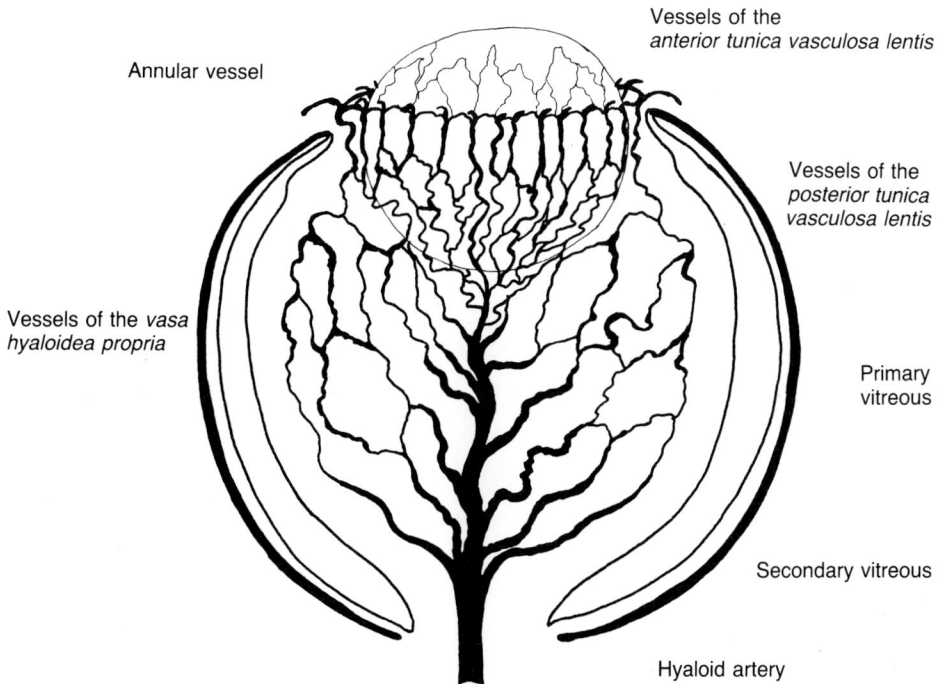

Fig. 2.22 Schematic diagram of the intraocular vasculature in a fetus of about eight weeks.

and together with mesenchymal tissue, forms the pupillary membrane (Fig. 2.18). According to Ko *et al.* (1985), this does not reach its maximum development until 25 weeks.

The primary function of the hyaloid vascular system is to provide the essential oxygen and nutrients for the rapidly developing lens. At approximately 16 weeks the lens diameter reaches its maximum relative to that of the eyeball, and at this point the hyaloid system begins to regress (Ko *et al.*, 1985), although Balazs *et al.* (1980), put it earlier, at 11 to 12 weeks.

The vasa hyaloidea propria regresses first (Fig. 2.23), followed by the capillaries of the tunica vasculosa lentis, and finally the hyaloid artery itself, so that at the ninth month the regression of the hyaloid vascular system is almost complete.

At birth, occasional vascular remnants or empty 'ghost' vessels indicate the previous existence of this system of vessels.

The atrophy of the hyaloid artery is accompanied by the retraction of the primary vitreous, in which the vessels were growing. The secondary avascular vitreous (Fig. 2.22) has been developing meanwhile between the retina and primary vitreous, and is thought to be complete by about three months

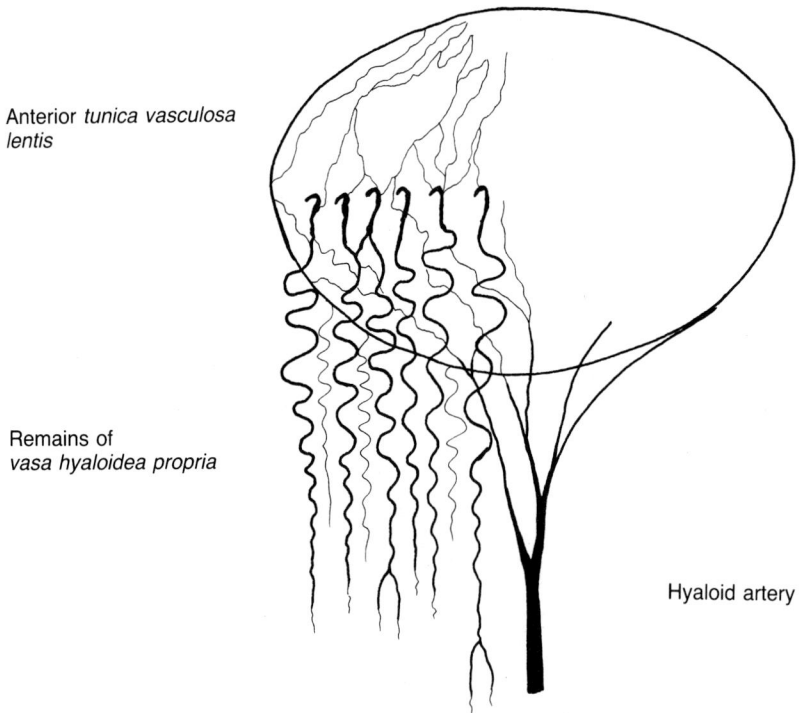

Fig. 2.23 Schematic diagram to show the regression of the intraocular vasculature (after Mann, 1964).

(Duke-Elder & Cooke, 1963). Gloor (1972), suggested that the first cells of the secondary vitreous are derived from the primary vitreous, and not from the retina or ciliary body as previously suggested (see Duke-Elder & Cooke, 1963, pp. 141–4 for review of the early literature).

As the hyaloid system regresses, the primary vitreous shrinks and condenses concomitantly, leaving an axial column surrounding the degenerating hyaloid artery. At birth, the remnants of the artery, still attached to the posterior pole of the lens, can often be seen floating in what is then termed Cloquet's canal. After four or five years of age, gravity causes the artery remnants to hang vertically, corkscrew-like behind the lens, where they remain throughout life.

Anteriorly the pupillary membrane also regresses, but not totally as part of it persists within the iris. As the margin of the optic cup grows forward, forming the ciliary body and iris, the central loops of the pupillary membrane shrink and recede, but the more peripheral arcades remain and form the minor iridic circle. Furthermore, the vessels peripheral to these arcades also persist and form the radial superficial vessels of the fully formed iris (Duke-Elder & Cooke, 1963). Like the hyaloid artery, remnants of the central arcade vessels may sometimes be seen in the adult eye, stretching across the pupil. This is referred to as a persistent pupillary membrane.

2.7.2   Retinal circulation

Retinal vessels are absent in the embryo, appearing only in the fourth month. Some controversy exists over the formation of the vessels.

Michaelson (1948), considered that the retinal arteries were the result of budding from the hyaloid artery at the disc, but several authors including Nilausen (1958), and Ashton (1970), failed to confirm this theory, suggesting a continuous differentiation of primitive mesenchymal cells into vascular endothelium over the retina from which the adult retinal vessels evolve (see Ashton, 1970 for review).

Whichever is the case, the retinal arteries are supplied in the fetus by the hyaloid artery, which following its degeneration in the vitreous, persists in the optic nerve to form the central retinal artery.

The retinal veins drain initially into two venous channels running alongside the hyaloid artery (Mann, 1964), the venous channels uniting somewhere behind the optic disc to form the central retinal vein.

2.8   Development of the adnexa

2.8.1   Eyelids

The upper and lower lids develop from the proliferation of the ectoderm and underlying mesoderm above and below the eyeball. The ectodermal growth is

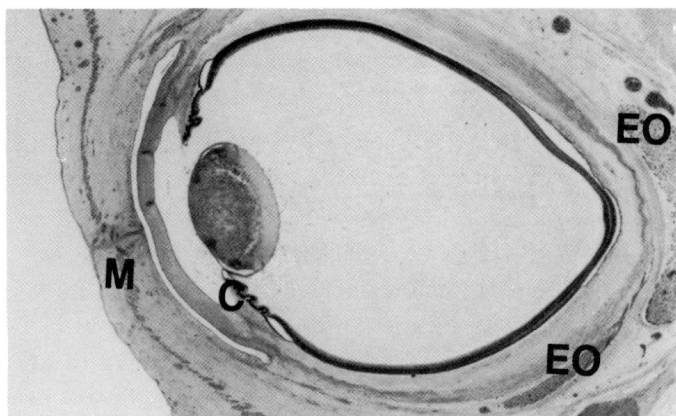

Fig. 2.24 Sagittal section through a fetal eye at approximately 20 weeks. The line of fusion of the eyelids can be seen, along with the developing Meibomian glands (M). EO = developing extraocular muscles; C = ciliary body.

first seen at around five weeks or 12 mm (Andersen *et al.*, 1965). According to Pearson (1980), the two eyelids first meet at the lateral end of the palpebral fissure, so establishing the outer canthus at 16.5 mm. The inner canthus is established at approximately 18 mm. The lid margins contact each other in a horizontal plane during the third month (35–40 mm), and fuse, or adhere together, soon after. The lids remain fused until shortly before birth (5–6 months), glands and lashes forming while the lids are fused. Separation of the lids does not occur until these structures are completed (Mann, 1964). The anlage of the cilia first appear at 41 mm by epithelial proliferation, and the Meibomian gland anlage (Fig. 2.24) at 80 mm (Andersen *et al.*, 1965).

2.8.2 Lacrimal gland

At six to seven weeks (25 mm) the lacrimal gland begins to form from epithelial buds of the conjunctiva covering the upper temporal fornix (Ozanics & Jakobiec, 1982). The gland is small at birth and is not fully developed until three to four years postnatally.

2.8.3 Extraocular muscles

Early authors, for example Gilbert (1952), and Mann (1964), suggested that the extraocular muscles arise from muscle plates (mesodermal condensations) surrounding the head cavities, which migrate forward into the orbits. The condensations destined to become the four muscles served by the oculomotor nerve are apparent by 26 days, that destined to be the lateral rectus by 27 days, and the superior oblique precursor by 29 days. Nervous supply is established by growth from the brain to the muscles in the following sequence: III and VI at 31 days, and IV at 33 days (Gilbert, 1957). The levator palpebrae superioris forms from the superior rectus muscle at 22–30 mm and is complete during the fourth month (Mann, 1964) (see Fig. 2.24).

The above information is disputed however by Sevel (1981a), who used serial sections to examine 54 human specimens from 8 mm to term. He found that the insertion, belly and origin of the extraocular muscles developed simultaneously, and that there was no forward migration of these structures in the orbit.

2.8.4   Bony orbit

During the third month, the orbital walls are differentiated, but are not ossified until the sixth and seventh month (Ozanics & Jakobiec, 1982). The angle between the orbital axes increases during development, starting at 160°, diminishing to 105° at three months, and reaching 71° at birth. The average adult condition is 68°.

2.8.5   Nasolacrimal apparatus

The entire nasolacrimal apparatus, i.e. canaliculi, lacrimal sac and nasolacrimal duct develop contemporaneously according to Sevel (1981b). The apparatus forms from a core of surface epithelium entrapped between the maxillary and frontonasal process at approximately 32 days (8–9 mm).

Partial canalization of the apparatus is observed during the fourth month according to some authors and the lacrimal puncta open after separation of the eyelids, but Adenis *et al.* (1983), found that in the majority of fetuses they examined, the lacrimal punctum was open at four months.

Sevel (1981b) reported that the lacrimal duct opening into the nose is patent in only 30% of newborn children, but becomes patent during the first month postnatally.

2.9   References

Adenis, J.P., Lebraud, P., Leboutet, M.J., Loubet, R. and Loubet, A. (1983) 'Embryology of human lacrimal pathways. A study of ten cases'. *J. Fr. Ophtalmol.*, **6**, 351–7.

Andersen, H., Ehlers, N. and Matthiessen, M.E. (1965) 'Histochemistry and development of the human eyelids'. *Acta Ophthalmol.*, **43**, 642–68.

Anderson, J.R. (1939) *Hydrophthalmia or Congenital Glaucoma: its Causes, Treatment and Outlook.* Cambridge University Press, London.

Ashton, N. (1970) 'Retinal angiogenesis in the human embryo'. *Br. Med. Bull.*, **26**, 103–106.

Balazs, E.A., Toth, L.Z. and Ozanics, V. (1980) 'Cytological studies on the developing vitreous as related to the hyaloid vessel system'. *Albrecht Von Graefes Arch. Klin. Exp. Ophthalmol.*, **213**, 71–85.

Bartelmez, G.W. and Blount, M.P. (1954). 'The formation of the neural crest from the primary optic vesicle in man'. *Contrib. Embryol., Carnegie Institution*, **35**, 55–71.

Burian, H.M. and Braley, A.E. (1956) 'A new concept of the development of the angle of the anterior chamber of the human eye'. *Arch. Ophthalmol.*, **55**, 439.

Duke-Elder, S. and Cooke, C. (1963) 'Normal and abnormal development', in *System of Ophthalmology, Vol. 3, Part 1, Embryology*. (S. Duke-Elder, ed.) C.V. Mosby, St Louis.

Gilbert, P.W. (1952) 'The origin and development of the head cavities in the human embryo'. *J. Morphol.*, **90**, 149–87.

Gilbert, P.W. (1957) 'The origin and development of the human extraocular muscles'. *Contrib. Embryol., Carnegie Institution*, **36**, 59–78.

Gloor, B.P. (1972) 'Zur Entwicklung des Glaskörpers und der Zonula'; and 'Glaskörperzellen wahrend Entwicklung und Ruckbildung der Vasa hyaloidea und der Tunica vasculosa lentis'. *Albrecht Von Graefes Arch. Klin. Exp. Opthalmol.*, **186**, 311–28.

Grädinger, M.C. and Leuenberger, P.M. (1973) 'Zur Frage der Kollagensynthese durch corneales Epithel. II. Biochemische und elektronmikroskopische Untersuchungen an kultivierten Epithelzellen der Kaninchenhornhaut'. *Albrecht Von Graefes Arch. Klin. Ophthalmol.*, **187**, 183–200.

Hay, E.D. and Revel, J.P. (1969) 'Fine structure of the developing avian cornea', in *Monographs in Developmental Biology, Vol. 1.* (A. Wolsky & P.S. Chen, eds). Karger, New York.

Heimann, K. (1972) 'The development of the choroid in man: choroidal vascular system'. *Ophthalmic Res.*, **3**, 257–73.

Hendrickson, A.E. and Yuodelis, C. (1984) 'The morphological development of the human fovea'. *Ophthalmology*, **91**, 603–612.

Imaizumi, M. and Kuwabara, T. (1971) 'Development of the rat iris'. *Invest Ophthalmol.*, **10**, 733–44.

Ko, M-K., Chi, J.G. and Chang, B-L. (1985) 'Hyaloid vascular pattern in the human fetus'. *J. Pediatr. Ophthalmol. Strabismus*, **22**, 188–93.

Lai, Y-L. (1972) 'The development of the dilator muscle in the iris of the albino rat'. *Exp. Eye Res.*, **14**, 203–207.

Magoon, E.H. and Robb, R.M. (1981) 'Development of myelin in human optic nerve and tract. A light and electron microscopic study'. *Arch. Ophthalmol.*, **99**, 655–9.

Mann, I. (1960) *The Development of the Human Eye*. Grune and Stratton Inc., New York.

Mann, I. (1964) *The Development of the Human Eye*, 3rd edn. British Medical Association, London.

Maumenee, A.E. (1959) 'The pathogenesis of congenital glaucoma: a new theory'. *Amer. J. Ophthalmol.*, **47**, 827.

Michaelson, I.C. (1948) 'The mode of development of the vascular system of the retina with some observations on its significance for certain retinal diseases'. *Trans. Ophthalmol. Soc., UK*, **68**, 137–80.

Müller, F. and O'Rahilly, R. (1985) 'The first appearance of the neural tube and optic primordium in the human embryo at stage 10'. *Anat. Embryol.*, **172**, 157–69.

Mund, M.L., Rodrigues, M.M. and Fine, B.S. (1972) 'Light and electron microscopic observations on the pigmented layers of the developing human eye'. *Amer. J. Ophthalmol.*, **73**, 167–82.

Nassbaum, M. (1893) 'The anatomical contributions to the knowledge of the eye muscle'. *Anat. Anz.*, **8**, 298.

O'Rahilly, R. (1966) 'The early development of the eye in staged human embryos'. *Contrib. Embryol. Carnegie Institution*, **38**, 1–42.

O'Rahilly, R. and Müller, F. (1984) 'Embryonic length and cerebral landmarks in staged human embryos'. *Anat. Rec.*, **209**, 265–71.

O'Rahilly, R. and Müller, F. (1987) 'Developmental stages in human embryos'. *Carnegie Institution of Washington, Publication No. 637*.

Ozanics, V. and Jakobiec, F.A. (1982) 'Prenatal development of the eye and its adnexa', in *Ocular Anatomy, Embryology and Teratology*. (F.A. Jakobiec, ed.). Harper and Row Publishers Inc., Philadelphia.

Pearson, A.A. (1980) 'Development of the eyelids. (1) External features'. *J. Anat.*, **130**, 33–42.

Provis, J.M., Van Driel, D., Billson, F.A. and Russell, P. (1985) 'Human fetal optic nerve: overproduction and elimination of retinal axons during development'. *J. Comp. Neurol.*, **238**, 92–100.

Remé, C. and Lalive d'Epinay, S. (1981) 'Periods of development of the normal human chamber angle'. *Doc. Ophthalmol.*, **51**, 241–68.

Rhodes, R.H. (1978) 'Development of the human optic disc: light microscopy'. *Amer. J. Anat.*, **153**, 601–615.

Rhodes, R.H. (1979) 'A light microscopic study on the developing human neural retina'. *Amer. J. Anat.*, **154**, 195–210.

Ruprecht, K.W. and Wulle, K-G. (1973) 'Licht und elektronmikroskopische Untersuchungen zur Entwicklung des menschlichen Musculus sphincter pupillae'. *Albrecht Von Graefes Arch. Klin. Exp. Ophthalmol.*, **186**, 117–30.

Rytkola, T. (1952) 'Über die Entwicklung des Kammerwinkels der menschlinchen'. *Feten. Suomalaisen Tiedeakatemian Toimituksia Annales Academiae Scientiarum Fennicae.* Suomalanen Tiedakatemia, Helsinki.

Sadler, T.W. (1985) *Langman's Medical Embryology*, 5th edn. Williams and Wilkins, Baltimore.

Sattler, C.H. (1915) 'Über die Makscheidenentwicklung im Tractus opticus. Chiasma und Nervus opticus'. *Albrecht Von Graefes Arch. Ophthalmol.*, **90**, 271–98.

Seefelder, R. (1910) 'Das Verhalten der Kammerbucht und ihres Gerustwerkes bis zur Geburt', in *Handbuch der gesamten Augenheilkunde*, 2nd edn. (A. Graefe & T. Saemisch, eds). Wilhelm Engelmann, Leipzig.

Sellheyer, K. and Spitznas, M. (1987) 'Ultrastructure of the human posterior vasculosa lentis during early gestation'. *Graefes Arch. Clin. Exp. Ophthalmol.*, **255**, 377–83.

Sellheyer, K. and Spitznas, M. (1988a) 'Development of the human sclera. A morphological study'. *Graefes Arch. Clin. Exp. Ophthalmol.*, **226**, 89–100.

Sellheyer, K. and Spitznas, M. (1988b) 'Surface morphology of the human ciliary body during prenatal development. A scanning electron microscopic study'. *Graefes Arch. Clin. Exp. Ophthalmol.*, **226**, 78–83.

Sevel, D. (1981a) 'Reappraisal of the origin of human extraocular muscles'. *Ophthalmol.*, **88**, 1330–8.

Sevel, D. (1981b) 'Development and congenital abnormalities of the nasolacrimal apparatus'. *J. Pediatr. Ophthalmol. & Strabismus*, **18**, 13–20.

Sevel, D., Bothwell, L., Hiss, P., Isaacs, R. and Miller, D. (1985) 'A reappraisal of the development of the anterior chamber'. *Ophthalmic Paediatr. Genet.*, **6**, 17–23.

Smelser, G.K. and Ozanics, V. (1971) 'The development of the trabecular meshwork in primate eyes'. *Amer. J. Ophthalmol.*, **71**, 366–85.

Spira, A. and Hollenberg, M.J. (1973) 'Human retinal development: Ultrastructure of the inner retinal layers'. *Developmental Biol.*, **31**, 1–21.

Streeten, B.W. (1982) 'Ciliary Body', in *Ocular Anatomy, Embryology and Teratology*. (F.A. Jakobiec, ed.). Harper and Row Publishers Inc., Philadelphia.

Streeter, G.L. (1945) 'Developmental horizons in human embryos. Description of age-group XII, embryos about 4mm or 5mm long, and age-group XIV, period of indentation of the lens vesicle. *Contrib. Embryol., Carnegie Institution*, **31**, 27–63.

Sturrock, R.R. (1987a) 'Development of the meninges of the human embryonic optic nerve'. *J. Hirnforsch*, **28**, 603–613.

Sturrock, R.R. (1987b) 'Changes in the number of axons in the human embryonic optic nerve from 8 to 18 weeks. *J. Hirnforsch.*, **28**, 649–52.

Szilli, A. (1901) 'Zur anatomie und Entwickelungageschichte der hintern Iris schichten, mit besonderer Berucksichtlgung des Musculus sphincter iridis des Menschen'. *Anat. Anz.*, **20**, 161.

Trelstad, R.L. and Coulombre, A.J. (1971) 'Morphogenesis of the collagenous stroma in the chick cornea'. *J. Cell Biol.*, **50**, 840–58.

Tripathi, B. and Tripathi, R. (1989) 'Embryology of the anterior segment of the human eye', in *The Glaucomas*. (R. Ritch, M.B. Shields & T. Krupin, eds). C.V. Mosby, St Louis.

Weale, R.A. (1982) *A Biography of the Eye*. Lewis, London.

Wulle, K-G. (1972) 'The development of the productive and drainage system of the aqueous humor in the human eye'. *Adv. Ophthalmol.*, **26**, 296–355.

Wulle, K-G. and Richter, J. (1978) 'Electron microscopy of the early embryonic development of the human corneal epithelium'. *Albrecht Von Graefes Arch. Klin. Exp. Ophthalmol.*, **209**, 39–49.

Yamada, E. and Ishikawa, T. (1965) 'Some observations on the submicroscopic morphogenesis of the human retina', in *Eye Structure, II Symp.* (J.W. Rohen, ed.). Schattauer-Verlag, Stuttgart.

Yanoff, M. and Fine, B.S. (1975) *Ocular Pathology: A Text and Atlas*. Harper and Row, New York.

Acknowledgements

I would like to thank the Carnegie Institution of Washington for allowing the reproduction of eight photomicrographs from O'Rahilly, 'The Early Development of the Eye in Staged Human Embryos', published originally in contributions to *Embryology* **38**, 1966 (Institution's Publication No. 625). The photographs appear in the present text as Figs 2.1 to 2.6, and 2.8 and 2.17. Figs 2.12 to 2.16 in this text are published courtesy of *Ophthalmology* (Hendrickson and Yuodelis, 1984; **91**, 603–612). Figs 2.9 to 2.11 are reproduced with permission from *Developmental Biology* (Spira & Hollenberg, 1973; **31**, 1–21). Figs 2.19 and 2.20 are reproduced with permission from Sellheyer & Spitznas, *Graefes Arch. Clin. Exp. Ophthalmol.* (1980; **226**, 78–83).

I would also like to thank Professor Remé for kindly donating an original photomicrograph (Fig. 2.18) for inclusion in this chapter.

CHAPTER 3

Child Visual Development

Annette Grounds

3.1 Introduction

This chapter is mainly concerned with the way the normal visual system develops. It is essential that good quality sensory input is available to a child to ensure adequate development of the normal visual system. Normal development can be prevented by biased inputs. One of the problems that can occur when sensory development is impeded is amblyopia (see Chapter 4).

At birth some visual functions are already quite well-developed, while others are in a very immature state, rendering them particularly vulnerable to inferior-quality input.

Much of our knowledge of visual development has been obtained from investigations using animals. In recent studies, the monkey has been favoured for comparison with human infants because, amongst the animal kingdom, the visual system of the monkey is the closest to that of humans. Many behavioural and anatomical studies suggest major similarities in development. Visual development in the monkey has been found to proceed approximately four-times faster than in human infants. For example, if a visual function first appears at about three weeks in the monkey this would correspond to approximately three months for human infants.

3.2 Anatomical changes in the eye

In comparison with the rest of the body, the size of the eye changes only slightly from birth to adulthood, with an approximately two- to three-fold increase in volume. Further, most of the growth of the eye takes place during the first two years of life. It should be remembered, however, that postnatal growth patterns are not equal in all structures of the eye.

The anterior surface of the cornea increases in area by approximately 50%, while the interior surface area of the retina more than doubles from 590 mm^2 to 1250 mm^2 (Scammon & Wilmer, 1950). The overall two- to three-fold increase in the volume of the eye can dramatically affect retinal image size, being particularly affected by the associated increase in axial length. Gordon & Donzis

43

(1985), carried out an extensive study of 148 normal eyes with an age range from premature newborns to adults. They found that a full-term newborn eye had a mean axial length of 16.8 mm, a mean corneal power of 51.2 D spherical equivalent, and a mean lens power of 34.4 D. These compared with adult mean values of axial length of 23.6 mm, corneal power of 43.5 D and lens power of 18.8 D. The axial length therefore increased by approximately 7 mm, requiring a reduction in total refracting power of the order of 30 D to maintain a comparable ocular refraction.

During growth the vertebrate eye achieves a close match between the power of its optics and its axial length, with the result that, in a large proportion of eyes, images of distant objects are sharply focused on the retina without accommodative effort.

The quality of the optical system of the newborn human or monkey infant is quite good when compared with non-primates such as the cat. The media of cats are cloudy at birth, while those of humans and primates are clear. The line-spread function has been assessed in infant monkeys and demonstrates that optical quality for well-focused retinal images is good at birth, and rapidly reaches adult levels by about nine weeks after birth. No line-spread functions are available for human infants but ophthalmoscopy shows good media clarity within a few days of birth.

3.3 Refractive development

Studies on early refractive development have shown the average newborn term infant to be hypermetropic with a mean refractive error of around 2 D (SD 2 D). Further, hypermetropia usually increases from birth, peaking at around six months of age, and thereafter tends to gradually decrease towards emmetropia (emmetropization) by approximately age six years. The most rapid decline in hypermetropia occurs between six months and two years in normally developing eyes. Infant monkey eyes are similarly hypermetropic and also move towards emmetropia during the first few months postnatally (Neuringer *et al.*, 1984). Premature babies have been shown to be less hypermetropic, with a mean value of about 1 D, but with a greater variation (SD 2.5 D). In some studies, very premature babies have shown high levels of myopia of up to 12 D.

Children who develop strabismus do not generally appear to show emmetropization. Instead, they demonstrate either increasing hypermetropia or their refractive error remains unchanged. In cases where hypermetropia increases, the most marked rise is within the first three years, which coincides with the period in which accommodative esotropia most frequently becomes manifest. Aurell & Norrsell (1990) showed that infants who were hypermetropic by 4 D or more at six months showed two trends. One group became progressively less hypermetropic and none developed strabismus. A second group showed no reduction in hypermetropia and all developed esotropia and amblyopia. Similar trends were found by Dobson & Sebris (1989).

Medina (1987) has proposed a mathematical model for the emmetropization process. The model implies a feedback mechanism that causes a reduction of refractive errors in all forms of ametropia. Over the past decade evidence has suggested that refractive error is controlled by the quality of visual input and that deficient visual input, or faulty neural transmission, cause failure of emmetropization.

There are two schools of thought as to why emmetropization occurs. One suggests that eye growth is actively regulated, and that visual experience guides the refractive state towards emmetropia (Banks, 1980; Medina, 1987; Young, 1977). An alternative theory suggests that the postnatal changes are a continuation of genetically determined embryological processes that, in combination with the physical constraints on eye growth, result in the eye achieving normal size and shape (Sorsby, 1979).

It has been suggested that the changes in shape of the lens occurring during accommodation cause increased intraocular pressure (IOP), which may lead to stretching of the eye, and an increased axial length. This idea is given further credence as a rapid decrease in hypermetropia has been found to be a presenting sign of juvenile aphakic glaucoma. Therefore, increased IOP may be linked with increasing myopia. It should also be noted that there is a higher incidence of open angle glaucoma among high myopes.

In a study by Hendrickson & Rosenblum (1985), four groups of kittens were examined. Group one was the control group; kittens in group two were made anisometropic by monocular radial keratotomy. Both groups showed a trend towards emmetropia over time, and in group two a reduction in the level of anisometropia was found. Group three kittens had daily atropine instilled monocularly, while in group four bilateral keratotomy was performed plus daily instillations of atropine monocularly. Anisometropia resulted in both these groups, with greater hypermetropia remaining in the atropinized eye. The eyes that could accommodate showed longer axial lengths, and shorter than normal focal lengths of the crystalline lens. They interpreted this as demonstrating that accommodation leads to a tendency towards myopia and away from hypermetropia.

Troilo & Wallman (1991) similarly assessed emmetropization in chicks and found that the major shift towards emmetropization was effected by adjustment of the vitreous chamber depth. They identified an additional factor, a slow change produced by 'shape-related mechanisms' that regulated eye size and shape to give normal appearance. They examined the possible role of accommodation by making lesions in the Edinger–Westphal nucleus in order to block the motor output of the accommodative system. The results led them to dispute the common assumption that accommodation was a guiding factor. They concluded, however, that even if accommodation was not involved in the control of eye growth the stimuli that drive accommodation may also drive the visually guided emmetropization mechanism. In an earlier study, (Wallman *et al.*, 1981) the amount of myopia induced by visual form deprivation was reduced by cutting the short ciliary nerves, thereby blocking the final motor pathway of accommodation. Clearly more research is required to resolve the controversy surrounding the possible effects of accommodation on emmetropization. In a study by Parssinen *et al.* (1989) the progression of myopia was assessed in myopic school children aged nine to eleven years. They were randomly split into three groups. Group one wore their full myopic correction constantly, group two used spectacles for distance only, and group three were issued with bifocals with a +1.75 addition. Their aim was to investigate if the reduction in the accommodative effort for close work required in groups two and three would reduce the trend towards increased myopia. However, it emerged that the extent of myopic progression was strongly correlated to the amount of close work undertaken, but that no significant difference in the rate of myopic progression was found among the three groups. One point of interest, observed when the author has deliberately underminused in the consulting room, is that young myopes tend to reduce their working distance. They seem to have a preference for a given amount of accommodative effort. This would effectively eliminate any potential advantage from underminusing and may in fact induce further problems by upsetting the AC/A ratio.

Astigmatism is commoner in infants than in adults and remains so during most of the preschool years. Gwiazda *et al.* (1984) and Dobson *et al.* (1984) found a mean level of astigmatism of 1 D in early infancy. Below the age of three-and-a-half years the astigmatism was more commonly against-the-rule, while after three-and-a-half years it was more commonly with-the-rule (Dobson *et al.*, (1984)). One proposed reason for the change from against- to with-the-rule is that pressure exerted by the lids causes corneal distortion. Howland (1982), using photokeratometric measurements, showed that an infant's astigmatism is highly correlated with the curvature of the infant's cornea. Astigmatism reduces between one-and-a-half and four years of age. It has generally been considered that astigmatism does not require correction prior to approximately three years of age.

3.4   Anatomical and physiological development of the visual system

3.4.1   Anatomical development of the retina

In the primate retina, ganglion cells and bipolar layers have already thinned in the macular region at the time of birth, leaving a characteristic foveal depression similar in gross histological appearance to that of an adult. There is incomplete migration of the ganglion cells and inner nuclear layers out of the foveal region. It also possesses only a single layer of short, thick immature cones. Yuodelis & Hendrickson (1986), studying human cadaver neonate retinas, showed that before birth the foveal region is over 1000 μm in diameter, but that it starts to narrow after birth reaching 650 to 700 μm by 45 months. This is due to cone migration towards the centre of the fovea, thus increasing their packing density from 18 cones/100 μm^2 in neonates to 42 cones/100 μm^2 in adulthood. Cone development postnatally shows maturation, elongation and increased packing density. Cone diameters are shown to be 7.5 μm at five days postnatally changing to 2 μm by 45 months. However, although foveal width and cone diameter have reached the adult developmental stage by 45 months the packing density at this age is still approximately half the adult level. Electro-oculography results have shown 'electrical activity' in the cones of newborns indicating that function is present despite the immaturity.

Amacrine, bipolar and ganglion cells also migrate as the foveal pit starts to form during the first four months postnatally. Due to these changes the information entering the eye will be detected by a changing array of receptor cells. In order that confusion does not result, plasticity of the visual centres must be present to enable continual recalibration.

The more peripheral areas develop faster than the foveal region. The peripheral retina at birth is structurally quite mature. However, studies have shown that, despite the immaturity of the foveal region, it still has superior resolving capacity compared to the periphery.

Myelination of the optic nerve begins first for those cells which subserve the fovea, and is complete for all ganglion cell areas by the beginning of the sixth postnatal month.

In general, the primary postnatal changes in the retina concern differentiation of the macular region.

3.4.2 Sensory development of the retina

Visual perception depends most directly on the retinocortical pathways. The first sensory cells of importance are the retinal ganglion cells. These cells fall into three different classes with different functions.

The basic receptive field organization of all three types of ganglion cell is circular, with centre and surround regions responding in opponent fashion. Some cells respond with an excitatory response when light stimulates the centre of the field and show an inhibitory response for the annular surround, while others respond with an inhibitory response in the centre and have excitatory surrounds.

Table 3.1 below summarizes some of the differences of the three retinal ganglion cell subgroups.

Table 3.1   Distinguishing features of ganglion cells.

Properties	X-Type	Y-Type	W-Type
Size	Medium	Large	Variable
Dendritic spread	Small	Medium	Large
Response characteristic	Brisk sustained	Brisk transient	Sluggish sustained
Conduction velocity	Medium	Fast	Slow
Receptive field size	Small	Medium	Large
Projection	LGN parvocellular	LGN magnocellular	LGN
Cortical destination	Temporal lobe	Parietal lobe	
Temporal condition for maximum response	Static targets/low frequency flicker	Moving targets/high frequency flicker	

3.4.3   Anatomical development of the LGN

The LGN is a laminated structure, with the left and right eye afferents already segregated into separate laminae at birth (Hitchcock & Hickey, 1980). The main difference between the infant and adult is the size of the geniculate cell bodies, with the cell bodies in the infant LGN being smaller. The time required for cell bodies to reach adult size varies in the magnocellular (transient, Y system) and parvocellular (sustained, X system) laminae. Cells in both laminae undergo a rapid increase in cross-sectional area during the first few months postnatally. Neurones in the parvocellular layers of the LGN grow rapidly over the early postnatal months and reach adult size near the end of the first year. The neurones in the magnocellular layers show continued rapid growth throughout the first year, but adult size is not reached until at least 24 months postnatally.

In terms of dendritic morphology, however, there is some evidence that both parvocellular and magnocellular neurones in the human LGN are adult-like by the end of the ninth postnatal month (Garey & De Courten, 1983).

3.4.4   Sensory development of the LGN

The LGN has a preponderance of spines and filopodia on the dendrites of immature neurones. The number of spines increases after birth to peak at around four months postnatally, and declines to adult levels by about nine months in humans (Garey & De Courten, 1983). A number of significant developmental events occur at around four months in the human visual system. It may be that these changes are linked to the alterations in the number of spines in the LGN and cortex.

The spatial resolution of LGN X-cells with receptive fields in the central fovea increases six-fold between birth and adulthood, while the increase is only two-fold in the peripheral retina beyond 10° eccentricity. It can be seen from this that, relative to that of the adult, the fovea at birth is more immature than the periphery. Despite this the newborn fovea is still capable of greater resolving power than the periphery. Blakemore and Vital-Durrand (1980) using Rhesus monkeys showed that recordings in the LGN at birth indicated that their foveas can resolve gratings equivalent to Snellen acuities of between 6/32 and 6/72 These estimates compare quite favourably with behavioural estimates of acuity obtained from newborn humans although the human results are generally lower. However, it is known that at birth the human retina is less mature than that of the monkey.

3.4.5 Anatomical and sensory development of the visual cortex (VC)

As in the LGN an overabundance of spines is found in the immature striate cortex. These spines initially increase in number, and are subsequently pruned back to adult levels over a similar time-course to that in the LGN. It appears that, early in development, neurones connect with all possible neighbours, perhaps as an aid to making the right connections.

During the first few weeks of postnatal development the geniculocortical projections from the two eyes overlap extensively in layer IV of the monkey visual cortex (Hubel *et al.*, 1977). This early overlap is similar to that found in the LGN prenatally. Segregation occurs in the last three weeks prenatally and this represents the first step in the development of ocular dominance columns.

Many properties of the receptive fields seem to be established in the newborn Macaque monkey. Cells can be classified as simple, complex or hypercomplex and they demonstrate orientation tuning and binocular input.

In the mature primate striate cortex the most striking feature is its organization into ocular dominance columns, where the input from the two eyes is segregated into discrete bands. At birth, ocular dominance columns are present and segregation is complete by about six weeks of age. This would suggest completion of ocular dominance columns in human infants by about six months old.

Deprivation of one eye while the columns are developing causes a shift in favour of the non-deprived eye, resulting in an increase in column size in the non-deprived eye and shrinkage in the deprived eye. Changes in ocular dominance column widths can only occur during the critical period of development (see Chapter 4, Section 4.3). In normal development about 80% of cortical neurones respond to binocular stimulation.

Visually evoked potential studies have suggested that in the human VC certain types of cortical inhibitory interactions do not appear until six months of age. Many sensory functions including orientation, spatial tuning and binocular interactions are critically dependent on inhibitory interactions in the cortex.

There are no electrophysiological findings from human infants, but single-cell recordings in the newborn monkey cortex reveal activity that is fairly mature. Cells have been shown to respond to visual stimulation, displaying orientation selectivity and ocular dominance. Further, the simple and complex field responses are similar to those of the mature monkey. There is some evidence from VEP recordings that the cells in the human VC are also capable of some function at birth.

3.5   The development of spatial vision

The ability to resolve detail is a basic attribute of form vision that can be assessed from the measurement of spatial resolution, visual acuity (VA) and by the measurement of the contrast threshold or contrast sensitivity function (CSF).

3.5.1   The development of visual acuity

Several studies have assessed infant visual acuity using a variety of techniques. Detailed discussion of these techniques is beyond the scope of this chapter. However, a brief résumé of the main methods will be given below, with details of expected normal visual acuity levels for different ages in Table 3.2.

One of the most popular methods for visual acuity evaluation in early infancy is preferential looking (PL). This method capitalizes on the natural tendency

Table 3.2   Variation in visual acuity and contrast sensitivity with age.

Age	Visual Acuity	Contrast Sensitivity Function (Peak Response)
Birth	≅6/300	Unknown
1 month	between 6/200 and 6/90	≅6/90 at 2 months
3 months	≅6/90 to 6/60	≅6/60
6 months	≅6/60 to 6/36	
9 months	≅6/36 to 6/24	≅6/12 equivalent grating
1 year	≅6/24	≅6/9 grating acuity
$1\frac{1}{2}$ years	≅6/18 to 6/12	≅6/6 grating acuity
2 years	≅6/12 to 6/9	≅6/6 grating acuity
3 years	≅6/9 to 6/6	Continues to improve in overall sensitivity
5 years	6/6 to 6/5 angular, and possibly morphoscopic	Approaches adult levels
6 years up to 12 years	6/6 to 6/5 Morphoscopic acuity has been shown to take up to 10 years to reach adulthood	True adult levels reached between 6 to 12 years of age

of an infant, even at birth, to look longer at a patterned stimulus than an unpatterned one. Two displays are viewed simultaneously by an infant, one containing a pattern of equal-width black and white bars (square-wave grating), the spatial frequency of which can be varied. The other display is a homogeneous grey of matched mean luminance. When an infant views the grating for 75% of the time it is deemed to have been resolved. A variation on this method is known as forced-choice PL (Dobson *et al.*, 1978b), in which an adult views directly the infant's viewing pattern through a hole between the two stimuli. The adult must decide on which side the grating is placed by observing the viewing behaviour of the infant. This method allows the observer to take other factors of infant behaviour into consideration. In older infants the two methods give similar visual acuity assessments, but in very young infants measurements of VA are higher with forced-choice PL.

An alternative method of VA assessment relies on the infant's natural tendency to track moving objects until they disappear, at which point a flick (saccade) occurs, moving the eyes back to the midline. This is known as optokinetic nystagmus (OKN). It is commonly observed when a person riding in a train views objects such as telegraph poles. The OKN reflex can be observed directly in infants, but most results have been obtained using an electrophysiological recording method, known as the electro-oculogram (EOG), in which electrodes are placed at the lateral canthi of each eye.

A third method measures the visually evoked potential (VEP) which is obtained with suitably placed scalp electrodes. The stimulus used varies. Sokol (1978) used flashing checkerboards, and made an estimate of the smallest check size that would elicit an identifiable electrophysiological response.

Ossenblok *et al.* 1992, using checkerboard onset evoked potential, found that the adult waveform is not obtained before the age of puberty.

While there is generally good agreement between the VA obtained by the assessment methods of PL and OKN, the results obtained using VEP methods generally give higher acuity estimates. VEP acuity approaches adult levels by about one year of age, while the other methods show a much slower time-course. This discrepancy has not yet been fully resolved.

Allen *et al.* (1992), measured the luminance-dependent nature of infants' grating acuity using forced-choice PL, steady-state VEP and sweep VEP. The relative improvement in performance with increasing luminance is slightly greater for forced-choice PL than for VEP. This may be related to the relationship between contrast sensitivity and grating acuity, which is also luminance dependent.

It has been shown, by Brown *et al.* (1987), that infant and adult spatial vision can be rendered identical if infants are tested at a brighter light level than adults. Therefore infant acuity-versus-luminance plots, once shifted leftward by a suitable amount, will superimpose on the adult plots.

Cannon (1983), devised an experiment to assess the correlation between the VEP and psychophysical estimates of VA. He measured both VEP and psychophysical detection thresholds, but presented exactly the same stimulus in both tasks – a sine-wave grating, phase reversing 20 times per second. The VEP thresholds were consistently higher than the psychophysical estimates.

Shimojo *et al.* (1984) used a variant of forced PL to measure vernier acuity from infants two to nine months of age. They found that the smallest detectable offset was less than three minutes of arc by six months. Furthermore, the growth curve for vernier acuity was different from that for grating acuity.

It is probable that hyperacuity develops at later ages than those predominantly studied to date. It may indeed coincide with the late development of finely sampled foveal high spatial frequency mechanisms in the cortex. What is important is that vernier and grating acuity appear to have a different developmental time-course until they reach adult levels of performance. In a more recent study, Zanker *et al.* (1992), who investigated 271 infants and children, found that vernier acuity develops gradually, but more rapidly than grating acuity and is adult-like by five years of age. It should be noted (see Chapter 4, Section 4.3.2) that strabismic and anisometropic amblyopes show different relative losses of grating and vernier acuity. This led Ciuffreda *et al.* (1991), to propose the intriguing question, or 'whether strabismus and anisometropia exert their effects on the developing visual nervous system at different times of development'.

At birth and through the first few postnatal months acuity is quite poor. Furthermore, the acuity of pre-term babies is even poorer than that of full-term babies of the same postnatal age (Dobson & Teller, 1978). However, if pre-term and full-term babies are age-matched from conception then similar acuity levels are recorded. The results from studies using variations of PL have generally found an acuity estimate of one cycle/deg (approximately 6/200 Snellen equivalent) at one month of age, improving to six cycles/deg (6/36) at six months.

Most studies have concentrated on acuity development up to about six months of age, though a few studies have extended the range. Gwiazda *et al.* 1980, studied infants up to 58 weeks of age, finding the acuity at one year to be equivalent to 6/18 to 6/24. Mayer & Dobson (1982), extended the measurements to age five years and found adult-like acuity of 6/6. This is in agreement with studies reviewed by Mayer & Dobson (1982) which show that similar results are found in preschool children with Allen cards, the E Game, and Snellen Letters. However, Atkinson & Braddick (1983), found that when Snellen charts (morphoscopic acuity) are used visual acuity does not reach adult levels until up to ten years of age.

It is considered that visual performance in infants approximates to the best possible, considering the state of neural development. Foveal cone separation decreases postnatally in humans, so receptor spacing contributes to age related changes. A broad range of neural mechanisms may also constrain acuity in early life. The spatial tuning of neurones at different levels of the visual system and the size of the neurones' receptive fields will limit spatial resolution. The size of retinal ganglion cell receptor fields decreases significantly postnatally in cats, therefore acuity will increase.

The spatial resolution of cortical and LGN neurones also improves postnatally in cats and monkeys (Blakemore & Vital-Durrand, 1980). There are no electrophysiological data on receptive field size development in humans, but there is evidence suggesting that it is similar to that in Macaque monkeys.

3.5.2 The development of contrast sensitivity

Contrast sensitivity measures the amount of contrast required to detect the presence of a grating of different spatial frequencies, from coarse to fine. Spatial frequency is measured in cycles per degree. A grating of one cycle/deg means that one dark and one light bar subtend 1° at the eye. Therefore, 10 cycles/deg would be 10 alternating light and dark bars which together subtend 1° at the eye.

Peak sensitivity is achieved at around four cycles/deg. This grating can be resolved with only approximately 1% contrast. More contrast is required for higher and lower spatial frequencies. At the high spatial frequency end the contrast for detection must be greatly increased, until the point when the grating is beyond the resolving power of the visual system and no detection is elicited even at a maximum 100% contrast, see Fig. 3.1.

The development of contrast sensitivity has been studied in infants and young children by several researchers. The peak of the CSF shifts towards higher spatial frequencies with age. The low spatial frequency fall-off characteristic of adult's CSFs is not found at one month. This suggests that lateral inhibition, which is considered to be responsible for the effect, must develop postnatally, see Fig. 3.2. Compared to the adult CSF curve the infants' curve is shifted to a lower band of spatial frequencies. Infants also appear to have a substantial deficit of overall contrast sensitivity when compared to adults.

In preschool and schoolchildren the shape of the CSF is essentially adult-like, although the overall sensitivity is less than that of adults until between six to twelve years of age (Atkinson & Braddick, 1981). This implies that more contrast is required if young children are to resolve detail. So a young child wishing to cross a road in foggy conditions may not see the emerging details of a light coloured car as easily as an adult, an important point to consider.

CSFs have been obtained longitudinally from infant monkeys from five to 60 weeks postnatally (Boothe *et al.*, 1980). Sensitivity increased monotonically (increases continually with time) at all spatial frequencies but the sensitivity

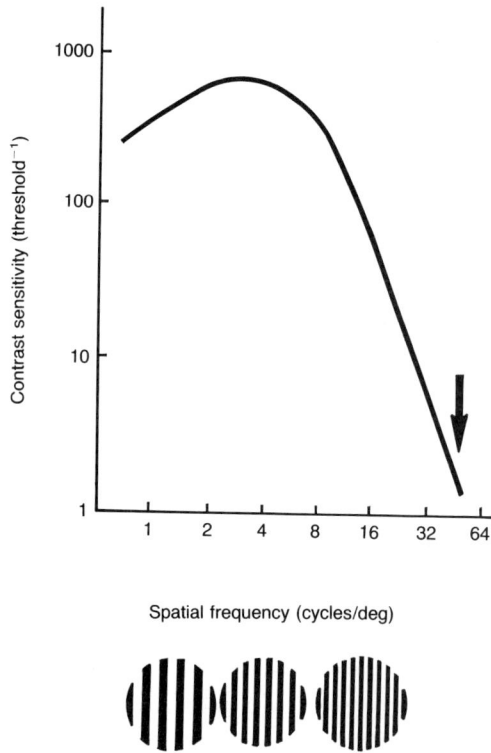

Fig. 3.1 A typical contrast sensitivity function.

to low spatial frequencies becomes adult-like earlier than that for the high frequency range. For example, sensitivities for one to five cycles/deg have reached adult levels by 20 weeks while sensitivities for gratings greater than fifteen cycles/deg are still improving at 40 weeks. Qualitatively, these changes consist of shifts of the CSF curve upwards, due to increasing sensitivity, and a shift of the peak response to the right, corresponding to higher spatial frequencies.

Any visual function will develop four times faster in a monkey than in a human infant. Based on this knowledge, a useful rule-of-thumb, known as the 4:1 rule, has been devised, and it allows results obtained from monkey subjects to be related to human visual development. For example, a function first worked at one week in monkeys will develop at four weeks in human infants.

When the CSF development curves for monkeys and human infants are appropriately scaled, following the application of the 4:1 rule, marked developmental similarity is displayed.

The developmental changes that occur in visual resolution and CS can be understood by considering the changes taking place in the retina and cortex.

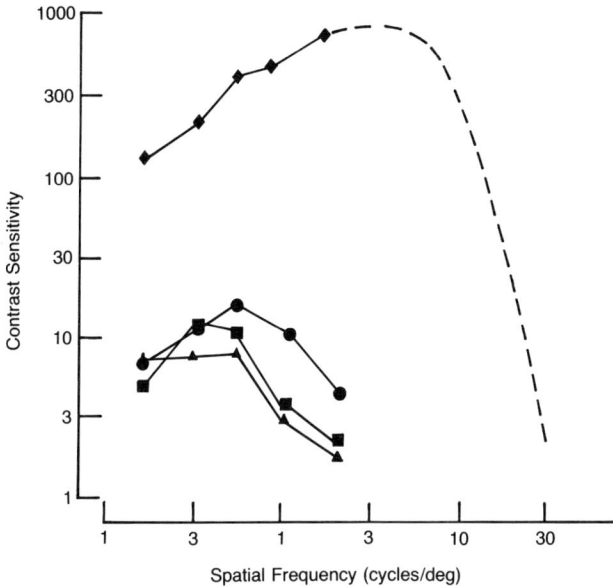

Fig. 3.2 Contrast sensitivity functions of human infants at one, two, and three months of age. Data gathered by preferential looking procedures for large sine-wave gratings. Data for adults were obtained on the same apparatus. Adapted from Banks and Salapatek, 1978, with permission from the publishers.

Wilson (1988), suggested that the migration of foveal cones produces a change in spatial scale and therefore a progressive shift of mechanisms tuned towards higher spatial frequencies, while the growth of the foveal cone outer segments causes an increase in mechanism sensitivity.

3.5.3   Orientation selectivity

Human infants can discriminate between different stimulus orientations during the first two postnatal months, but there is no evidence for variations in acuity with orientation in non-astigmatic infants less than six months of age (Dobson *et al.*, 1978a). In older infants and young children, results show slightly better acuity for vertical and horizontal gratings than for oblique gratings. This is also true for adults, although there is considerable variation between individuals. The variation in acuity with orientation may be the result of different amounts of exposure to stimulus orientation in our normal environment. It could also be affected by astigmatism. In a study by Manny (1992), orientation selectivity of three-month-old infants was similar to that of adults tested with the same stimulus parameters.

However when adults are tested with stimulus parameters selected to optimize their VEP response instead of those which optimize the infant's response, the orientation discrimination of adults improves by a factor of two.

A study by Braddick *et al.* (1986) showed that oblique orientation sensitivity is not found until six weeks of age. However, orientation selective cells have been recorded in newborn monkeys. There are two possible explanations for this discrepancy. Firstly, vertical and horizontal gratings were used in these latter studies, not oblique, and it is possible that sensitivity to oblique directions does develop later. Secondly, there is evidence that the human visual system is more immature at birth than that of primates.

3.6 Other aspects of visual perceptual development

It is not within the scope of this chapter to deal with all aspects of visual perceptual development. Therefore, details of changes in visual function such as wavelength discrimination, spectral sensitivity and absolute visual threshold are omitted, as are critical flicker fusion frequency and temporal visual development. Investigations have shown that these functions are essentially adult-like by about three months of age, if not earlier, and tend to imply that visual experience exerts little influence over them. In two recent studies, by Hansen & Fulton (1991) and Fulton *et al.* (1991), it was shown that there are post-receptoral immaturities in rod-mediated function in ten-week-old infants.

Wattam-Bell (1991), assessing the development of motion-specific cortical responses in infancy, found that directional responses were first found for low speed velocities at an approximate age of ten weeks. By 13 weeks of age directional responses were found for velocity speeds four times as fast. However, the VEP amplitudes were significantly greater for the lower velocity speeds. It was concluded that the development of directional sensitivity starts at low velocities, and extends to higher velocities with age. Human infants as young as two to three months possess adult-like photopic and scotopic sensitivity functions and their absolute visual thresholds are within an order of magnitude of those of adults. Infants as young as one month old have shown that they can make certain wavelength discriminations in the absence of luminance cues, which establishes that they are at least dichromatic. By three months of age, infants are demonstrably trichromatic. Evidence for the essentially innate development of colour vision is given by trichromacy being evident in monkeys dark reared from two weeks to threee months of age. Further details on colour vision are found in Chapter 10.

3.7 Motor aspects of visual development

The visual system relies on several sophisticated motor mechanisms to orient the receptors and optimize quality of information available for perceptual analysis.

In adults, control of ocular fixation, accommodation and pupil size constrain the quality of visual information available to the retina. As a result any inefficiency in visuomotor control may lead to a loss of visual information.

Maturity of these motor systems in infants may also affect the quality of visual information. Therefore, age-related improvements attributed to sensory or perceptual systems may be based, at least in part, on improvement in motor control.

3.7.1   Development of accommodation

The focus of the retinal image is determined by the accuracy of accommodation to a stimulus at different viewing distances. Infants are generally somewhat hypermetropic, therefore, accommodation will be required for viewing even at distance. This low level of accommodation should not pose problems once the accommodative system has developed accuracy. Early studies of infants aged one month suggested that their accommodation was fixed at one level (Haynes *et al.*, 1965). More recently Banks (1980), showed that this is not true if the stimulus used is of sufficient size to be resolvable by the immature visual system at all testing distances. Under these conditions the infants' responses were close to those of adults by two or three months. The results still, however, showed a marked postnatal improvement during the first three months. Similar findings have been reported by using photorefraction to obtain details of the accommodative change. Experiments have indicated that the infant's visual system is less susceptible to blur, suggesting that the stimulus for accommodation is less efficient.

Acuity in young infants is not significantly affected in the first few weeks of life by blur induced by lenses of up to 6 D, while by about six months the level of dioptral blur which does not affect acuity has to be 2 D or less. There would appear to be little functional advantage in accurate accommodation until the sensitivity to high spatial frequencies emerges around the sixth to seventh month postnatally. When adults are deliberately blurred by plus lenses, rendering them effectively myopic to a varying degree, their CSF shows a drop-off at high spatial frequencies similar to that found in early infancy. The low to medium ranges are unaffected, except when very high degrees of blurring are used.

The failure of high spatial frequencies to develop may be the reason why amblyopic eyes show a lag of accommodation and microfluctuations, with the result that the eye may remain in an immature accommodative state, see Chapter 4.

Another important factor is depth of focus. Compared with adults, children have small eyes and, in particular, small pupil diameters, leading to a greater depth of focus. Banks (1980), provided evidence that the accommodative inaccuracies of young infants at one to three months of age were within the estimated depth of focus of the infant visual system. It would appear therefore, that the infant's control of accommodation can be accounted for largely by sensory rather than motor factors.

Motor factors are not, however, irrelevant to the control of accommodation. In a study by Sokol *et al.* (1983), the latency of the adult VEP increased with increasing blur. In infants, even two dioptres of induced hypermetropia, which require two dioptres of accommodation, caused increases in the VEP latencies, indicating that infants do not use the accommodative capacity available to them. The effect of high ametropia on the accommodative response of infants is important. Brookman (1983), using similar experimental details to those of Banks (1980), also measured the refractive errors of infants at 20 weeks of age by cycloplegic retinoscopy. He found one infant who had a high hypermetropic refractive error at 20 weeks. This infant showed very little accommodative response. Following refractive correction this infant showed normal accommodative responses at 22 weeks.

Those with high refractive errors, either hypermetropic or myopic, are more likely to develop accommodative inaccuracies with a resultant loss of acuity and contrast sensitivity. There is some controversy as to whether accommodation or refractive error is the mediating factor in these losses. It may well be that both have a part to play. In some cases a reduced amplitude of accommodation may mean that even low hypermetropes would be put at risk.

3.7.2   The pupillary response

Video recording techniques have shown a sluggish pupillary response to light in infants, giving larger latencies and reduced amplitude changes in pupil diameters, as compared to adults.

Pupillary response improvements that occur between birth and adulthood are thought to be due to improvements in the motor system itself. In studies of infants' resting pupil size it has been found that the average pupil size increases with increasing age. In normal infants the consensual response to light is present from birth. Failure of development of a brisk consensual response in one eye is generally an indicator of possible amblyopia.

3.7.3   Eye movements

As the foveal and para-foveal areas of the retina are responsible for good resolution, the main role of the ocular motor system is to accurately move and align the central region with the object of regard.

The saccadic system

The function of the saccadic system is to move both eyes together (conjugate movement) in order to bring the stimulus of interest onto the foveal region. An important aspect of saccadic eye movements is that their neural programming is ballistic, i.e. once the ocular motor nucleus has initiated the neural response to move the eyes, it cannot be cancelled or modified until after the eyes have taken up their new position.

'Saccades' consist of an acceleration of the eyeball by a very brief neuro-muscular pulse, and deceleration by the dampening characteristics of the eyeball within the orbital tissue. The saccadic system in adults is remarkably accurate. For example, if a target under view is suddenly moved by 40°, there is a short latency of 200–250 millisecond, after which a saccade with velocity of up to 900°/second will place the eye within 5 to 10% of the desired position. This is followed by one or two small saccades to accurately foveate the target. By contrast, a two-month-old infant performs a series of fixed amplitude saccades at regular intervals until foveation is reached. Studies on saccadic locations in infants have been carried out by many research groups. Their results have shown the following trend: firstly, the probability of initiating a directionally-appropriate first saccade to a peripheral target decreases with increasing retinal eccentricity; secondly, the probability of accurate peripheral target location increases with increasing postnatal age. Infants are capable of making large saccades because they frequently do so in the dark. It appears that in early infancy the visual system is actually programming a sequence of small fixed amplitude saccades, probably due to an underlying sensory or motor constraint. Infants may be unable to control finely enough the duration of the neural pulse that the oculomotor system can reliably initiate. Thus, it may be more efficient to programme a minimum pulse duration, one that leads to a predictable outcome, rather than attempting to programme a variable pulse duration whose outcome cannot be controlled accurately.

The saccadic system in infants undergoes marked development during the first three months of postnatal life. However, truly efficient adult-like saccades are not found until the fifth postnatal month.

The pursuit system

This controls the ability of the eye to make smooth pursuit movements, moving the eyes conjugately with a velocity which matches that of the moving visual stimulus. When an object is tracked until it moves out of the visual field then a saccade moves the eye in the opposite direction which gives a whole field movement. This saccade, which follows smooth pursuit movement, is known as optokinetic nystagmus (OKN).

Smooth pursuit

In early quantitative studies the EOG was used to record infant tracking. The results tended to show that tracking was purely saccadic until about the end of the second month. However it has been suggested that the EOG lacked accuracy. More recent studies, using an infra-red video based recording system, have been used to measure smooth tracking. These results show a purely saccadic response in infants up to six weeks of age. Smooth pursuit was found after eight weeks of age but only for low velocities (less than 16°/second). By ten weeks of age, infants are able to catch up with the moving target and follow it quite well. However, at higher speeds, e.g. 40°/second, which would cause no problems to an adult, the infant is unable to follow at all. Between infancy and adulthood the smooth pursuit system clearly develops significantly. Aslin (1987), has proposed that a possible explanation of the saccadic inaccuracy, and failure of accurate pursuit in young infants, might be due to the migration of retinal photoreceptors towards the developing fovea in early infancy. Thus, assuming a proportional increase in the optical properties of the developing eyeball, a target located 10° from the fovea at an early age will stimulate a set of photoreceptors that will eventually be closer to the fovea on maturation. Therefore if there is an innate link between retinal locus and extraocular muscle output this would result in smaller saccades in early infancy. Similarly, the pursuit system will underestimate the movement of a target from the fovea to the periphery. Further work on kittens has shown similar results, and there seems to be an innate sensory or motor linkage between retinal locus and the direction and magnitude of saccades.

Optokinetic nystagmus (OKN)

OKN has been observed in newborn infants a few hours after birth. The smooth pursuit phase of OKN increases dramatically during the first few months of life. Atkinson & Braddick (1981), and Naegele & Held (1982), showed that there is asymmetry in the temporalward versus nasalward monocular OKN. This is due to an earlier onset for OKN elicited by nasalward stimulus movement than to temporalward movement. Naegele & Held (1982) used EOGs to record binocular and monocular OKN elicited by stripes that moved nasalward or temporalward and found that symmetry was approached gradually and was achieved at about five months in the normally developing visual system. It is possible that under binocular viewing conditions the moving stripes would move nasalward in one eye but temporalward in the other, and this may interfere with the programming of symmetrical conjugate OKN found in older infants and adults. Hainline *et al.* (1984) showed that infants and adults were able to elicit accurate vertical OKN equally in each eye. It appears therefore, that no vertical asymmetry is present.

It has been suggested that failure of the development of symmetry by three to four months is a possible indication of problems in visual development.

3.7.4 Development of the vergence system

The vergence system

Vergence eye movements are driven by two different types of visual information, diplopia (fusional vergence) and blur (accommodative vergence) and these are difficult to vary independently.

Fusional vergence

The attainment of fusion despite dual retinal inputs from a single visual target is attributed to corresponding retinal points. All possible pairs of corresponding points define a surface called the horopter, which intersects the point of bifoveal fixation. As such, it represents the locus of points in space around which stereoscopic processing is possible. Thus, if a single target stimulates a pair of corresponding retinal points, the target is perceived as single or fused. However, to either side of the horopter is a small area in which non-corresponding points can still be fused and perceived as single; this is known as Panum's fusional area. Outside this area diplopia will occur.

Adults have precise control over their vergence eye movements and will adjust to realign the two foveae onto a single visual target, provided the target is fusable.

Infant studies are hampered by the relative divergence of the two eyes due to non-alignment of the mid-pupillary axis and the foveal axis. Slater & Findlay (1975), have shown that the centre of the pupil is not the best estimate of the line of sight, and find a discrepancy of as much as 8–10° between the two, which declines with age, and in adults is only 3–4°. However, despite this it is still possible to use corneal reflections to measure relative convergence or divergence to the target distance. Aslin (1977), studied the vergence of 12 two- and three-month-old infants for a target that moved from 50 cm up to 15 cm. Corneal photography was used to assess binocular fixation, and the visual target itself created the corneal reflection. In this way consistent binocular fixation could be indicated by an invariant relationship between the centre of the two pupils and each corneal reflex. These studies showed that, at best, infants binocular fixation is intermittent, especially for near targets. By three months of age, changes in vergence are magnitude appropriate.

If a prism is placed base out in front of one eye while viewing a target binocularly, adults will make a vergence movement. In infants this was not consistently found until between four-and-a-half and six months of age. The most likely cause is the larger size of Panum's areas in young infants, as a result of which diplopia does not occur. In older infants and adults diplopia does occur and stimulates vergence.

Therefore, diplopia will be absent as long as the level of non-correspondence is within Panum's area. It has been shown that Panum's area is larger in adults for low spatial frequency stimuli. Therefore, the shrinkage may be linked with the infant's gradually increasing sensitivity to higher spatial frequencies.

Another possibility for explaining inaccurate binocular fixation of near targets, is the migration of photoreceptors towards the fovea. If the migration is linked to the eventual position (i.e. is preprogrammed), then it would result in an underestimate of the angular displacement of a target from the line of sight.

Accommodative vergence

Even when one eye is occluded both eyes will converge if a target is moved closer to the eye. This is caused by accommodative vergence.

If accommodative factors influence the accuracy of vergence movements in maintaining binocular fixation, then young infants may show poor vergence movements because their accommodative system is inaccurate. Accommodative accuracy does improve with age. It has been found that infants between the age of two and six months show convergence to a near target under monocular viewing conditions.

The most likely explanations for the inaccuracies of vergence eye movements among young infants are, firstly, the larger Panum's fusional area and, secondly, an inaccurate accommodative system that fails to trigger accurate vergence eye movements via accommodative vergence.

3.7.5   Depth perception

Depth perception is the process by which the distance of objects is gauged. It is obviously crucial for determining the spatial layout, but may also be important for object recognition. How do we see things three-dimensionally? The retinal surface on which images are projected is two-dimensional, so it can only indicate the direction of the stimulus but not its distance. In order to convert this two-dimensional representation into a three-dimensional one, different information sources are used by the visual system. These can be divided into three classes each of which contain multiple cues to depth: (1) binocular information; (2) monocular static information; and (3) kinetic information. The multiplicity of depth cues is essential, as different cues are required for different situations. For example, binocular disparity is a powerful depth cue for objects at close range, while aerial perspective which shows changes in hue towards blue and loss of contrast with increasing distance, is only applicable to very distant objects. A number of researchers have shown that infants can discriminate between two-dimensional and three-dimensional stimuli. Fantz (1961), for example, presented a disc and a sphere to one-month-old infants and found a preference for the sphere.

Stereoscopic depth perception

Stereopsis is the appreciation of the relative distance of objects by binocular disparity alone. Disparity detectors are cells that respond most to simultaneous binocular stimulation of small but precise deviations from exactly corresponding retinal points. With binocular deprivation such units are absent.

Development of disparity detection

Infant stereoscopic development has been studied by variations of three techniques: (a) behavioural responses to line stereograms; (b) behavioural responses to random dot stereograms; and (c) VEPs elicited by random dot stereograms. Data from the three different techniques agree well, showing that few infants respond to disparity cues at two months, but virtually all respond by five to seven months. Fox *et al.* (1980), employed random dot stereograms combined with a preferential looking procedure on a number of infants who were followed up longitudinally. Their results indicated that stereopsis emerges sometime between three-and-a-half and six months of age. Similar findings emerge from other studies. Also, infants were capable of discriminating convergent crossed disparities at a mean age of twelve weeks, while divergent uncrossed disparities emerge later, at approximately seventeen weeks. Braddick *et al.* (1986), produced a dynamic random dot pattern stimulus and recorded results via the VEP. The whole display alternates between two phases, correlated, which is seen by an individual with binocular vision as a single coherent depth plane, and uncorrelated, which has a woolly appearance without a clear localization in depth. In an individual without binocular vision, the two phases are indistinguishable 'snowstorms' of continuously changing dots, and no VEP waveform is obtained. A VEP response was elicited in infants at seventy-four days of age, but not in infants of sixty days. Therefore, stereoscopic vision arises somewhere between these two ages.

In addition to documenting the age of onset of stereopsis, Held *et al.* (1980) also timed the subsequent development of stereoscopic acuity, which improves very rapidly. After about three to four weeks, following the onset of stereoscopic discrimination, infants were shown to be able to detect disparity of one minute of arc.

Ciner *et al.* (1991), assessed stereoacuity development in 180 young children between the ages of 18 and 65 months. The greatest improvement in stereoacuity occurred between 18 and 30 months, when they found the mean value improved from 225 to 125 second of arc. They felt the overall steady improvements in stereoacuity appear to be the result of the developmental changes in the variability of responses rather than actual neurophysiological changes within the visual system. Figure 3.3 shows the average stereoacuities found at different ages. Note the increased variability of the values obtained before the age of 30 months.

Held (1984), compared the developmental time-course of these binocular functions with the segregation of ocular dominance columns found in the monkey, and suggested that the two develop together. Further, in young kittens it is particularly noteworthy that the period of rapid improvement of binocular depth perception coincides with the time-course of fine tuning of binocular cells in the visual cortex to retinal disparity.

In summary, the ability to detect binocular disparity, the adequate stimulation for stereopsis, seems to emerge between three and six months of age and to improve rapidly thereafter. Table 3.3 shows the average value for given ages as assessed by clinical methods.

Depth-appropriate responses to stereoscopic displays

The studies discussed above do not tell us with certainty whether infants at a given age actually experience the true depth perception specified by binocular disparity. One can investigate this by determining when depth-appropriate responses, such as reaching or avoidance, can be elicited by stereoscopic displays.

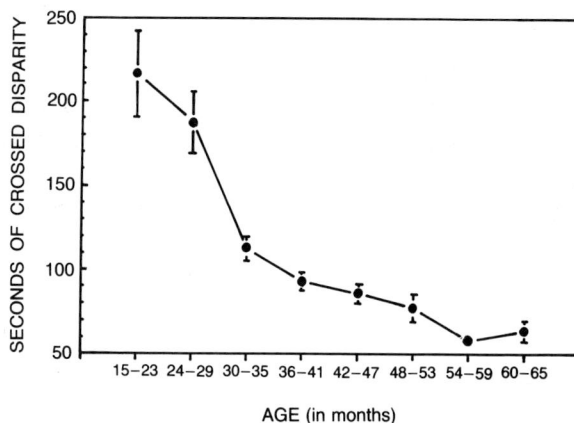

Fig. 3.3 Scatterplot of individual data points for stereoacuity thresholds (Reproduced with permission of the publishers from Ciner *et al.*, 1991).

Table 3.3   Variation in stereoacuity with age. Data from the Colchester Primary Ophthalmic Clinic (CPOC) Pediatric Clinic were obtained using the Frisby, Lang and Titmus tests for children older than two years, while the Frisby test was used predominantly for those up to age two years. Results of the different methods in the older age-groups are comparable. In the right hand column are listed the results, displayed in Fig. 3.3, of Ciner *et al.* (1991). The CPOC results increase with age in a similar fashion, but show better stereoacuity at all ages.

	Stereoacuity (seconds)	
Age	CPOC Pediatric Clinic	Ciner et al.
6 months	≅600	
9 months	≅400 to 300	
1 year	≅300 to 200	
18 months	≅170 to 150	≅220
2 years	≅100 to 85	≅180
3 years	≅85 to 55	≅100
4 years	≅40 to 30	≅80
5 years	≅30 to 20	≅60

Experiments have shown that infants reached appropriately to stereoscopic displays by five to seven months of age. This is also shown in some infants at six to seven months using the Frisby stereotest.

Yonas (1981) used a stereoscopic display which made the stimulus appear to approach the infant on a collision course. At five months of age infants were more likely to exhibit fixation, reaching, head withdrawal and blinking, on trials in which the virtual object loomed towards the face, than when the object remained at a constant distance. Infants of three-and-a-half months did not show these responses. However, the failure to observe evidence of these behaviour patterns at three to three-and-a-half months may be the result of an inability to appreciate stereoscopic depth, but could also be due to immaturity of the development to reach, or make avoidance movements, as these mechanisms may develop later.

A substantial number of studies point to the emergence of binocular processing between three and six months that is consistent with the segregation of inputs from the two eyes to form dominance columns in the striate cortex.

In general, infants under three months

(1)   fail to respond to binocular stimuli,
(2)   fail to demonstrate stereopsis,
(3)   fail to show aversion to rivalrous stimuli,
(4)   have asymmetric OKN.

Both stereopsis and binocular rivalry probably play an important role in cortical inhibition.

Monocular depth cues

In addition to binocular information, depth information can also be gained from monocular depth cues. Some monocular depth cues require motion (kinetic depth cues), while others do not (static depth cues).

Static depth cues include linear perspective, texture gradients, relative and familiar size and aerial perspective. Yonas *et al.* (1978), investigated sensitivity to linear perspective and found that infants of seven months are able to appreciate linear perspective cues. Below the age of five months appropriate responses to linear perspective were not shown. Therefore, it is reasonable to conclude that the utilization of linear perspective develops between five and seven months of age.

Kinetic depth information is produced by changes over time in the retinal image. These can be created by movement of the observer's head (motion parallax), or by movement of the objects in the environment, as in optical expansion when the object appears to approach the observer's face.

Kinetic depth development has been examined in infants by Yonas and co-workers. Three conditions were presented to infants from one to nine months of age. Firstly, symmetrical optical expansion of a solid form which specified a direct collision. Secondly, asymmetrical expansion of the same object specifying a miss and thirdly, a rising contour of a non-expanding form which did not specify collision. They concluded that infants do not appreciate impending collision specified by symmetrical optical expansion until four to six months of age. However, it should be noted that younger infants may possess the same perceptual knowledge but may simply not exhibit it.

In summary, infants exhibit sensitivity to all three types of depth information. Kinetic information sensitivity appears at about the same time as binocular, which is followed by monocular static information sensitivity.

3.8   Other aspects of visual performance in infancy

Even at birth, babies will search for patterns and inspect novel displays. If newborn infants are placed in total darkness they can be observed to open their eyes wide and broadly search the potential field moving their eyes two or three times per second. Thus, from birth, babies are capable of searching out detail and are not constrained to a stimulus response existence. If homogeneous displays without pattern details are placed in the field of view, the neonate continues to search broadly. However, if a patterned display is presented the neonate will restrict search and engage in eye movements which continually cross the edges of the pattern. This aids continued stimulation of the neurones' receptive fields, so the infant is effectively pre-programmed to maximize visual activity through scanning behaviour. This system provides maintenance of useful neural connections that would otherwise atrophy.

Once infants are able to move on their own, certain striking differences in their perceptive abilities arise in comparison with infants of the same age who are still immobile. This has been studied using the visual cliff experiment, which consists of a clear acrylic plastic panel suspended by edge supports, under which a red-checked tablecloth is placed; half being at full height and half appearing three feet below, creating an impression of a drop-off at the centre, a 'chasm'. Infants who were lifted onto the panel over the chasm showed heart rate deceleration, indicating interest. However infants of the same age, approximately nine months, who crawled onto the panel showed heart rate acceleration, denoting fear. Therefore, the studies show that the interpretation of depth as potentially dangerous is related to the onset of self motility.

Benson & Uzgiris (1985), demonstrated a relationship between the appreciation of spatial relations and infants' mobility. The infants were placed behind a plastic barrier and watched someone place a toy under one of two tablecloths. The infants were then allowed to walk or crawl round, or were carried if not mobile. It was found that those who were carried round were not as successful at retrieving the object as those who crawled or walked.

3.9   Conclusion

It is important for the pediatric optometrist to know at what ages different visual functions first appear, because delay in the start of a particular function, for example, stereoscopic vision, may be an indication of the development of amblyopia. New testing methods for use in early infancy show that sensory maladaptations can appear after strabismus has arisen. This indicates that congenital esotropia can be the primary cause of strabismus, while amblyopia and stereoblindness are secondary.

In very early-onset congenital esotropia, stereopsis can arrive on schedule between three to five months, provided the wearing of prisms or corrective surgery are carried out, and normal retinal correspondence can result. However, if not treated within this period stereoblindness occurs rapidly, followed more slowly by the onset of amblyopia, detectable by about nine months in unilateral esotropia.

An important point to remember is that an infant cannot develop a defect in any particular function prior to the normal age of onset of that function. Cortical awakening generally occurs between three to six months postnatally, and it is generally immediately after this age that occlusion therapy begins to alter acuity, or, more generally, when any restricted input to one eye causes reduction of acuity to begin. This is generally considered to be the start of the critical period of development in human infants.

We have seen that some visual functions seem to progress innately, for example colour vision, which is shown to be normal by about two months (see Chapter 10). Further, in a monkey model, dark reared from birth, normal trichromacy was found at three months. Therefore, environmental factors exert little influence on colour vision development.

Other functions are quite mature at birth but need stimulation to prevent atrophy, e.g. orientation-selective cells. In cats and primates numerous orientation selective cells are found at birth, but following total binocular deprivation for several months very few remain.

The characteristic visual scanning of newborns discussed in the previous section is designed to maximize stimulation of receptors by constantly moving across contours. At birth, or soon after, human infants show orientation selectivity for horizontal and vertical directions. The oblique direction matures slightly later at about one-and-a-half months. In adults sensitivity to horizontal and vertical gratings is greater than for oblique gratings, indeed this may reflect the greater prevalence of horizontal and vertical directions, over oblique, in our normal environment.

Finally, some functions are relatively immature at birth but progress rapidly, while others are immature and develop slowly over many years. An example of the former is accommodation, which becomes relatively mature by about three months of age, but still undergoes refinement up to about six to seven months as the sensitivity to higher spatial frequencies develops. It appears that final adjustment is caused by the increasing acuity, making stimulus blur more apparent thus increasing accommodative accuracy.

Visual acuity and contrast sensitivity development have a very long time-scale, taking up to six to twelve years to become truly adult-like. The developmental changes for both VA and CSF are most rapid in the earlier stages up to about three years, and then gradually reach maturity. The CSF curve has an adult shape by about three years of age, but more contrast is required by the younger child. An important point to remember, however, is that there is considerable variation in the maturing of VA and probably also CSF (see Table 3.4 below for more details).

Aslin (1987), has suggested infants' acuity is predictable on anatomical grounds. Further, he suggests that several functions which are inaccurate in early infancy may be due to photoreceptor migration. As cells migrate to form the foveal pit the information received will be detected by a changing array of receptors. If the visual system is pre-programmed for the final position of the photoreceptors, then in early infancy the distance to a stimulus will be underestimated. Aslin feels this may be the cause of small amplitude saccades in early infancy, vergence errors and the failure of smooth pursuit.

On average the refractive error at birth is approximately one to two dioptres of hypermetropia with up to one dioptre of astigmatism. However, there are considerable variations. Myopia is more common in premature babies (approximately 16%) and even higher in those who have retinopathy of prematurity.

Atkinson *et al.* (1984), estimated that approximately 11% of infants have some form of significant refractive error, including myopia, anisometropia, astigmatism, and hypermetropia of 3.5 D or more. Other estimates have varied between 6% and 12%. Further, with hypermetropia of 3.5 D or more, 40–48% show amblyopia and/or strabismus. Aurell & Norrsell (1990), and Dobson & Sebris (1989) found that with hypermetropia of 4 D or more, two distinct groups emerged. The first reduced their hypermetropia, and did not develop amblyopia or strabismus. The second either remained unchanged or became more hypermetropic during the first few years of life, and did develop strabismus and/or amblyopia.

Aurell and Norrsell suggest that approximately 50% of these infants reduce their level of hypermetropia and avoid amblyopia and/or strabismus. This reduction in refractive error is known as emmetropization and is largely controlled by change in the vitreous chamber depth, in response to the presence of ametropia.

From the author's clinical data, as yet unpublished, of some 3500 infants, those who at three to four months of age showed moderate to high hypermetropia, but who did emmetropize, often showed very marked refractive change over subsequent months. One particular case of note was an infant who when first examined at three months had +7.5 D of hypermetropia but at age nine to ten months had reduced to +3.0 D, having lost 4.5 D of hypermetropia in six to seven months. On the other hand, infants who show normal levels of hypermetropia initially, say of 2 D at three to four months, are often still around 1.5–2 D at nine to ten months. It appears that the higher the refractive error the more rapidly emmetropization occurs. Unfortunately, not all infants emmetropize, for reasons that are not fully understood, although hereditary factors are certainly important.

The author has found one interesting prognostic guide to emmetropization. Infants whose negative fusional ability (the ability to turn the eyes out while maintaining binocular viewing) is good, generally emmetropize. Those with poor negative fusion are more likely to retain or increase their existing level of hypermetropia. A possible explanation is that in order to gain a clear image when moderate hypermetropia is present the infant must accommodate, producing a convergence (due to the AC/A ratio) which would generally lead to diplopia. However, if good negative fusion is present this may counteract the convergence tendency, avoiding diplopia, therefore making accommodative effort viable. This explanation would, however, link accommodation with emmetropization and there is some controversy as to whether such a link exists, or whether common triggering factors control both functions.

Equal quality visual input to each eye is essential to prevent a shift in ocular

Table 3.4 Visual development at different ages.

AGE	Orientation selectivity	Accommodation	Pupil responses	Saccades	OKN	Smooth pursuit	Fusional vergence	Accom. vergence	Stereopsis	Appropriate responses to stereopsis	Mono. static depth cues	Mono. kinetic depth cues
BIRTH	Present for vertical and horizontal.		Small pupil sluggish responses.		Present from birth.							
1 MONTH		Inaccurate but in appropriate direction.	Increased pupil size. Responses improve.	Up to 2 months fixed amplitude responses.	Asymmetry of monocular OKN up to 3 months of age.	No smooth pursuit, just series of fixed saccades.	Binocular fixation intermittent.	Immature up to 2 months.	Can discriminate between a disc and a sphere.	Not present.	Not present.	Not present.
2 MONTHS	Present by 2 months for oblique.	Increased accuracy by 3 months.										
3 MONTHS			Between 3 and 5 months responses become adult-like.	Undergo marked improvement between 3 and 4 months.		Smooth pursuit first noticed for low speeds.	Changes are magnitude appropriate.	Starts to mature.	Earliest start of stereopsis.			
4 MONTHS		Undergoes fine adjustment.			Between 3 and 4 months symmetry appears.	Responses continue to improve. Essentially adult-like by 6 months of age.	Between 4 and 6 months responses mature.	Slight improvement continues up to 6 months.	Crossed disparities appear first; between 4 and 7 months uncrossed disparities arrive. Stereopsis is generally present by 7 months.			First appreciation of kinetic depth cues between 4 and 6 months.
5 MONTHS		Matures between 5 and 7 months.		Become adult-like between 5 and 6 months.	Normal infants should show symmetry between 5 and 6 months.					Appreciation of depth relations specified by disparity occurs between 5 and 7 months.	Mono. static depth cues first appear between 5 and 7 months.	
6 MONTHS												
7 MONTHS								Adult-like by 7 months.				

dominance. Therefore, when one eye is receiving an inferior image (e.g. due to anisometropia) then a correction should be given to equalize the clarity of the two images. Furthermore, the correction of high ametropia, particularly high hypermetropia, has been shown to improve accommodative ability, and thus possibly aid emmetropization (Brookman, 1983). Motor activities such as eye movements, reaching, avoidance of obstacles or anticipating the impending location of a moving target are all behaviours that involve correlation of motor responses with sensory stimulation. Table 3.4 gives a brief résumé of visual development at different ages.

The pediatric optometrist needs to be aware of the time-scale and expected developmental level of different visual functions with age, particularly those functions that can be assessed relatively easily in the clinic. For clinical discussion of the best methods for assessing these visual functions in different age groups, the reader is referred to Section 2 of this book.

3.10 References

Allen, D., Bennett, P.J. and Banks, M.S. (1992) 'The effects of luminance on FPL and VEP acuity in human infants'. *Vis. Res.*, **32**, 2005–2012.

Aslin, R.N. (1977) 'Development of binocular function in human infants'. *J. Exp. Child Psychol.*, **23**, 133–50.

Aslin, R.N. (1987) 'Motor aspects of visual development in infancy', in *Handbook of Infant Perception, 1. From Sensation to Perception.* (P. Salapatek & L.B Cohen, eds). Academic Press, London, 43–113.

Atkinson, J. and Braddick, O. (1981) 'Acuity, contrast sensitivity, and accommodation in infancy', in *The Development of Perception 2: The Visual System.* (R.N. Aslin, J.R. Alberts & M.R. Petersen, eds). Academic Press, New York.

Atkinson, J. and Braddick, O. (1983) 'Assessment of visual acuity in infancy and early childhood'. *Acta. Ophthalmol. [Suppl.]*, **157**, 18–26.

Atkinson, J., Braddick, O.J., Durden, K., Watson, P.G. and Atkinson, S. (1984) 'Screening for refractive errors in 6–9 month old infants by photorefraction'. *Brit. J. Ophthalmol.*, **68**, 105–12.

Atkinson, J., French, J. and Braddick, O. (1981) 'Contrast sensitivity function of preschool children. *Brit. J. Ophthalmol.*, **65**, 525–9.

Aurell, E. and Norrsell, K. (1990) 'A longitudinal study of children with a family history of strabismus: factors determining the incidence of strabismus'. *Brit. J. Ophthalmol.*, **74**, 589–94.

Banks, M.S. (1980). 'The development of visual accommodation during infancy'. *Child Develop.*, **51**, 646–66.

Banks, M.S. and Salapatek, P. (1978) 'Acuity and contrast sensitivity in one-, two- and three-month-old human infants'. *Invest. Ophthalmol. Vis. Sci.*, **17**, 361–5.

Benson, J.B. and Uzgiris, I.C. (1985) 'Effect of self-initiated locomotion on infant search activity'. *Dev. Psychol.*, **21**, 923–31.

Blakemore, C. and Vital-Durrand, F. (1979) 'Development of the neural basis of visual acuity in monkeys. Speculation on the origin of deprivation amblyopia'. *Trans. Ophthalmol. Soc. UK*, **99**, 363–8.

Boothe, R.G., Williams, R.A., Kiorpes, L. and Teller, D.Y. (1980) 'Development of contrast sensitivity in infant *Macaca nemestrina* monkeys'. *Science*, **208**, 1290–92.

Braddick, O.J., Wattam-Bell, J. and Atkinson, J. (1986) 'Orientation-specific cortical responses develop in early infancy'. *Nature*, **320**, 617–19.

Brookman, K.E. (1983) 'Ocular accommodation in human infants'. *Am. J. Optom. Physiol. Optics*, **60**, 91–9.

Brown, A.M., Dobson, V. and Maier, J. (1987) 'Visual acuity of human infants at scotopic, mesopic and photopic luminances'. *Vis. Res.*, **27**, 1845–58.

Cannon, M.W. (1983) 'Contrast sensitivity: psychophysical and evoked potential methods compared'. *Vis. Res.*, **23**, 87–95.

Ciner, E.B., Schanel-Klitsch, E. and Scheiman, M. (1991) 'Stereoacuity development in young children'. *Optom. & Vis. Science.*, **68**, 533–6.

Ciuffreda, K.J., Levi, D.M. and Selenow, A. (1991) In *Amblyopia: basic and clinical aspects*. Butterworth-Heinemann, Boston.

Dobson, V., Fulton, A.B. and Sebris, S.L. (1984) 'Cycloplegic refractions of infants and young children: the axis of astigmatism'. *Invest. Ophthalmol. Vis. Sci.*, **25**, 83–7.

Dobson, V. and Sebris, S.L. (1989) 'Longitudinal study of acuity and stereopsis in infants with an at-risk for esotropia'. *Invest. Ophthalmol. Vis. Sci.*, **30**, 1146–58.

Dobson, V. and Teller, D.Y. (1978) 'Visual acuity in human infants: a review and electrophysiological studies'. *Vis. Res.*, **18**, 1469–83.

Dobson, V., Teller, D.Y. and Belgum, J. (1978a) 'Visual acuity in human infants assessed with stationary stripes and phase-alternated checkerboards'. *Vis. Res.*, **18**, 1233–8.

Dobson, V., Teller, D.Y., Lee, C.P. and Wade, B. (1978b) 'A behavioral method for efficient screening of visual acuity in young infants: 1. Preliminary laboratory development'. *Invest. Ophthalmol. Vis. Sci.*, **17**, 1142–50.

Fantz, R.L. (1961) 'The origin of form perception'. *Sci. Am.*, **204**, No. 4, 66–72.

Fox, R., Aslin, R.N., Shea, S.L. and Dumais, S.T. (1980) 'Stereopsis in human infants'. *Science.*, **207**, 323–4.

Fulton, A.B., Hansen, R.M., Yeh, Y-L. and Tyler, C.W. (1991) 'Temporal summation in dark-adapted 10-week-old infants'. *Vis. Res.*, **31**, 1259–69.

Garey, L.J. and De Courten, C. (1983) 'Structural development of the lateral geniculate nucleus and visual cortex in monkey and man'. *Behav. Brain Res.*, **10**, 3–14.

Gordon, R.A. and Donzis, P.B. (1985) 'Refractive development of the human eye'. *Arch. Ophthalmol.*, **103**, 785–9.

Gwiazda, J., Brill, S., Mohindra, I. and Held, R. (1980) 'Preferential looking acuity in infants from two to fifty-eight weeks of age'. *Am. J. Optom. Physiol. Optics*, **57**, 428–32.

Gwiazda, J., Scheiman, M. and Held, R. (1984) 'Anisotropic resolution in children's vision'. *Vis. Res.*, **24**, 527–31.

Hainline, L., Lemerise, E., Abramov, I. and Turkel, J. (1984) 'Orientational asymmetries in small-field optokinetic nystagmus in human infants'. *Behav. Brain Res.*, **13**, 217–30.

Hansen, R.M. and Fulton, A.B. (1991) 'Electroretinographic assessment of background adaptation in 10-week-old human infants'. *Vis. Res.*, **31**, 1501–1507.

Haynes, H., White, B.L. and Held, R. (1965) 'Visual accommodation in human infants'. *Science*, **148**, 528–30.

Held, R. (1984) 'Binocular vision, behavioural and neural development', in *Neonate Cognition: Beyond the Blooming Buzzing Confusion.* (J. Mehler & R. Fox, eds). Erlbaum, New Jersey, 38–44.

Held, R., Birch, E. and Gwiazda, J. (1980) 'Stereoacuity of human infants'. *Proc. Nat. Acad. Sci. USA*, **77**, 5572–4.

Hendrickson, P. and Rosenblum, W. (1985) 'Accommodation demand and deprivation in kitten ocular development'. *Invest. Ophthalmol. Vis. Sci.*, **26**, 343–9.

Hitchcock, P.F. and Hickey, T.L. (1980) 'Ocular dominance columns: evidence for their presence in humans'. *Brain Res.*, **182**, 176–9.

Howland, H.C. (1982) 'Infant eyes: optics and accommodation'. *Current Eye Res.*, **2**, 217–24.

Hubel, D.H., Wiesel, T.N. and Le Vay, S. (1977) 'Plasticity of ocular dominance columns in monkey striate cortex'. *Philos. Trans. R. Soc. London. Ser. B.*, **278**, 377–409.

Manny, R.E. (1992) 'Orientation selectivity of 3-month-old infants'. *Vis. Res.*, **32**, 1817–28.

Mayer, D.L. and Dobson, V. (1982) 'Visual acuity development in infants and young children, as assessed by operant preferential looking'. *Vis. Res.*, **22**, 1141–51.

Medina, A. (1987) 'A model for emmetropization: predicting the progression of ametropia'. *Ophthalmologica*, **194**, 133–9.

Naegele, J.R. and Held, R. (1982) 'The postnatal development of monocular optokinetic nystagmus in infants'. *Vis. Res.*, **22**, 341–6.

Neuringer, M., Conner, W.E., Van Petten, C. and Barstad, L. (1984) 'Dietary omega-3 fatty acid deficiency visual loss in infant rhesus monkeys'. *J. Clin. Invest.*, **73**, 272–6.

Ossenblok, P., Reits, D. and Spekreijse, H. (1992) 'Analysis of striate activity underlying the pattern onset EP of children'. *Vis. Res.*, **32**, 1829–35.

Parssinen, O., Hemminki, E. and Klemetti, A. (1989) 'Effect of spectacle use and accommodation on myopic progression: final results of a three-year randomised clinical trial among school children'. *Brit. J. Ophthalmol.*, **73**, 547–51.

Scammon, R.E. and Wilmer, H.A. (1950) 'Growth of the components of the human eyeball. Comparison of the calculated volumes of the eyes of the newborn and of adults, and their components'. *Arch. Ophthalmol.*, **43**, 620–37.

Shimojo, S., Birch, E.E., Gwiazda, J. and Held, R. (1984) 'Development of vernier acuity in infants'. *Vis. Res.*, **24**, 721–8.

Slater, A.M. and Findlay, J.M. (1975) 'Binocular fixation in the newborn baby'. *J. Exp. Child Psychol.*, **20**, 248–73.

Sokol, S. (1978) 'Measurement of infant visual acuity from pattern reversal evoked potentials'. *Vis. Res.*, **18**, 33–9.

Sokol, S., Hansen, V.C., Moskowitz, A., Greenfield, P. and Towle, V.L. (1983) 'Evoked potential and preferential looking estimates of visual acuity in pediatric patients'. *Ophthalmol.*, **90**, 552–61.

Sorsby, A. (1979) 'Biology of the eye as an optical system', in *Refraction and Clincal Optics.*, (A. Safir ed.). Harper & Row, Philadelphia.

Troilo, D. and Wallman, J. (1991) 'The regulation of eye growth and refractive state: an experimental study of emmetropization'. *Vis. Res.*, **31**, 1237–50.

Wallman, J., Adams, J.I. and Trachtman, J.N. (1981) 'The eyes of young chickens grow toward emmetropia'. *Invest. Ophthalmol. Vis. Sci.*, **20**, 557–61.

Wattam-Bell, J. (1991) 'Development of motion-specific cortical responses in infancy'. *Vis. Res.*, **31**, 287–97.

Wilson, H.R. (1988) 'Development of spatiotemporal mechanisms in infant vision'. *Vis. Res.*, **28**, 611–28.

Yonas, A. (1981) 'Infants' responses to optical information for collision', in *The Development of Perception 2: The Visual System.* (R.N. Aslin, J.R. Alberts & M.R. Petersen, eds). Academic Press, New York.

Yonas, A., Cleaves, W.T. and Pettersen, L. (1978) 'Development of sensitivity to pictorial depth'. *Science*, **200**, 77–9.

Young, F.A. (1977) 'The nature and control of myopia'. *J. Am. Optom. Assoc.*, **48**, 451–7.

Yuodelis, C. and Hendrickson, A. (1986) 'A qualitative and quantitative analysis of the human fovea during development'. *Vis. Res.*, **26**, 847–55.

Zanker, J., Mohn, G., Weber, U., Zeitler-Driess, K. and Fahle, M. (1992) 'The development of vernier acuity in human infants'. *Vis. Res.*, **32**, 1557–64.

CHAPTER 4
Amblyopia
Annette Grounds

4.1 Introduction

Functional amblyopia was described by Von Graefe as a condition 'in which the observer sees nothing and the patient very little'. Over the years many different definitions have been put forward which elaborate somewhat on the above. Taking all the known factors into account a suitable definition might be: 'Functional amblyopia refers to deficiency predominantly of form vision affecting either one or both eyes, occurring generally before the age of seven years, which cannot be corrected purely by accurate refraction. Further, it should not be associated with any recognizable pathological cause, but should be attributable to an amblyogenic (amblyopia-causing) factor'.

This chapter is concerned with functional amblyopia. Other types that have been identified are:

(1) Organic amblyopia
(2) Idiopathic or congenital amblyopia
(3) Toxic amblyopia
(4) Nutritional amblyopia
(5) Psychogenic amblyopia

Towards the end of the chapter a table will summarize the main clinical distinguishing features of these amblyopias, together with the functional type, but apart from this they will not be considered in any greater detail.

4.2 The prevalence of amblyopia

Amblyopia is generally thought to occur in 2–4% of the general population. It is interesting that, in the population under the age of 20 years, amblyopia is ten times more common a cause of visual loss than all others taken together, whether caused by trauma or disease.

It is important to note that the prevalence of both squint and amblyopia increase when associated with other conditions. For example, Down's syndrome children are ten times more likely to have squints and/or amblyopia, while brain-damaged infants are approximately 50–60% more likely to have these problems. Squints and/or amblyopia are more frequently found in premature babies, where the prevalence rises to about 18%. The prevalence also rises in difficult and traumatic births. Hereditary factors also cause significant increase in the prevalence of squint and amblyopia. When there is a family history of either squint, amblyopia or high refractive error, there is a dramatic increase in the chance of an infant being similarly affected. It has been estimated that if one parent has suffered from a squint or amblyopia there is a 35–46% chance of an infant being similarly affected, while if both parents have suffered from a squint or amblyopia this figure rises to 78–90%.

4.3 The classification of amblyopia

Over the past 20 years amblyopia has been investigated in both animal (mainly cats and primates) and human subjects.

Most forms of amblyopia are associated with ocular problems which produce disruption of normal visual input. The three main categories of functional amblyopia are:

(1) Strabismic amblyopia, in which the visual system is deprived of simultaneous corresponding images from the two eyes.
(2) Refractive amblyopia (including anisometropia, iso-ametropia, and monocular and binocular astigmatism) caused by optical defocus, which removes predominantly high spatial frequencies (fine detail) from the retinal limage.
(3) Deprivation amblyopia, the causes of which include dense cataract and ptosis, and which can lead to a complete loss of spatial (visual) detail in the retinal image.

4.3.1 Strabismic amblyopia

Strabismus involves non-alignment of the two eyes resulting in diplopia and confusion. This causes binocular rivalry and leads to suppression by cortical inhibition (von Noorden, 1980). There are two types of strabismics: those with constant monofixational squint, and those who alternate fixation. It is only in monofixation strabismus that amblyopia occurs. When alternating strabismus occurs, loss of binocular function and stereoblindness are generally found, but no amblyopia should be present unless associated with other amblyogenic factors such as anisometropia. However, the level of anisometropia must be low, except when one eye is myopic, or there would be no need for alternation. Hence, alternating strabismics rarely have acuity which is reduced by more than one line in the worst eye. Ikeda *et al.* (1978), and Hubel & Wiesel (1965), found that with a squint, regardless of type, the number of binocularly-driven cortical cells is reduced, but amblyopia was only found in monofixational strabismus.

According to a study by Shapero (1971), there is a 3:1 ratio of esotropic to exotropic amblyopia. However, in order to assess this finding there should be no anisometropia present in the subjects. Shapero did not exclude anisometropia and this leaves some doubt as to whether primary exotropia exists as an amblyogenic factor. Exotropia is generally considered to be an effect secondary to anisometropia or trauma, or a consecutive divergence following surgical overcorrection of primary esotropia.

Anomalous retinal correspondence

In strabismic amblyopia, due to the non-alignment of the eyes, anomalous retinal correspondence (ARC) often results. This occurs when a retinal area that is outside the normal foveal area in the deviating eye forms a neural association with the foveal region of the normal (non deviating eye). Further discussion of ARC is beyond the scope of this chapter, but see Chapter 8). Rutstein *et al.* (1991), who studied the change in retinal correspondence following surgical re-alignment of the eyes, found that normal retinal correspondence (NRC) which was present prior to surgery remained after surgery. Of 20 patients who had ARC prior to surgery, 13 retained ARC following surgery, while 7 developed NRC. In all the patients who developed NRC, the direction of the squint was reversed. They concluded that following squint surgery a change from ARC to NRC was more likely if the squint was overcorrected.

4.3.2 Refractive amblyopia

Anisometropic amblyopia

This form of amblyopia can occur in uncorrected refractive error when one eye has a higher error than the fellow. It is difficult to state with certainty what refractive difference constitutes an amblyogenic factor. For example, in some studies one dioptre difference has been cited as significant. However, at this level of anisometropia amblyopia is unlikely if one or both eyes are myopic, because the more myopic eye would be favoured for near while the fellow would be favoured for distance. If both eyes are hypermetropic, for example R + 2.00 and L + 1.00 then the left eye would be favoured at all distances, resulting in the right eye continually receiving an out of focus image, which could cause a mild degree of amblyopia.

Ciuffreda *et al.* (1991), showed that the prevalence of anisometropic amblyopia is 100% with anisometropia greater than 6.5 D difference if both eyes are myopic. They found 100% prevalence of amblyopia associated with a difference of 3.5 D if both eyes are hypermetropic. A 50% prevalence of amblyopia was found with anisometropia of 5 D in myopes, and anisometropia of 2 D in hypermetropes.

In the general population, anisometropia is more prevalent in myopes than in hypermetropes. However, amblyopia is much more common with hypermetropic anisometropia.

There is evidence of a correlation between the prevalence and depth of amblyopia and the magnitude of the anisometropia (Kirlin & Flynn, 1981; Tanlamai & Goss, 1979; Boothe *et al.*, 1982; Harwerth *et al.*, 1983).

Suppression in anisometropia is more variable in area than in strabismus, and the suppression is generally lighter than the well-defined form usually found in strabismus.

Iso-ametropic amblyopia

This occurs secondary to significant bilateral uncorrected refractive error. The effects of bilateral loss of clear form vision are not as damaging as asymmetrical visual input. Consequently, the depth of iso-ametropic amblyopia, and its resistance to therapy, is less.

Such cases are generally amenable to treatment and they often get 6/6 VA following vision therapy, even in adulthood (Selenow & Ciuffreda, 1986). The therapy that is generally effective is based on exercises that improve accommodation and ocularmotor function.

Again, myopic iso-ametropia has less amblyogenic effect than hypermetropic, because a clear image will be focused on the retina for near objects. Iso-ametropic amblyopia is common in very high hypermetropia, because the accommodative effort needed to focus an image is too great to be worthwhile. Lower levels of bilateral hypermetropia will generally lead to secondary esotropia. Amblyopia is also more common when bilateral astigmatism is present.

Suppression characteristics are different from those of anisometropic and strabismic amblyopes. Pratt-Johnson *et al.* (1967) investigated suppression characteristics of five iso-ametropic amblyopes. Three had no suppression scotomas, one had suppression scotomas in both eyes, and the fifth had a suppression scotoma in one eye only, but a microtropia may have been present in this case.

Astigmatic (meridional) amblyopia

In high bilateral astigmatism iso-ametropic amblyopia is quite common, giving rise to bilateral meridional amblyopia.

The uncorrected astigmatic eye is unable to focus simultaneously on the retina lines that are parallel to both of its principal meridians. If the eye is hyper-metropic in both principal meridians one set of lines will be out of focus for both distance and near vision. The development of acuity for lines in the 'in-focus' meridian will be normal, while that for lines in other directions will be impaired and may lead to amblyopia. In myopic astigmatism, it may be possible for each principal meridian to be in focus for a different near working distance, thus reducing meridional amblyopia.

If high astigmatism is not corrected within the sensitive period then meridional amblyopia results, and subsequent correction of the astigmatism does not rectify the poor acuity. Human adults who were not optically corrected as children often show acuity and contrast sensitivity differences for stimuli of different orientations which are predictable from the axis and degree of their astigmatism (Freeman & Pettigrew, 1972; Mitchell *et al.*, 1973; and Cobb & McDonald, 1978). Similar results have been found in monkeys (Harwerth *et al.*, 1980, 1983; Boothe & Teller, 1982).

As has already been discussed in Chapter 3, astigmatism does not appear to have a detrimental effect on acuity before about three years of age. However, the author's clinical experience suggests that the age at which uncorrected astigmatism causes amblyopia is related to the degree of astigmatism. High levels of astigmatism can cause lowered acuity earlier than three years of age. A study is under way to test this hypothesis.

4.3.3   Deprivation amblyopia

Deprivation amblyopia can occur due to ptosis, dense cataract or even due to long periods of occlusion for therapeutic reasons. Deprivation can occur either monocularly or binocularly and results in pattern deprivation and loss of spatial detail in the retinal image.

Binocular deprivation

Binocular deprivation can be accomplished in two ways, by dark rearing or by bilateral lid suturing. These two deprivation methods differ in several respects. Dark rearing removes all visual stimulation and inhibits visual development leaving the visual cortex in an immature state (Mower *et al.*, 1981, 1982). Cellular recordings show a reasonable proportion of visually responsive cells, but with ill-defined properties. There is evidence that for short periods anatomical segregation of ocular dominance columns proceeds normally, indicated by the high proportion of binocular cells found in cats, while synaptic development proceeds at a reduced rate. However, long periods of dark rearing cause deterioration of cortical function rather than arrest of development. Following short periods of dark rearing of up to four months, visual acuity has been shown to eventually recover to normal levels after a period of normal stimulation. Dark rearing for short periods would appear to be more harmful to binocular function than to visual resolution, for, despite the high proportion of binocular cells found in the cortex, stereopsis does not seem to recover.

Bilateral lid suturing prevents pattern vision, while moderately reducing light. The resultant diffuse visual stimulation through closed eyelids results in partial development of the visual cortex, and the effects of deprivation are much less easily reversed than with dark rearing. Mower *et al.* (1981, 1982), showed that in cats and monkeys, following four months of lid suturing only partial acuity recovery occurs, in contrast to the full recovery following the same period of deprivation caused by dark rearing.

Both forms of binocular deprivation cause the cortex to show reduced responsiveness, but lid suturing gives a higher proportion of unresponsive cells.

Monocular deprivation

Awaya *et al.* (1973, 1979 and 1980) have shown that infants who receive monocular patching for only one week following entropion surgery show long-standing visual deficits. Also, they noted that when both eyes are treated in sequence, the second eye shows greater loss of acuity. After consideration of this and the previous section, it is clear that bilateral surgery or bilateral occlusion, when required, will minimize the visual deprivation as compared with monocular intervention. Changes in surgical procedures with regard to cataract are discussed below. When patching lasts for longer than one week the acuity deficit becomes greater and is harder to eliminate. Von Noorden (1981b) has reported that, even in a five-year-old, several months of monocular occlusion can cause insuperable acuity loss.

Studies of monkeys and cats who have received monocular pattern deprivation within their sensitive period have shown extremely poor acuity and contrast sensitivity (von Noorden *et al.*, 1970; Hendricksen *et al.*, 1977; Harwerth *et al.*, 1981, 1983).

Even periods of monocular lid suture as short as two weeks, performed during the most sensitive period of development, are sufficient to cause severe loss of spatial resolution. Further, von Noorden (1973) found little recovery following extended periods of reverse suturing. However, Hendrickson *et al.* (1977), did report some recovery after several months of lid suturing, and also that deliberate damage to the normal eye speeded up the recovery of the amblyopic eye.

In the previous section on binocular deprivation it was shown that there were often quite high numbers of binocularly driven cells in the cortex even though stereopsis was not present. With monocular deprivation electrophysiological recordings show few binocularly driven cells, hence binocular function is not present.

The commonest cause of image deprivation in human infants is congenital cataract. Recently, with increased knowledge from animal experimentation the visual outcome for such infants has improved. The main changes in strategy are outlined below, but it should be remembered that these changes have not been universally adopted:

(1) The cataract is extracted very early, often before 8 weeks of age.
(2) If a bilateral extraction is required, there should be a short interval between the extractions (often 48 hours or less).
(3) Total bilateral occlusion should be used between the operations.
(4) There should be early bilateral correction of aphakia, usually with extended wear contact lenses (fitted within one week of surgery).

It should always be remembered that amblyopia is more severe with monocular rather than binocular cataract.

The other important factors that influence the levels of amblyopia caused by image deprivation resulting from cataract are:

(1) the age at which the cataract developed;
(2) the length of time the cataract has been present;
(3) the child's age at the time of the extraction;
(4) the time interval between the operation and optical correction;
(5) the presence of a squint, either before or after the cataract is removed.

Occlusion amblyopia in human infants is now well established. Even short periods (less than one week) of direct occlusion in a young amblyope can result in a dramatic change in monocular acuities, with a trade-off between the acuities of the two eyes (Thomas *et al.*, 1979; Awaya *et al.*, 1979; Levi, 1976).

Awaya *et al.* (1979), looked at 100 cases of stimulus deprivation amblyopia. Poorest recovery from amblyopia was found when degradation occurred between six and nine months of age. Recovery of visual acuity was good when degradation occurred after the eighteenth month of age.

Optometrists are more likely to encounter infants and children with anisometropic or strabismic amblyopia than with deprivation amblyopia.

4.4   The development of amblyopia

In behavioural studies of lid-sutured monkeys (Harwerth *et al.*, 1981) evidence was provided for several sensitive periods for different visual functions. Early lid suturing, between the ages of three and six months, had a marked influence on scotopic and photopic spectral sensitivity, and essentially abolished both pattern and binocular vision. When lid suturing was started between six and 25 months there was no effect on spectral sensitivity, but reduced contrast sensitivity occurred to high spatial frequencies, as did reduced binocular summation. Lid suturing beyond 25 months had no effect on contrast sensitivity, but disrupted binocular functioning. Any visual function will develop four times faster in a monkey than in a human infant (i.e. a function first noted at one week in monkeys will develop at four weeks in human infants). If this 4:1 rule is applied, in human infants the influences on scotopic and photopic spectral sensitivity, and the abolition of pattern and binocular vision, would occur between one and two years of age. Reduced contrast sensitivity to high spatial frequencies would occur between two and eight years of age. No effects on contrast sensitivity would be found on children following total occlusion commencing after eight years of age, but disruption of binocular function could still occur.

Clearly, different visual functions develop at different rates. In general, those which develop earliest seem the most robust to the influences of pattern deprivation, while those which develop later are at risk, and remain at risk, for longer.

Binocular connections are most susceptible at about 18 months of age and remain so up to about seven years. Not surprisingly, the susceptibility to strabismus and anisometropic amblyopia has a similar time-scale.

4.4.1   Sensory processing in amblyopia

Consideration will now be given to different visual processes in amblyopia.

The light sense

This is essentially normal in amblyopia. It should be noted that some amblyopes do report small differences in perceived brightness between the two eyes. In some cases the amblyopic eye's image is slightly dimmed, as if the target is seen through a filter. However, this is not a generally observed phenomenon, and indeed some amblyopes report the opposite effect. This 'sunglasses' effect may be more common in anisometropic amblyopia.

Colour vision

Colour vision is not affected in amblyopia.

Increment threshold spectral sensitivity

Amblyopes demonstrate anomalies in their increment threshold spectral sensitivity function. This is measured by superimposing a test spot on a bright uniform white background (Harwerth & Levi, 1977). The observer's task is to distinguish the test spot from the background. However, these anomalies can be explained by the generally reduced contrast sensitivity curves of amblyopes. Bradley *et al.* (1986), showed that the contrast sensitivity of the amblyopic eye is similarly reduced for chromatic and achromatic sine wave gratings. This suggests that the reduction in increment threshold spectral sensitivity can be understood in terms of its reduced spatial contrast sensitivity. Amblyopia is essentially a loss of 'form sense'.

4.4.2   Spatial vision in amblyopia

Visual acuity

Clinically, visual acuity is generally recorded as a Snellen acuity. There are other accepted methods for recording VA and, since the results for different methods vary in amblyopes, they will be outlined briefly below:

(1)   Minimum visible acuity (detection of a feature).
(2)   Minimum resolvable acuity (resolution of a feature).
(3)   Minimum recognizable visual acuity (identification of features in a target).

Minimum visual acuity is the detection of a line on a uniform background. The width of the line is altered until it is just visible. The angle subtended by this line in normal vision would be 0.5 min of arc. It is believed that this method may be highly sensitive to the amblyopic deficit.

Minimum resolvable acuity refers to the smallest angular separation between neighbouring targets. Grating acuity is a form of this type of acuity measure. Although in amblyopia grating acuity is reduced, it tends to be better when assessed by this method than by the other two. A normal result for this VA assessment method would be 1 min of arc, i.e. 6/6 acuity.

Minimum recognizable acuity is the type of measurement obtained with Snellen charts; a normal result is between 0.5 and 1 min of arc, i.e. 6/3 to 6/6. Generally, VA is on average better with anisometropic amblyopia than with strabismic. However, when both forms of amblyopia are present together the VA has the poorest average level, which may indicate an additive effect.

Hyperacuity

When clinically assessed, acuity is generally considered in terms of Snellen acuity, but the visual system is actually capable of much finer spatial discrimination. For example, relative position, size and orientation can, in normal vision, be judged to a level of three to six seconds of arc. This is five to ten times finer than either the cut-off spatial frequency or the intercone spacing (foveal cone separation is about 30 seconds of arc). This exceptional spatial discrimination is termed hyperacuity (Westheimer, 1975).

It is believed that hyperacuity tasks reflect cortical processing, and that the mechanisms underlying this have the more general task of form and shape analysis. Not surprisingly, in amblyopia hyperacuity is markedly degraded (Buckingham *et al.*, 1990). In fact vernier hyperacuity is not found, and vernier acuity is either equal or inferior to the amblyope's grating acuity (Murphy & Mitchell, 1991).

Hyperacuity tasks have also provided evidence which suggests that the neural losses of strabismic and anisometropic amblyopes are fundamentally different.

4.4.3   Spatial contrast sensitivity

Amblyopia is generally defined by the smallest high-contrast stimuli that can be detected. However, in everyday life, we are generally more concerned about our ability to discriminate in low contrast situations. The visual system is more sensitive to contrast for objects of a certain size than for others.

It is well known that the loss of contrast sensitivity at high spatial frequencies increases with the severity of the amblyopia. The high spatial frequency cut-off (i.e. the highest spatial frequency that can be detected at 100% contrast) provides a measure of the resolving capacity of the eye. This cut-off is around 40 to 50 cycles per degree (equivalent to a Snellen VA of about 6/4.5). In an amblyope with a best VA of 6/18 the cut-off would be expected to be between 10 to 12 cycles per degree.

Levi & Klein (1982), compared grating acuity versus Snellen acuity for subjects with anisometropic amblyopia, strabismic amblyopia and with both. For anisometropia alone the results for the two methods are similar. However with either strabismic alone, or anisometropia and strabismus together, Snellen acuity is worse than grating acuity. Therefore, Snellen acuity is affected to a greater degree than grating acuity if strabismus is present. This finding shows that grating acuity can underestimate the Snellen acuity loss, and this highlights one of the drawbacks of the contrast sensitivity approach.

In anisometropic amblyopia the grating and Snellen acuities are similar. Therefore, the reduced Snellen acuity equates to their reduced resolution, and hence to their contrast sensitivity. Thus there is an extra loss, beyond simple resolution, in the visual system of strabismics that contributes to the poor Snellen acuity. The reduced CSF in amblyopia represents a loss of foveal function.

The loss of photopic contrast sensitivity (CS) at high spatial frequencies in central vision appears to be one of the defining features of both strabismic and anisometropic amblyopia.

Wali *et al.* (1991) showed that inter-eye correlations of CS at different spatial frequencies were found in even very deep amblyopia, which suggests continued interocular interactions and binocularity. Also, during occlusion therapy both the amblyopic and dominant eyes showed improved CSF. This suggests that the amblyopic eye may influence CS in the dominant eye through interocular interactions. This process may serve to minimize CSF differences between the two eyes and maximize binocular vision.

Hess & Pointer (1985), among others, have investigated the CS of amblyopes as a function of retinal location. In strabismic amblyopia they found sparing of the peripheral region of one or both hemifields. The presence or absence of asymmetrical CS loss depended on the depth of strabismic amblyopia. In mild amblyopes marked asymmetries were found, though confined to the central 30°. It has been noted that where asymmetrical CS loss occurs, the greatest loss is in the temporal field in esotropia and nasal field in exotropia, which suggests that this is associated with prolonged binocular suppression.

In anisometropic amblyopes these results are consistent with the defocus hypothesis, however, this is not the whole story because when both eyes are equally defocused, marked amblyopia does not result. The essential difference is in retinal image clarity between the two eyes. It is therefore likely that binocular competition, induced by monocular blur, results in the loss of CS in the amblyopic eye.

When CS was measured in both the monocular and binocular fields of the amblyopic eyes of anisometropic subjects the deficit, which extended over 50–55° of binocular field, was found to disappear when the monocular field was tested. This lends strong evidence for the idea that binocular competition plays an important role in amblyopia. The main conclusions to emerge from these results are, firstly, that the strabismic deficit is not explained purely by defocus; and, secondly, that the pattern of binocular competition differs in strabismic and anisometropic amblyopia.

It has long been known that visual acuity will remain constant, or improve, if a 2.0 log unit neutral density filter is placed in front of an eye with strabismic amblyopia. However, in anisometropic amblyopia and normals the acuity will drop, usually by about two lines. Hess *et al.* (1980) measured contrast sensitivity functions under progressively lower background luminances. In an eye with strabismic amblyopia there is a point at which responses become normal under mesopic or scotopic conditions (normalization), and this point is frequency-dependent. They suggested that in normal vision the reduction of luminance biases detection progressively towards more peripheral receptors, thus normal and amblyopic responses should converge. Similar results were found when an artificial scotoma was placed in front of a normal eye and contrast sensitivity was measured under reduced background luminance. This supports the retinal locus-specific hypothesis proposed by Hess and co-workers. That is, that strabismic amblyopia is restricted to a central region while in anisometropia the deficit spreads over a greater retinal locus, thus normalization does not occur.

4.4.4   Supra-threshold contrast perception

In normal everyday vision, stimuli have variable contrast levels, some of which will be well above the threshold level, thus it is important to consider what happens in amblyopia at these supra-threshold levels.

While amblyopes often demonstrate normal contrast perception at supra-threshold contrast levels, they demonstrate several abnormalities of supra-threshold contrast processing. These include reduced contrast discrimination, reduced evoked potential gain, prolonged reaction times, and abnormalities in discerning the phase or polarity of a target. Moreover, some amblyopes report perceptual distortions of supra-threshold stimuli (Hess *et al.*, 1978).

4.4.5   The spatial sense

Amblyopia is characterized by marked spatial uncertainty or imprecision. This inability of amblyopes to judge relative position, width and orientation is most marked under conditions where normal observers perform best, that is when the features of the object of regard are close together. Anisometropic amblyopes show a loss of positional information that is commensurate with the reduced acuity and contrast sensitivity of the amblyopic eye. However, strabismic amblyopes show an additional loss in hyperacuity, often accompanied by distortion of space perception. The losses in the precision of spatial judgements are closely linked with the amblyope's Snellen acuity.

In anisometropic amblyopia, it is hypothesized that the reduced hyperacuity and resolution share a common basis, that is, the reduced contrast sensitivity (signal-to-noise ratio) of the spatial filters of the amblyopic eye. In strabismic amblyopia, it is more likely that sparse spatial sampling due to loss of neurons or scrambling of their signals accounts for the high degree of intrinsic positional uncertainty.

It is likely that the high precision of spatial judgements in normal foveal vision is the consequence of mechanisms which are involved in form and pattern discrimination.

4.4.6 Amblyopia and peripheral vision

It has now been shown, in a variety of detection and resolution tasks, that central and peripheral vision are similar when the dimensions are appropriately scaled.

For example, when considering vernier acuity, and its associated crowding phenomenon, results are similar in central and peripheral vision, when scaled according to the cortical magnification factor (i.e. the number of millimetres of cortex devoted to each degree of visual space). This similarity is only true when the same form of visual assessment is carried out. It does not apply to measurements of acuity that assess different visual tasks, e.g. hyperacuity and grating acuity.

When comparing grating versus hyperacuity in amblyopes, the data from strabismic amblyopes are similar to those from the normal periphery, while data from anisometropic amblyopes are not.

Why is there this similarity between central vision in strabismic amblyopia and normal peripheral vision? In both cases, hyperacuity is worse than would be predicted from the reduced resolution, contrast sensitivity or supra-threshold contrast response, and cannot be simply mimicked by optical blurring. Moreover, both show similar benefit from additional sampling, suggesting that both these visual systems may be sparsely sampled. In the normal periphery, sparse sampling has its basis in the reduction of cone density and the reduction in cortical magnification with eccentricity. In strabismic amblyopia similar functional losses may result from a loss of cortical neurons and/or scrambling of their connections, as a consequence of abnormal binocular interaction.

4.4.7 Temporal processing in the visual system

The abnormalities in spatio-temporal processing found in amblyopes can be largely understood in terms of the reduced spatial contrast sensitivity of the amblyopic eye. They show minimal or no losses to large uniform fields, or targets of low spatial frequency flickering rapidly (i.e. high temporal frequency). In contrast, they show reduced sensitivity to small fields and high spatial frequencies, losses that are more marked at low temporal frequency. In addition, amblyopes show normal velocity discrimination for high speed targets, but poor velocity discrimination for slow speed targets.

On the basis of developmental changes in the VEP it has been suggested that the higher temporal frequency mechanisms develop early, while the lower temporal frequency mechanisms (which have superior spatial resolution) develop later. Thus, selective losses at high spatial and low temporal frequencies may reflect neural deficits that depend on the age of onset of the amblyopia.

Reaction time is also affected. Latencies are greater in amblyopia, with the most prolonged reaction times being associated with the poorest acuities. Reaction time decreases as the stimulus contrast increases. Increased reaction time may not simply reflect a fixed neural delay, but also the contrast deficit of the amblyopic eye.

4.5 The effects of the amblyogenic process on different levels of the geniculostriate pathways

4.5.1 The retina

The results of psychophysical and electrophysiological experiments suggest that the basic retinal receptor processes (rods and cones) of the amblyopic eye are essentially normal.

There has been some evidence from electrophysiological recordings (Ikeda & Tremain, 1979) that X-ganglion cells show reduced spatial resolution in strabismic kittens. Also abnormal ERG responses have been elicited by pattern stimuli in humans with strabismic amblyopia (Arden et al., 1980). However, other researchers have been unable to confirm these findings. In fact, there is little hard evidence for a primary retinal abnormality in amblyopia. Although some amblyopes may show retinal anomalies, they do not appear to be a general feature of amblyopia. Further, there is no direct relationship between retinal and psychophysical abnormalities. These retinal abnormalities may be the result of retrograde degeneration due to long standing amblyopia. In Ikeda's work, very radical surgical procedures were used in order to obtain the squint. Such surgery could result in immobilization of the eye, which others have found can cause deficits.

4.5.2 The lateral geniculate nucleus (LGN)

In a post-mortem examination of the dorsal LGN of a human anisometropic amblyope, cell shrinkage was found in the parvocellular layers which received input from the amblyopic eye (von Noorden et al., 1983). Similar results were found by von Noorden & Crawford (1992), in a human strabismic amblyope. Cell shrinkage was most marked in the ipsilateral LGN. Similar cell shrinkage occurs in monkeys reared with either lid suture, chronic atropinization or surgically induced squint. Despite these well-documented anatomical effects on the LGN, the functional effects are less clear. In primates at least, even lid suture from birth seems to cause little or no change in functional properties of the LGN neurons (Blakemore & Vital-Durand, 1979).

4.5.3 The striate cortex (SC)

The most profound and consistent effects of the amblyopic process are found in the striate cortex.

In amblyopia produced by either lid suture, prism rearing or surgically induced strabismus, a massive loss of binocular neurons results (Baker *et al.*, 1974; Crawford & von Noorden, 1979a, 1979b).

Hubel & Wiesel (1962), showed that about 80% of cortical neurons respond to stimulation of either eye, i.e. they are binocularly driven. In monocular strabismus there is a marked shift in ocular dominance, such that most cells are driven through the normal eye. Similar effects also occur in animals reared with monocular deprivation, which results in few binocular cells and few monocular cells driven through the amblyopic eye. The effects are most profound when deprivation occurs in early life. When deprivation occurs later on in development the cell loss for both binocular and monocular cells is less marked, and once the pathways have matured no effect on cortical cells will result, even following several years of monocular deprivation.

Loss of functional binocularity and stereopsis is associated with loss of binocularly-driven cells, while loss of monocular cells results in reduced spatial resolution (amblyopia).

Cellular recordings from neurons driven by the anisometropic or strabismic eye have lower optimum spatial frequencies, poorer spatial resolution, and lower contrast sensitivity than the neurons driven by the normal eye. This results in a shift of ocular dominance towards the non-deprived eye.

Cells preferring relatively low spatial frequencies are generally unaffected in amblyopic animals, while those preferring high spatial frequencies show large interocular differences. This may result in normal binocular interaction at low spatial frequencies. This supports the psychophysical findings of Holopigian *et al.* (1986).

Visual evoked potentials (VEPs)

Neither strabismic nor anisometropic amblyopes show deficits in VEPs when no spatial structure is used in the test stimuli. However, when spatially structured stimuli are used, marked changes in the response are found. These losses, like those found psychophysically, depend on the pattern size, its spatial frequency and retinal location, and are most profound for small stimuli positioned within the central part of the visual field.

Binocular competition

The vastly different effects of binocular and monocular deprivation amblyopia on the visual cortex in monkeys led Hubel & Wiesel (1965), to propose that the functional integrity of the cortex depends not only on the total afferent activity from the two eyes but also on a competitive interaction between the pathways from the two eyes. The effects in the visual cortex suggest that these afferent paths compete for control of cortical cells. This results in the non-deprived eye having a competitive advantage, and enables it to gain functional control of neurons in the cortex, to the detriment of the deprived eye. It was suggested that the site of competitive interaction was at the cortex.

There is also evidence for binocular competition in human amblyopia. The work of Hess & Pointer (1985), showed that the amblyopic eye in anisometropic amblyopes had reduced contrast sensitivity across the binocular visual field, but showed normal contrast sensitivity in the monocular segment of the visual field.

A striking feature of the normal mature primate striate cortex is the alternate pattern of ocular dominance columns as revealed by auto-radiographic techniques (Hubel *et al.*, 1977). If one eye gains competitive advantage due to the fellow receiving inferior input prior to the maturation of the dominance columns, then only the afferent pathways of the deprived eye will retract. This results in the normal eye gaining neural territory that would otherwise have been kept by the deprived eye. It is this process of binocular competition that leads to the expansion of cortical territory subserving the non-deprived eye and shrinkage of the ocular dominance columns of the deprived eye.

Binocular inhibition (suppression)

Interocular suppression mechanisms have been assumed to play an important role in the development of amblyopia. These mechanisms are thought to exert an influence on the vision of the amblyopic eye well beyond the 'sensitive' period. Evidence for such tonic suppression is the observation that following the loss of a non-deprived eye due to disease or injury the acuity of the amblyopic eye will often increase. Harwerth *et al.* (1986) demonstrated that the enucleation of the non-deprived eye resulted in an immediate increase in the number of cells that can be driven through the deprived eye.

Although it has been traditionally assumed that suppression leads to amblyopia, recent research shows that deep amblyopes may have less suppression than alternating strabismics with good visual acuity, which suggests a negative correlation between the depth of amblyopia and the degree of suppression.

In studies of amblyopes using the drug bicuculline, which acts as an antagonist to the inhibitory neurotransmitter 8-aminobutyne acid (GABA), very dramatic evidence for binocular suppression is shown. Sillito *et al.* (1981), found that roughly one-third of the cells initially dominated by the non-deprived eye became responsive to the deprived eye during the application of bicuculline. Even more marked alterations were noted in ocular dominance columns in the normal visual cortex, suggesting that GABA mediated intracortical inhibition plays an important role in normal vision.

Levodopa is a drug which acts like the neurotransmitter dopamine, which is found in retinal amacrine and interplexiform cells, and is thought also to be involved in information processing to the brain. Investigations have shown the involvement of dopamine in various visual functions. In patients with Parkinson's disease levodopa has caused changes in contrast sensitivity, electroretinograms and visually evoked potentials. Gottlob *et al.* (1992) showed that after the administration of levodopa to human amblyopes for only one week, visual acuities improved and scotomas in the central visual field reduced. These effects persisted after the patients stopped receiving the drug.

Hess (1991) suggested that suppression was likely to occur at the site of adaptation rather than before or after it. The site for adaptation is known to be in the striate cortex. The competitive advantage held by one eye in monocular cataract or anisometropia is clear, but it is less obvious in some cases of strabismus. Because, if strabismus precedes amblyopia what gives one eye competitive advantage? Why do some strabismics develop alternation and avoid amblyopia while others do not? In some strabismic amblyopes a degree of anisometropia is also found, so it is easy to see why one eye gains competitive advantage. However, approximately 30% have no significant anisometropia. Of these some will have lower levels of isometropia, while others may be essentially emmetropic. Obviously, with low to moderate bilateral hypermetropia if accommodative amplitude is normal, then over-convergence will result when the eyes try to improve focus. So it is easy to see why a squint might arise, but what decides which eye becomes the squinting eye, is suppressed and therefore becomes amblyopic?

An alternative hypothesis for these amblyopes is that the afferents from one eye reach target neurons in the LGN and cortex first, thus gaining a competitive advantage. Thus both the strabismus and the amblyopia may result from a common cause. It is not yet clear why the afferents from one eye arrive first.

In normal subjects one can usually demonstrate a dominant or referent eye, and this is generally associated with a general dominant side, i.e. right-eyed, right-handed and right-footed. So it may be that afferents from the naturally dominant eye will always arrive very slightly ahead of the non-dominant eye. Obviously, this does not result in a squint in normal observers, but where there is a congenital muscle weakness, or over-convergence due to accommodative effort in bilateral hypermetropia, this may be sufficient to start the process of competitive inhibition. To take this argument a stage further, some people show a very weak dominance or even a lack of dominance (very common in subjects with learning difficulties such as dyslexia) and they may favour alternation. Further evidence for such a possibility is shown in dyslexic children who often show marked convergence insufficiency, and often alternate spontaneously during reading.

It would be interesting to establish if visually normal observers with very strong ocular dominance show any minor amblyopic effects in their non-dominant eyes.

4.6   Eye movements

The main functions of the human eye movement system are to provide accurate tracking and to stabilize the retinal image. This allows the object of regard to be maintained within the central foveal area, enabling precise localization and high resolution of detail.

When an object moves with a simple lateral motion it is tracked by versional (conjugate) eye movements. However, when a depth component is added, vergence (disjunctive) movements are involved. In everyday vision both eye movement systems are activated simultaneously. Various effects which amblyopia and strabismus may have on the eye movement system are now discussed.

4.6.1   Increased drift

This refers to an abnormally large and/or rapid smooth drift amplitude found in amblyopic eyes during attempted maintained monocular fixation. It has been shown by Ciuffreda *et al.* (1980), that amblyopia, and not strabismus, is the cause of increased drift amplitude.

4.6.2   Saccadic intrusions

These are small eye movements which occur without any functional purpose. They are observed in individuals with strabismus, with or without amblyopia, and are therefore a functional effect of strabismus.

4.6.3   Latent nystagmus

This is only present with monocular fixation. It appears as a conjugate jerk nystagmus. Latent nystagmus can also be produced by shining a bright light into one eye.

Latent nystagmus is reduced by the use of a parasympathomimetic ocular drug. This can be a useful aid during occlusion therapy to treat amblyopia in such patients. Latent nystagmus is generally associated with strabismus.

4.6.4 Saccadic eye movements

These are the predominant eye movements during reading and scanning the visual scene. In amblyopic eyes increased latency is the main feature found. Increased latency refers to the delay in time between the change in stimulus direction and the initiation of a saccadic eye movement. Amblyopia is a necessary condition for these increased latencies, but strabismus is not. Although amblyopes without strabismus show the delay, non-amblyopic strabismics do not. Further, increased latencies were shown to be related to the degree of amblyopia; the greater the amblyopia the greater the delay in response. These increased latencies suggest a slowing in the sensory pathways that process visual information used subsequently by the oculomotor system in generating saccadic eye movements.

Fukushima & Tsutsui (1984), showed that the increased latencies were attributable to visuosensory rather than visuomotor factors. They measured saccadic latencies for visual and auditory evoked saccades, and showed that delays were only found with visually evoked saccades. From this Fukushima & Tsutsui suggested that these increased saccadic latencies were the result of a visual processing delay.

Abnormal tracking properties have also been found in amblyopic subjects.

4.6.5 Pursuit eye movements

The ability to follow a smoothly moving target requires an intact pursuit system. Pursuit allows stabilization of the retinal image, with the addition of saccades to give foveation of the detailed information. For very fast-moving objects a combination of smooth pursuit and saccades are required. In amblyopic eyes three abnormalities of smooth pursuit are found, reduced gain, directional asymmetries, and abnormal saccadic substitution.

Reduced gain

This means that the target speed which can be followed by smooth pursuit alone is slower than the normal level.

Asymmetric pursuit (directional asymmetries)

This is when pursuit is smooth in one direction but breaks down to saccadic pursuit in the opposite direction.

Schor (1975), suggested that marked directional impairment, with the gain being grossly reduced for nasalward versus temporalward target movement on the retina, was due to hemi-retinal suppression reducing velocity sensitivity over the nasal retina.

Amblyopes with asymmetric pursuit and asymmetric nystagmus have the poorest prognosis for the recovery of binocular function.

Abnormal saccadic substitutions

In normal individuals, when a target velocity becomes too great for smooth pursuit, saccades are added to the pursuit movement to reduce an accumulating positional error. The amplitude of the saccade is always less than the displacement of the target. However, in amblyopic eyes, saccades having amplitudes of up to four times greater than the displacement of the target can occur, particularly over small spatial extent, up to a maximum of 2°, resulting in an overshoot.

4.6.6   Asymmetric optokinetic responses (OKN)

It was suggested by Schor & Levi (1980b), that asymmetric optokinetic nystagmus was due to the incomplete development of binocular vision. Cortical mechanisms, particularly those which mediated temporally driven OKN, were most affected. Schor (1983), also implicated subcortical pretectal mechanisms as underlying this abnormal response. Mein (1983), reported asymmetric OKN only in subjects who also had strabismic nystagmus and dissociated vertical divergence. When nystagmus was absent the OKN asymmetry disappeared.

One interesting point is that OKN asymmetries have been found in both eyes of amblyopes. This has been explained by the fact that asymmetric OKN is due to a combination of reduced cortical input to subcortical structures, and binocular cortical suppression effects in the amblyopic eye.

4.6.7   Vergence eye movements

Disparity vergence is not found within the central suppression area present in amblyopia, because this area blocks the disparity input to the ocular motor system. However, outside this central area of binocular suppression the disparity input can be processed, resulting in disparity vergence responses.

In animal models with strabismus and amblyopia there is a reduction of cortical binocular cells. If there is also a reduction of cells which process and code disparity information this would explain the reduced vergence response capability.

4.6.8 Accommodative vergence

No changes are found in slightly to moderately amblyopic eyes, but a drop in accommodative vergence amplitude is found when the visual acuity is less than 6/120.

4.6.9 Accommodation

There are several types of accommodative deficiency in the amblyopic eye under both static and dynamic testing conditions. These accommodative abnormalities include increased latency, increased response variability, reduced gain, and poorly sustained accommodation.

A common feature in amblyopes is the overall reduction in average response level, which is frequently found in conjunction with increased response variance. The sensory basis for these abnormalities and additional factors that contribute to the deficits are the same for both static and dynamic accommodation.

It has been argued that accommodative dysfunction is the result of a sensory deficit rather than a motor one. This is presumed to be due to the early, prolonged abnormal visual experience, which includes monocular contrast deprivation for high spatial frequencies in anisometropia, and suppression in strabismus.

4.7 The effect of orthoptic treatment (amblyopia therapy)

Some functions do improve following orthoptic therapy; these include increased drift, saccadic intrusions and accommodative deficits. These three functions in particular have shown quite marked improvements, even in older amblyopes.

Interestingly, some other ocularmotor findings such as abnormal saccadic substitutions, disparity vergence, saccadic latencies and smooth pursuit remain unchanged after orthoptic therapy.

4.8 The pupillary system

Several studies have shown that afferent pupillary defects are quite common in amblyopia, and are not found in strabismus without amblyopia.

If the light is shone into the eye centrally, in normal eyes the pupillary reflexes are brisk, while in amblyopes the response is more sluggish. Interestingly, in amblyopes when the light is shone onto the peripheral retina the response is brisker than when light is shone centrally. This suggests that in amblyopia a central sensory defect exists.

The general view is that a subtle afferent pupillary defect is present in many amblyopic eyes, as many as 80% in a study by Thompson *et al.* (1981). This gives rise to reduced pupillary response amplitude caused by diminished sensitivity, and increased pupillary response latency due to slower processing. However, the abnormal consensual response suggests also an efferent-pathway anomaly. There are no details of the pupillary-accommodative pathways.

There is evidence to suggest that pupillary responses can improve following intensive orthoptic therapy, indicating a reversible afferent defect of primarily non-cortical origin.

4.9   The main clinical features of the different types of amblyopia

These are summarized in Table 4.1.

4.10   Summary

Amblyopia is not simply a general amorphous loss of acuity and binocularity. Although all functional amblyopes have these two factors in common, research has revealed differences in deficits across the visual field, different results for threshold and supra-threshold testing, and for high and low spatial frequency gratings. Further, strabismic amblyopes, particularly, suffer from geometric distortion causing 'crowding' and pattern distortion. They also show poor localization and eye-tracking movements. Accommodation and pupillary responses are often abnormal, and there are increased latencies for the detection of elements in a multiple element pattern. Therefore, an amblyope may complain of difficulties out of proportion to those simply predicted by reduced acuity alone.

Different visual functions emerge at different times. Structures and functions that develop earliest are the most robust to the effects of abnormal visual input, while those which develop more slowly seem more susceptible. Thus the amblyopic visual system resembles in many ways the immature visual system. Both show normal or near normal receptoral function (light sense), relatively normal function at low spatial and high temporal frequencies, reduced acuity and contrast sensitivity, particularly at high spatial frequencies, and reduced hyperacuity.

The consequences of monocular occlusion can be particularly detrimental. Von Noorden (1981a), reported that following atropinization of the normal eye for amblyopia therapy between the ages of two and four years, amblyopia was produced in the formerly normal eye. Despite this, occlusion remains the best method for improving the acuity of an amblyopic eye. Preferential looking and VEP studies have shown that relative acuity differences between the two eyes can be rapidly and dramatically reduced with occlusion therapy. Full-time occlusion is no longer used. The amount of time required daily for effective

Table 4.1 Summary of clinical findings in the various types of amblyopia.

Test used	Type of amblyopia					
	Strabismic	Anisometropic	Deprivation 'occlusion'	Organic, idiopathic and congenital	Toxic and nutritional	Psychogenic
Morphoscopic VA *'Crowded' optotype*	Reduced	Reduced	Reduced	Reduced; can be bilateral.	Reduced, bilaterally, not always equally.	Reduced, variable; inconsistent with test distance; susceptible to suggestion.
Angular VA	> morphoscopic	= morphoscopic; sometimes slightly > morphoscopic	> morphoscopic	= morphoscopic	= morphoscopic	Variable
VA with 2.0 ND filter	> or = morphoscopic	morphoscopic	> or = morphoscopic	Usually slightly < morphoscopic	< morphoscopic	Variable
Fixation	Sometimes eccentric; can be variable.	Central; unsteady in high errors.	Generally no deviation; unsteady fixation may be noted.	Normal	Normal	Normal
Cover test	Non-alignment of one eye; sometimes alternation.	Normal or may show unequal phorias with high errors.	Generally no deviation; unsteady fixation may be noted.	Normal	Normal	Normal
Amsler charts	Lang's one-sided scotoma in microtropia.	May show large central blur.	No details; probably similar to anisometropia.	Small central scotoma may be present.	Central defect, especially for red.	Usually normal
Visual fields	Normal, except when suppression is very dense.	Normal	Normal	Central defect is sometimes found.	Raised macular threshold; defect worse for red.	Defect not physiologically possible. Sometimes star or spiral defect.
Others	Generally obvious on inspection except for microtropias.	Refractive error present at least in one eye.	May report relevant histroy i.e. ptosis or cataract.	Macular disturbance with poor or absent foveal reflex.	Possible systemic signs, symptoms, or history i.e. ptosis or cataract.	Has underlying psychological cause; may have detached attitude or be unconcerned.

treatment with occlusion therapy is dependent on the age of the infant. In early infancy occlusion is only required for short periods, say one to one-and-a-half hours per day, but as you near the close of the sensitive period of acuity development this will increase to several hours per day. Mitchell *et al.* (1986) found that occlusion for 50% of the time was the optimum therapy regime in cats, giving improvement in acuity in the amblyopic eye without loss of acuity in the fellow eye. Clinical data obtained from occlusion therapy has shown that maximum improvement in acuity occurs between fourteen and eighteen months in human infants. The efficiency of occlusion reduces steadily with increasing age, until little effect is obtained when nearing the end of the sensitive period at around seven to eight years. However, as with all developmental processes, there will be variability between individuals. The author suggests, from unpublished studies, that when a higher-than-average amplitude of accommodation is found in older children, or even adults, occlusion therapy can still have beneficial effects. So amplitude of accommodation may be a useful prognostic guide as to the likely efficacy of amblyopia therapy.

The author suggests that infants should be screened immediately following 'cortical awakening' at about six months of age, particularly those who fit categories known to have a higher incidence of squints and/or amblyopia (see Section 4.2), and that subsequent management of refractive anomalies significantly reduces the prevalence of amblyopia.

4.11   References

Arden, G.B., Carter, R.M., Hogg, C.R., Powell, D.J. and Vaegan, J.W. (1980) 'Reduced pattern electroretinograms suggest a preganglionic basis for non-treatable human amblyopia'. *J. Physiol.*, **308**, 82–3.

Awaya, S., Miyake, Y., Imaizumi, Y., Shiose, Y., Kanda, T. and Komuro, K. (1973) 'Amblyopia in man, suggestive of stimulus deprivation amblyopia'. *Jpn. J. Ophthalmol.*, **17**, 69–82.

Awaya, S., Sugawara, M. and Miyake, S. (1979) 'Observations in patients with occlusion amblyopia. Results of treatment'. *Trans. Ophthal. Soc. UK*, **99**, 447–54.

Awaya, S., Sugawara, M., Miyake, S. and Isomura, Y. (1980) 'Form vision deprivation amblyopia and the results of its treatment – with special reference to the critical period'. *Jpn. J. Ophthalmol.*, **24**, 241–50.

Baker, F.H., Grigg, P. and von Noorden, G.K. (1974) 'Effects of visual deprivation and strabismus on the response of neurons in the visual cortex of the monkey, including studies on the striate and prestriate cortex in the normal animal'. *Brain Res.*, **66**, 188–208.

Blakemore, C. and Vital-Durand, F. (1979) 'Development of the neural basis of visual acuity in monkeys. Speculation on the origin of deprivation amblyopia'. *Trans. Ophthalmol. Soc. UK*, **99**, 363–8.

Boothe, R.G., Kiorpes, L. and Hendrickson, A. (1982) 'Anisometropic amblyopia in *Macaca nemestrina* monkeys produced by atropinization of one eye during development'. *Invest. Ophthalmol. Visual Sci.*, **22**, 228–33.

Boothe, R.G. and Teller, D.Y. (1982) 'Meridional variations in acuity and CSFs in monkeys reared with externally applied astigmatism'. *Vis. Res.*, **22**, 801–810.

Bradley, A., Dahlman, C., Switkes, E. and De Valois, K. (1986) 'A comparison of color and luminance discrimination in amblyopia'. *Invest. Ophthalmol. Vis. Sci.*, **27**, 1404–1409.

Buckingham, T., Watkins, R., Bansal, P. and Bamford, K. (1990) 'Hyperacuity thresholds for oscillatory movement are abnormal in strabismic and anisometropic amblyopes'. *Optom. Vis. Sci.*, **68**, 351–6.

Ciuffreda, K.J., Kenyon, R.V. and Stark, L. (1980) 'Increased drift in amblyopic eyes'. *Brit. J. Ophthalmol.*, **64**, 7–14.

Ciuffreda, K.J., Levi, D.M. and Selenow, A. (1991) In *Amblyopia: Basic and Clinical Aspects.* Butterworth-Heinemann, Boston.

Cobb, S.R. and MacDonald, C.F. (1978) 'Resolution acuity in astigmats: evidence for a critical period in the human visual system'. *Brit. J. Physiol. Opt.*, **32**, 38–49.

Crawford, M.L.J. and von Noorden, G.K. (1979a) 'Concomitant strabismus and cortical eye dominance in young rhesus monkeys'. *Trans. Ophthalmol. Soc. UK*, **99**, 369–74.

Crawford, M.L.J. and von Noorden, G.K. (1979b) 'The effects of short-term experimental strabismus on the visual system in *Macaca mulatta*'. *Invest. Ophthalmol. Visual. Sci.*, **18**, 496–505.

Freeman, R.D. and Pettigrew, J.D. (1973) 'Alteration of visual cortex from environmental asymmetries'. *Nature*, **246**, 359–60.

Fukushima, M. and Tsutsui, J. (1984) 'Visually and auditory evoked saccadic reaction time in amblyopia', in *Strabismus 11*. (R.D. Reinecke, ed.). Grune and Stratton, New York, 443–9.

Gottlob, I., Charlier, J. and Reinecke, R.D. (1992) 'Visual acuities and scotomas after one week Levodopa administration in human amblyopia'. *Invest. Ophthalmol. Vis. Sci.*, **33**, 2722–8.

Harwerth, R.S., Crawford, M.L.J., Smith, E.L. and Boltz, R.L. (1981) 'Behavioural studies of stimulus deprivation amblyopia in monkeys'. *Vis. Res.*, **21**, 779–89.

Harwerth, R.S. and Levi, D.M. (1977) 'Increment threshold spectral sensitivity in anisometropic amblyopia'. *Vis. Res.*, **17**, 585–90.

Harwerth, R.S., Smith, E.L. and Boltz, R.L. (1980) 'Meridional amblyopia in monkeys'. *Expl. Brain Res.*, **39**, 351–6.

Harwerth, R.S., Smith, E.L., Boltz, R.L., Crawford, M.L.J. and von Noorden, G.K. (1983) 'Behavioural studies on the effect of abnormal early visual experience in monkeys: spatial modulation sensitivity'. *Vis. Res.*, **23**, 1501–1510.

Harwerth, R.S., Smith, E.L., Duncan, G.C., Crawford, M.L.J. and von Noorden, G.K. (1986) Multiple sensitive periods in the development of the primate visual system. *Science*, **232**, 235–8.

Hendrickson, A., Boles, J. and McLean, E.B. (1977) 'Visual acuity and behaviour of monocularly deprived monkeys after retinal lesions'. *Invest. Ophthalmol. Vis. Sci.*, **16**, 469–73.

Hess, R.F. (1991) 'The site and nature of suppression in squint amblyopia'. *Vis. Res.*, **31**, 111–17.

Hess, R.F., Campbell, F.W. and Greenhalgh, T. (1978) 'On the nature of the neural basis of human amblyopia: neural aberrations and neural sensitivity loss'. *Pflugers Archiv.*, **377**, 201–207.

Hess, R.F., Campbell, F.W. and Zimmern, R. (1980) 'Differences in the neural basis of human amblyopias: the effect of mean luminance'. *Vis. Res.*, **20**, 295–305.

Hess, R.F. and Pointer, J.S. (1985) 'Differences in the neural basis of human amblyopia: The distribution of the anomaly across the visual field'. *Vis. Res.*, **25**, 1577–94.

Holopigian, K., Blake, R. and Greenwald, M.J. (1986) 'Selective losses in binocular vision in anisometropic amblyopes'. *Vis. Res.*, **26**, 621–30.

Hubel, D.H. and Wiesel, T.N. (1962) 'Receptive fields, binocular interaction and functional architecture in the cat's visual cortex'. *J. Physiol.*, **160**, 106–54.

Hubel, D.H. and Wiesel, T.N. (1965) 'Binocular interaction in striate cortex of kittens reared with artificial squint'. *J. Neurophysiol.*, **28**, 1041–59.

Hubel, D.H., Wiesel, T.N. and Le Vay, S. (1977) 'Plasticity of ocular dominance columns in monkey striate cortex'. *Philos. Trans. R. Soc. London. Ser. B.*, **278**, 377–409.

Ikeda, H. and Tremain, K.E. (1979) 'Amblyopia occurs in retinal ganglion cells in cats reared with convergent squint without alternating fixation'. *Exp. Brain Res.*, **35**, 559–82.

Ikeda, H., Tremain, K.E. and Einion, G. (1978) 'Loss of spatial resolution of lateral geniculate nucleus neurones in kittens raised with convergent squint produced at different stages in development'. *Exp. Brain Res.*, **31**, 207–20.

Kirlin, J.D. and Flynn, J.T. (1981) 'Therapy of anisometropic amblyopia'. *J. Pediatr. Ophthalmol. Strabismus*, **18**, No. 5, 47–56.

Levi, D.M. (1976) 'Occlusion amblyopia'. *Am. J. Optom. Physiol. Opt.*, **53**, 16–19.

Levi, D.M. and Klein, S. (1982) 'Hyperacuity and amblyopia'. *Nature*, **298**, 268–70.

Mein, J. (1983) 'The OKN response and binocular vision in early onset strabismus'. *Austral. Orthoptic. J.*, **20**, 13–17.

Mitchell, D.E., Freeman, R.D., Millodot, M. and Haegerstrom, G. (1973) 'Meridional amblyopia: evidence for modification of the human visual system by early visual experience'. *Vis. Res.*, **13**, 535–58.

Mitchell, D.E., Murphy, K.M., Dzioba, H.A. and Horne, J.A. (1986) 'Optimization of visual recovery from early monocular deprivation in kittens: implications for occlusion therapy in the treatment of amblyopia'. *Clin. Vis. Sci.*, **1**, 173–7.

Mower, G.D., Berry, D., Burchfiel, J.L. and Duffy, F.H. (1981) 'Comparison of the effects of dark rearing and binocular suture on development and plasticity of cat visual cortex'. *Brain Res.*, **220**, 255–67.

Mower, G.D., Burchfiel, J.L. and Duffy, F.H. (1981) 'The effects of dark-rearing on the development and plasticity of the lateral geniculate nucleus'. *Brain Res.*, **227**, 418–24.

Pratt-Johnson, J.A., Wee, H.S. and Ellis, S. (1967) 'Suppression associated with esotropia'. *Canad. J. Ophthal.*, **2**, 284–91.

Rutstein, R.P., Marsh-Tootle, W., Scheiman, M.M. and Eskridge, J.B. (1991) 'Changes in retinal correspondence after changes in ocular alignment'. *Optom. Vis. Sci.*, **68**, 325–30.

Schor, C.M. (1975) 'A directional impairment of eye movement control in strabismic amblyopia'. *Invest. Ophthalmol. Vis. Sci.*, **14**, 692–7.

Schor, C.M. (1983) 'Subcortical binocular suppression affects the development of latent and optokinetic nystagmus'. *Am. J. Optom. Physiol. Opt.*, **60**, 481–501.

Schor, C.M. and Levi, D.M. (1980a) 'Direction selectivity for perceived motion in strabismic and anisometropic amblyopia'. *Invest. Ophthalmol. Vis. Sci.*, **19**, 1094–1104.

Schor, C.M. and Levi, D.M. (1980b) 'Disturbances of small-field horizontal and vertical optokinetic nystagmus in amblyopia'. *Invest. Ophthalmol. Vis. Sci.*, **19**, 668–83.

Selenow, A. and Ciuffreda, K.J. (1986) 'Visual function recovery during orthoptic therapy in an adult esotropic amblyope'. *J. Am. Optom. Assoc.*, **57**, 132–40.

Shapero, M. (1971) *Amblyopia*. Chilton, Philadelphia.

Sillito, A.M., Kemp, J.A. and Blakemore, C. (1981) 'The role of GABAergic inhibition in the cortical effects of monocular deprivation'. *Nature*, **291**, 318–20.

Tanlamai, T. and Goss, D.A. (1979) 'Prevalence of monocular amblyopia among anisometropes'. *Am. J. Optom. Physiol. Opt.*, **56**, 704–15.

Thomas, J., Mohindra, I. and Held, R. (1979) 'Strabismic amblyopia in infants'. *Am. J. Optom. Physiol. Opt.*, **56**, 197–201.

Thompson, H.S., Corbett, J.J. and Cox, T.A. (1981) 'How to measure the relative afferent pupillary defect'. *Surv. Ophthalmol.*, **26**, 39–42.

von Noorden, G.K. (1973). 'Experimental amblyopia in monkeys. Further behavioural observations and clinical correlations'. *Invest. Ophthalmol. Vis. Sci.*, **12**, 721–6.

von Noorden, G.K. (1980) In *Burian-von Noorden's binocular vision and ocular motility*. C.V. Mosby Co., St Louis.

von Noorden, G.K. (1981a) 'Amblyopia caused by unilateral atropinization'. *Ophthalmol.*, **88**, 131–3.

von Noorden, G.K. (1981b) 'New clinical aspects of stimulus deprivation amblyopia'. *Am. J. Ophthalmol.*, **92**, 416–21.

von Noorden, G.K. and Crawford, M.L.J. (1992) 'The lateral geniculate nucleus in human strabismic amblyopia'. *Invest. Ophthalmol. Vis. Sci.*, **33**, 2729–32.

von Noorden, G.K., Crawford, M.L.J. and Levacy, R.A. (1983) 'The lateral geniculate nucleus in human anisometropic amblyopia'. *Invest. Ophthalmol. Vis. Sci.*, **24**, 788–9.

von Noorden, G.K., Dowling, J.E. and Ferguson, D.C. (1970) 'Experimental amblyopia in monkeys. 1. Behavioural studies of stimulus deprivation amblyopia. *Arch. Ophthalmol.*, **84**, 206–14.

Wali, N., Leguire, L.E., Rogers, G.L. and Bremer, D.L. (1991) 'CSF interocular interactions in childhood amblyopia'. *Optom. Vis. Sci.*, **68**, 81–7.

Westheimer, G. (1975) 'Visual acuity and hyperacuity'. *Invest. Ophthalmol. Vis. Sci.*, **14**, 570–72.

SECTION 2

EXAMINATION OF THE CHILD

CHAPTER 5

Examination Techniques and Routines

Simon Barnard & David Edgar

5.1   Introduction

This chapter will discuss examination procedures and techniques that may be employed to assess the infant or child with a relatively normal medical and developmental history, and also offers a guide to examination routines at different age groups. In addition a number of special category patients are also discussed including the autistic, Down's syndrome and deaf child. Procedures such as assessing vision and visual acuity, colour vision, refraction and additional techniques related to binocular vision are covered in other chapters.

5.2   General considerations

For a child, a visit to the optometrist starts as he or she arrives at the practice. The waiting room should be bright and friendly. There should be books, comics, and safe, quiet toys easily visible and accessible. Toilet facilities should be readily available. It can be the practice policy for reception staff to greet the child as well as the parents, and for staff to avoid wearing white coats. One of the best investments a practitioner can make is to purchase a miniature table and chairs and place these in the waiting room with the toys. This will help a young child feel welcome and relaxed, and the table, chairs and toys often help to keep siblings occupied whilst the parents and patient are in the consulting room.

On a child's first visit it is generally preferable for the optometrist to greet the patient in the waiting room. On subsequent visits when the child knows the practitioner, and is probably looking forward to the eye examination, the patient and parents can be called or ushered into the consulting room, where the practitioner is waiting. It is easy for the optometrist to forget that it is the child who is the patient. However, as soon as the patient is old enough (about two years) it is the child that the practitioner should greet first, using the child's first name, followed by the parents.

With a very young or shy child the practitioner should crouch down, so that he and the patient are at eye level, and try to initiate a conversation. In the consulting room the child should be asked to sit on 'his own chair'. The importance of the child's role in the proceedings can be further emphasized at this stage by the practitioner pointing out to the child where the parents should sit. Parents usually take their cue from this conversation with the child. Most children enjoy a ride, especially if it is done by 'magic', and the chair inexplicably rises when the child points to the ceiling. The optometrist should attempt to obtain a positive verbal response as early as possible as this is a good sign that a rapport has been made and anxiety reduced.

One or, if preferred, both parents should be invited into the consulting room with the child. The benefits of having both parents present at the first visit are particularly great in cases where ongoing treatment is likely to be necessary and where the understanding and assistance of both mother and father may be helpful, for example when a child is likely to require orthoptic or vision therapy. All too often it is the mother alone who undertakes all health-care visits with her children – working with parents is discussed in Chapter 15.

A child of walking age can be invited to sit on the patient's chair by himself. Often the child will be happier if he or she can sit on the chair with a cuddly toy provided by the optometrist. The infant patient will need to be located on his or her parent's lap. Occasionally, a child beyond the infant stage will not sit on the chair by himself. Confrontation between the practitioner and child is to be avoided at all costs, and the child should be allowed to sit on his mother's lap until confidence is gained and a natural break in the routine allows the mother to move elsewhere. When talking with a child it is helpful if the clinician and the patient are as close to eye level as possible. This can be achieved by raising the patient's chair and, if necessary, by providing an extra cushion. The optometrist should not be in the position of physically looking down on the child. This helps to foster the development of friendship between the practitioner and his or her young patient. Mentally and/or physically handicapped children can usually be placed on the patient chair, and only on rare occasions will the child need to remain in a wheelchair.

The consulting room should have a friendly ambience, and it is advantageous for the room to be 5 metres or more in length to avoid the need for a mirror. This is because in smaller rooms a mirror must be used to achieve 5 m or 6 m viewing distances, and children are often confused if they have to view a chart imaged by a mirror. A variety of small, squeaky or otherwise interesting toys should be readily available to the practitioner, to help rescue the situation in the case of an uncooperative child. Toy animals can also be placed strategically around the room, but sweets or chocolates should never be given to a patient without the parents' permission. The practitioner can be uninhibited and feel free to whistle, make funny noises, sing and generally adapt his behaviour as required to build rapport and keep the child's attention. Whispering or speaking very softly whilst making eye contact is sometimes useful in helping to control a boisterous child.

Generally, the optometrist should be honest in his dealings with the young patient. For example, when instilling a topical ophthalmic drug it is wise to take time to show the child the size of the drop, commenting on how small it is, and to explain that, just as if the child is splashed in the eyes while in the bath, 'the drop will sting just a little bit, but not for very long'. If the practitioner adopts the more devious approach stating that 'this drop will not sting', the child is likely never to trust the practitioner again. Use of the words 'hurt' or 'pain' should be avoided. 'Make-believe' game play can be of great assistance with certain children for tests such as tonometry and ophthalmoscopy: however, under no circumstances should the practitioner bribe the child by making promises that cannot be met.

The practitioner should observe the child as he enters the consulting room. Obvious anomalies may be apparent, including squint, head tilt or turn, skull anomalies, hypertelorism or behavioural anomalies. The general state of well-being of the child should also be assessed, taking note of any signs of injury (see Chapter 14). The mentally or physically handicapped child is discussed later in this chapter.

5.3   History and symptomatology

Apart from the initial and continuing observation of the child's behaviour on the way to and in the consulting room, the examination routine begins with the taking of symptoms and history. Some practitioners provide parents or guardians with a questionnaire a few days prior to the examination, and this can be very useful when dealing with more complex cases such as the assessment of a child with learning difficulties. In the case of a very young child with a short span of attention, or a very 'active' child with behavioural difficulties, some history-taking may be left until later in order that the child's interest and limited concentration is utilized optimally. For the same reason, it is wise to carry out the most 'important' tests early in the routine, leaving the less important until later.

Generally, for children under the age of five or six years, the authors prefer to direct their history-taking to the parent or guardian. Occasionally the parent responds by asking the child to explain, and the practitioner should go along with this approach as far as is possible, returning to the parent as necessary. However, in this regard, preferences between individual optometrists may vary, some preferring to obtain information directly from the child and often without the parent in the room.

In most instances, the practitioner will want to elicit the primary reason for the child being brought for an eye examination. Possible reasons for this include:

- Routine check-up

- Family history of visual problems
- Failed vision screening or school vision check
- Referred by GP, pediatrician or teacher
- Signs noticed by parents
- Symptoms reported by child
- Visual assessment with particular reference to educational difficulties
- Further opinion sought.

5.3.1   History

Questioning should be directed to obtain relevant information concerning the following:

Birth history	Birth weight? Full-term or premature? Forceps delivery? Required oxygen? Prenatal history may also be important in some instances, e.g. maternal rubella, the use of systemic drugs.
Developmental history	Did the child crawl and walk at a 'normal' age? Are there any known motor coordination difficulties?
General health	What illnesses has the child had? Present general health? Current medications? History of ENT/ hearing problems? Are there any known allergies?
Educational progress	How is the child doing at school?
Family history	Is there a family history of squint or any eye disease?

5.3.2   Symptoms in the infant

For the infant, the presenting 'symptoms', if any, are actually 'signs' noticed by parents (see Table 5.1).

For children up to the age of about four or five years it is also usually observed signs rather than reported symptoms that cause parents to bring their children for optometric investigation. However, younger children occasionally complain of symptoms to their parents. It is worth remembering that whilst the practitioner might be an expert on eyes, parents tend to be experts on their own children! Grandmothers are particularly astute at noticing anomalies such as strabismus. They have had the benefit of many years of experience, and observations of this nature should be carefully noted. Many teachers are also excellent observers.

As with any history-taking, it is important to establish for how long symptoms or signs have been present. For example, more significance would be attached to

Table 5.1 Some common clinical signs noted by parents in infants.

Sign	Possible causes
'red spot in the eye'	Sub-conjunctival haemorrhage (also birth trauma; abuse)
'squint', 'eye turns'	Strabismus; epicanthus
'watering eye' (epiphora)	Poorly developed lacrimal duct; ectropion; buphthalmos; conjunctival/corneal anomaly
'one eye bigger than other'	Proptosis; ptosis; buphthalmos; Duane's retraction syndrome; lid retraction; anisocoria (idiopathic; CNS anomaly)
'keeps rubbing his eyes'	Entropion; conjunctival inflammation; binocular discomfort; buphthalmos
'uncomfortable in bright light'	Fair skin; albinism; buphthalmos; binocular vision anomalies; corneal/conjunctival anomalies

the information that a three-year-old developed a ptosis a week ago than to the information that the anomaly was present at birth.

Additional signs that are commonly noted by parents in children up to four years of age are shown in Table 5.2.

5.3.3 Symptoms in toddlers and older children

By the age of five or six years children may start to observe and report symptoms reliably. It should be noted, however, that a child will complain of pain at a much younger age, and serious pain will produce obvious distress at any age.

In a retrospective study of 1008 case records of children aged from birth to 16 years who attended an optometric practice specializing in pediatrics, 24% of the patients complained of symptoms or had signs noticed by the parents or teacher. Headaches and blurred vision were by far the most common presenting symptoms and signs, a complete list of which is given in Table 5.3. The youngest age at which a child reported symptoms was four years (Elkins, 1991).

Table 5.2 Some common clinical signs noted in the preschool child.

Sign	Possible causes
'sits close to television'	Ametropia; reduced vision; behavioural habit
'Not good with his colours'	Colour vision anomaly; immature development
'screws eyes up'	Refractive error; photophobia
'blinks a lot'	Behavioural/psychosomatic anomaly; conjunctival/corneal anomaly

Table 5.3 Presenting symptoms/signs of children attending a primary-care optometric practice, listed in order of prevalence (n = 1008) (Elkins 1991).

Symptom/sign	% of patients
Headaches	8.1
Blurred vision	7.0
Blinking	1.4
Eye ache	1.4
Suspected strabismus	1.3
Double vision	1.2
Watery eye	1.2
Screwing up eyes	1.1
Photophobia	0.7
Eye pain	0.4
Red eye	0.2
Total presenting with symptoms/signs	24

Headache

Although headache is one of the commonest presenting symptoms for a child, a visual or oculomotor etiology is uncommon. Whilst certain refractive errors and oculomotor anomalies can sometimes produce headaches in adults, a child is more likely to lose concentration and cease the visual task in hand before symptoms become apparent. Whilst the optometrist should ask the child about the headache symptoms, the child's responses are very often vague. Parents can sometimes offer some information as the child may have informed them of the characteristics of the headache. Careful history-taking alone will often provide clues as to the likelihood of a visual, ocular, neurological or psychosomatic etiology.

Questioning should include:

In which part of the head does the pain occur?

Do the headaches occur at any specific time of day, or after any particular task (e.g. watching television or reading)?

Are the symptoms associated with school?

Do they occur at weekends?

Does the child wake up with a headache in the morning?

For how long have they been occurring, and with what frequency?

For how long do they last?

What alleviates the symptoms?

In an analysis of 82 children complaining of headache, Elkins (1991), found symptom association as shown in Table 5.4, though it should be noted that some children described more than one association.

If a child is complaining of headache, and no obvious visual or oculomotor cause is found, then the patient should be referred to the general medical practitioner.

Migraine is a not infrequent cause of headache in children, and the associated symptoms may include scotomata, scintillating spots, or hemianopias. The fortification spectra suffered by adults are not common (Taylor, 1990). Transient mydriasis may also occur.

Blurred vision

Children are often completely unaware that their vision is blurred, and poor vision is frequently first noted at a preschool screening, at a school medical examination, or at a routine visit to the family optometrist. A child with poor vision in one eye only is even less likely to be aware of the problem or to exhibit signs, except possibly in the area of hand/eye coordination and depth perception skills. In the case of a child exhibiting binocular blurring the parents may be alerted because the child sits close to the television, or 'screws up' his eyes. A child who has become myopic may start to make mistakes whilst copying from the board at school, but occasionally clinicians will encounter a child who despite four or five dioptres of uncorrected myopia has no symptoms or signs of under-achievement.

Table 5.4   The association of the headache symptom in 82 children (Elkins, 1991).

Association	%
Unknown or not recorded	48.8
Study/reading	26.9
Present on awakening	13.4
Watching television	9.8
School in general	7.3
When 'tired'	7.3
At weekends	3.7
When listening to music	1.2
In sunlight	1.2
During hot weather	1.2

If a refractive error or an anomaly of binocular vision has been ruled out as the cause of reduced visual acuity, referral should be made for ophthalmological investigation. Any child reporting blurred vision associated with symptoms such as pain or redness of the eye should be examined by an ophthalmologist without delay.

Closing or covering one eye

This sign may provide an indication of the presence of an anomaly of binocular vision. In the case of recent onset strabismus, diplopia may be removed by closing one eye or turning the head. Intermittent squint or a poorly compensated heterophoria may also produce this sign. A child may read or write whilst covering one eye, and may even position his or her head so that it lies on his or her arm on a desk, in order to occlude the eye. Exotropia or poorly compensated exophoria often precipitates the closing of one eye (Wang & Chrysasanthou, 1988), particularly in sunlight.

Other possible reasons for covering one eye include discomfort, which may have a number of causes, including conjunctivitis and keratitis.

Diplopia

The clinician must establish whether the diplopia is *monocular* or *binocular*, vertical, horizontal or oblique. Binocular horizontal diplopia may be reported by an observant child becoming aware of physiological diplopia. Alternatively, it could be caused by a recent-onset concomitant or inconcomitant squint. Monocular diplopia suggests pathology of the ocular media or retina, occasionally a psychosomatic anomaly, or rarely abnormal exteroception from a deeply amblyopic eye (Mallett, 1988).

Frequent blinking

In the absence of any pathology such as dry eye, conjunctivitis, keratitis or corneal foreign body, the commonest cause of this sign, which is very common in primary-care optometric practice, is a psychosomatic disorder (see Chapter 20).

Micropsia and macropsia

By the age of three to four years, intelligent hypermetropic children may report seeing objects becoming smaller in size (micropsia). This is usually caused by a spasm of accommodation, or increased accommodation. Parents are often very worried by this symptom, and can be reassured, once this benign diagnosis has been made, by explaining the cause and remarking that it is usually intelligent, observant children who notice this phenomenon. Other possible causes of micropsia (and macropsia), which include retinal or macular disease, should be ruled out.

Ocular pain

As with adults, the practitioner must exclude the large variety of organic conditions that can produce pain. A child who has consistently reported pain of this nature should be referred to his general medical practitioner.

Asthenopia

Children do occasionally complain of tired, uncomfortable eyes, and the cause is often alleviated by the correction of hypermetropia, astigmatism or an oculomotor anomaly. However, it should be remembered that very often the child will not pursue a visual task long enough to produce the symptoms but rather will 'lose concentration' and stop what he is doing.

Photophobia

Possible causes of photophobia include exotropia or exophoria, corneal pathology, anterior uveitis, buphthalmos, aniridia, and albinism, or the complaint may be associated with fair skin. The investigation should be directed to determine the cause.

5.4   Examination of the orbit and external eye

This is done by observing with diffuse ambient light, and using gentle manipulation when necessary. The clinician should look for general symmetry of the eyes and orbit and note any proptosis, enophthalmos, epicanthus, ptosis, or lesions of the lids (see Chapter 12).

The interpupillary distance in the first three years of life is about 48–50 mm (Kasparek, 1981), and can be measured with a simple rule.

5.5   Examination of the cornea and anterior chamber

Although a direct ophthalmoscope will be routinely used, the *slit lamp biomicroscope* is the method of choice for examining the anterior segment in detail in patients in all age groups, including babies (see Fig. 5.1). An infant patient can be manoeuvred in a tummy-down, horizontal position with the chin supported by the parent. In the case of older children, a helping hand to keep the head

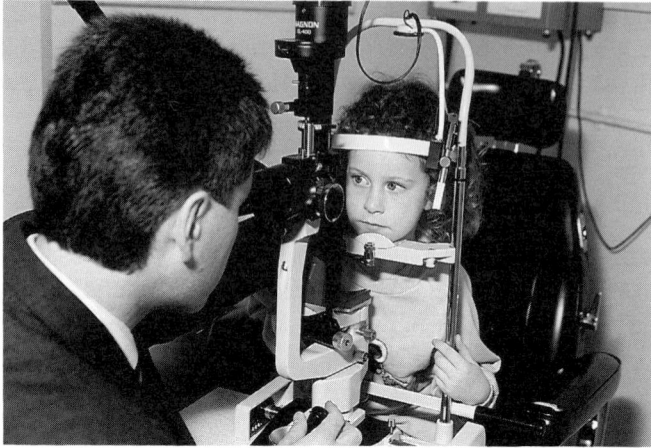

Fig. 5.1   Examining a young child with the slit lamp.

against the forehead rest is often required. Diagnostic stains can be used as necessary.

Keratometry can be carried out on children old enough to co-operate. On younger children and infants the use of a *placido disc* can provide useful information concerning corneal regularity.

5.5.1   Gonioscopy

Gonioscopy is rarely carried out in primary care optometric practice. The appearance of the angle of the anterior chamber of infants and young children does differ from that of an adult (see Hoyt & Lambert, 1990).

5.6   Examination of the iris, pupils and pupillary reflexes

The practitioner should initially observe the iris and pupils under normal room illumination. A direct ophthalmoscope, a hand-held lamp, or the slit lamp biomicroscope can then be used as required. The iris stroma of a neonate contains little pigment and will therefore usually appear blue. The development of iris colour will occur in the first twelve months. The neonate's pupil tends to be small (3 mm or less) and pupillary reflexes are sluggish for the first three to four months of life. Whilst anisocoria should be noted, a small difference (<2 mm) in pupil diameter is very common, and in the absence of other signs is not clinically significant.

Whilst gross direct and consensual pupillary reflexes can be readily assessed at all ages, it can be more difficult to determine the presence of a *relative* afferent defect unless accurate fixation is encouraged and maintained. The near reflex can be verified as soon as convergence can be elicited. A child with heterochromic irides who has not previously been investigated by a neurologist should be referred, to rule out active pathology of the sympathetic pathway. Unilateral hippus should also be referred.

5.7 Examination of the vitreous and fundus

Ophthalmoscopy should be routinely carried out, or at least attempted, on all patients in order to assess the ocular media and fundi, and is best performed under mydriasis, with the light pupil reflex abolished by an antimuscarinic drug. A completely dark room should be avoided as this can prove frightening to the child, who is always happier if he or she can see a parent. In primary-care practice in the UK routine mydriasis is not always carried out, and indeed is not always necessary. However, when ophthalmoscopy is carried out without pupil dilation, a full view of the fundus cannot be expected.

With infants, care must be taken to use the smallest dosage of drug possible to obtain the desired mydriatic effect. Such an approach helps to reduce the risks of adverse reactions. Sympathomimetics should not be used with premature neonates. Phenylephrine 10% is contra-indicated in children because of the risks of systemic toxicity; one drop of 2.5% solution may used, and it is not usually necessary to exceed this dosage. Instillation of the drops is made easier if the infant lies down on the mother's knee, and she can gently restrain little arms and legs. This position also aids ophthalmoscopy. Quietening the infant with a bottle or dummy is very useful (see Fig. 5.2).

Whilst *direct ophthalmoscopy* potentially provides a detailed view of important

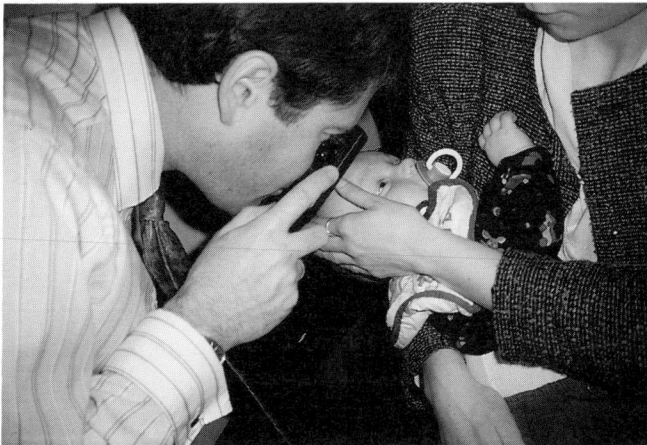

Fig. 5.2 Direct ophthalmoscopy on an infant.

features such as the optic nerve head and the macular region, very often, particularly with an infant, the only view obtained is that of the macula, because the infant tends to fixate the ophthalmoscope light. Occasionally, the practitioner is able to undertake ophthalmoscopy whilst the infant is asleep, gently opening the lids to view the eyes.

For older babies and young children, the use of toys positioned in various locations, or held by a parent, will often help the child maintain fixation. A child of thirty months and older will often respond well if asked questions such as 'can you see a little bird on the ceiling?', and will often describe the imaginary bird in great detail. Another widely employed trick is for the optometrist to tell the child that he wants to look in his eye to see what he had for breakfast or lunch.

Indirect ophthalmoscopy will give a much greater field of view at any one time than direct methods, and should be carried out to obtain an overall assessment of the state of the fundus. In primary-care practice not every child is routinely dilated, and the Reichert monocular indirect ophthalmoscope does give a wider field of view than a direct instrument under these circumstances.

Whenever an optometrist is suspicious of a fundus appearance, the child should be referred. An ophthalmologist will, when necessary, be able to undertake a fuller fundoscopy under sedation or general anaesthetic.

5.8　　Ophthalmic ultrasound (echography)

Ultrasound is a non-invasive technique that may be used for both diagnostics and biometry. Ophthalmic ultrasound generally uses frequencies of between 7.5 MHz (orbital examination) and 20 MHz (anterior segment examination). There are two main modes of examination. Firstly, 'A-Scan', in which a narrow beam of sound is directed along a desired path and the returning echoes from tissue interfaces are received and analysed. This technique is particularly useful for biometric measurements. However, 'standardized A-Scan echography' can, in expert hands, also be very precise in differentiating between different tissue types for diagnostic purposes. With the 'B-scan' mode of investigation the ultrasound transducer is oscillated to produce a sector of acoustic coverage so that a two-dimensional image is built up. For diagnostic work, a combination of A- and B-scans is useful. Ultrasound can be used for axial length measurement, for examination of the posterior eye in the presence of media opacities, and in cases of trauma. Standardized echography can also be used differentially to diagnose malignant melanoma of the choroid. For examination of anything other than anterior segment, the procedure can be carried out through the closed eyelid, and this poses few difficulties with a cooperative child or a quietened feeding infant. For further discussion the reader is referred to Storey (1988), Colman *et al.* (1977) and Ossoinig (1977).

5.9   Visual fields

Visual fields may be investigated in infants and babies using *kinetic perimetry* (Mohn & Van Hof-van Duin, 1986; Schwartz *et al.*, 1987). The technique requires the infant to be positioned on the mother's lap at a bowl perimeter, with the head gently restrained. The infant's fixation on the central target must be obtained and retained, and this can be facilitated by a second helper providing an auditory stimulus. A third assistant observes the infant's eyes as the perimetrist moves the stimulus from the periphery into the visual field. The infant will make an eye movement towards the stimulus as it enters the field. This technique is slow and laborious, and is not suitable in primary-care practice. However, for children between the ages of thirty months and five years, a modified form of kinetic perimetry may be employed in general practice, requiring no more equipment than a fixation target and a stimulus manipulated by the optometrist alone. This is termed *kinetic outline perimetry* (Barnard, 1989), and is a combination of *outline perimetry*, first described by Kestenbaum (1925), and the kinetic techniques discussed above.

5.9.1   Outline perimetry (Kestenbaum)

Kestenbaum noted that 'the visual field in the plane of the face corresponds with surprising exactness to the outline of the face when the eye is looking straight ahead'.

   Whereas in the 'confrontation' technique the field of the examiner serves as the control, in Kestenbaum's method it is the shape of the patient's face that serves this purpose.

Method

The examiner places a cover over one of the patient's eyes, and the patient fixates a target held by the practitioner at a distance of about 15 cm directly in front of the patient's open eye. A test stimulus is brought around the side of the patient's head in an arc, some 3–5 cm from the patient's head. The patient reports when he first notices the stimulus appearing in the field of vision. The test may be repeated in a number of different meridians, as in the 'confrontation test.' If the visual field is normal, the patient will report seeing the target appear as soon as it crosses the imaginary line drawn from the centre of the cornea to that part of the face around which the target is being moved. For example, on the nasal side the target will be seen as soon as it passes beyond the nose. Inferiorly, the limiting factor for the visual field is the cheek, and superiorly, the superior orbital bone and glabella. Comparison with the normal outline of the field enables an abnormal field to be recognized without difficulty. Because of the close working distance between the stimulus and the patient's eye, this technique is not suitable for assessing scotomatas within the visual field, but is most useful as a check on the normality of the peripheral extent of the visual field. Kestenbaum's technique can be usefully employed as a crude visual field screening test for patients over the age of six years.

5.9.2   Kinetic outline perimetry

Method

The practitioner asks the child to fixate on the practitioner's nose. This request needs to be repeated often, and the practitioner may even ask the child to touch his nose during the procedure. A miniature toy on the end of a wand is the ideal target, and the child is told that whilst he watches the practitioner's nose the toy is going to 'creep around the corner'. As in outline perimetry, the stimulus is moved in an arc about 3–5 cm from the patient's head, and the field is compared with the outline of the patient's face. The child is encouraged to tell the optometrist when the toy is first seen. However, it is unrealistic to expect a three- or four-year-old to respond solely verbally, and as the stimulus is moved into the field the child often makes a version movement to take up fixation. Such a response is shown in Figs 5.3 and 5.4. In Fig. 5.3 the child is shown fixating directly ahead, and in Fig. 5.4 he has made a version movement in the direction of the stimulus as soon as it entered his visual field.

  In addition to being useful for the thirty-month to five year age-group, this technique can be applied to other patient categories, including Down's syndrome children.

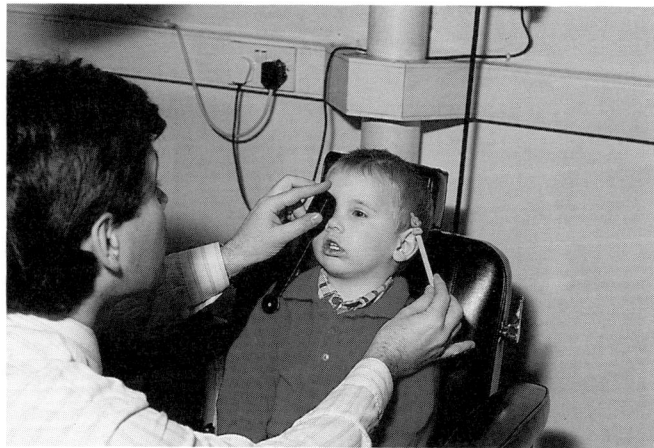

Fig. 5.3 Child fixing on practitioner's nose as the stimulus is moved in from the periphery.

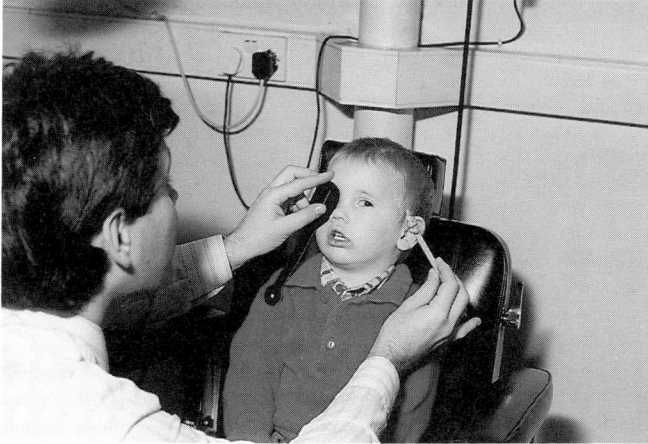

Fig. 5.4 As the stimulus enters the temporal visual field the child makes a kinetic response.

Static quantitative perimetry can be successfully carried out on bright co-operative five-year-olds and above. Dynamic perimetry can be employed with the slightly older child.

5.10 Tonometry

The ocular tensions of most infants and children can be readily measured using the Keeler Pulsair tonometer (Buscemi *et al.*, 1991; Evans & Wishart, 1992). This non-contact instrument has a number of advantages which make it suitable for pediatric practice; the instrument does not require a chin-rest, nor an anaesthetic, and the procedure is relatively comfortable. Pulsair measurements compare favourably with applanation tonometry in adults (Fisher *et al.*, 1988; Moseley *et al.*, 1989; Bricker *et al.*, 1990).

Whilst an average of four readings should ideally be taken, in practice with infants it is often only possible to obtain one reading before the young patient refuses to cooperate. With slightly older children, more than one reading can often be taken. In the case of an uncooperative or fidgety child, a useful ploy is to ask the child if he can see his favourite cartoon character hiding in the red fixation light, and to tell the child that if he does not keep very still the instrument will 'tickle' him. More than one reading can often be obtained using this trickery. However, a consolatory reward such as a badge or sticker should be given to the child to avoid the disappointment of not seeing the cartoon character.

Tonometry should be carried out whenever there are suspicious signs, symptoms or a family history that causes concern.

5.11 Assessment of accommodation

5.11.1 Amplitudes of accommodation

These should be assessed for two reasons. First, as part of the routine investigation of the health of the eye in general, and of the function of the oculomotor (3rd cranial) nerve in particular; and second, as part of the refractive/orthoptic investigation.

A reduced monocular amplitude of accommodation may be indicative of pathology, and alerts the clinician to carry out further diagnostic procedures. Amblyopia will also produce reduced amplitudes.

Push-up method

Amplitudes may be may be assessed on any child capable of providing a subjective response by using a fine target (N5 equivalent) on a push-up rule, such as the RAF rule. The child should be wearing the distance refractive findings. The practitioner should carefully explain that they want the patient to report when the target becomes blurred. The word 'blurred' can be explained by saying 'blurred means not clear'. The target should then be moved out slowly until it just becomes clear again. At this point, the amplitude is recorded in dioptres. This technique usually provides satisfactory results from the age of 5 years. For younger children a useful assessment can be made using a 'jump accommodation' technique. Here the practitioner takes a fixation stick on which there is very small line drawing, for example a teddy bear, the size of an N5 letter. This is suddenly placed about 8 cm from the patient's eye for a few seconds, and the child is asked to report what picture they have seen. A different picture should be used for each eye. Although crude, this technique works very well, and can provide an assessment of the amplitudes of accommodation in children as young as two years of age.

Increasing negative power to blur

An alternative method of measuring monocular amplitudes is to *increase negative power* whilst the patient views a near target (N5) until blurring is reported. An allowance must be made for the viewing distance and the patient should be wearing the distance refractive findings. When this technique is carried out binocularly a lower 'amplitude' is obtained as it gives a measure of positive relative accommodation. The procedure is most easily carried out using a phoropter with the near target placed at 40 cm.

Objective assessment

Objective investigations of both amplitudes and lag of accommodation can be carried out using dynamic retinoscopy.

5.11.2 Accommodative facility

This can be measured using a binocular lens flipper (Cooper, 1987). The flipper contains two pairs of lenses; a typical flipper would contain one pair of $+1.50\,D$ spherical lenses and one pair of $-1.50\,D$ spherical lenses. The patient is asked to focus on fine print at a distance of either 35 cm or at the Harmon distance. The pair of minus lenses is held in front of the patient's eyes, and the patient focuses on the print. As soon as the print is reported clear the flipper is twirled so that the patient is looking through the pair of positive lenses. Following this change, as soon as the print is reported clear again the procedure is repeated, and the number of cycles over a period of 60 seconds is recorded. Spherical lenses between $\pm1.00\,D$ spheres and $\pm3.00\,D$ spheres can be used in the flipper. Retinoscopy can be used during the procedure to verify the subjective responses (Eskridge, 1989). This technique is also usefully employed as a vision therapy exercise to develop accommodation.

5.12 Ocular motility

An assessment of ocular motility in infants of about three months and above is readily achieved by gently picking up and slowly rotating the baby, making no attempt to restrain the baby's head. The optometrist's face will be a strong stimulus to fixation, and the baby should rotate both head and eyes to keep fixation. This provides a useful assessment of horizontal gaze (Figs 5.5 and 5.6). Similarly, the baby can be tipped along the vertical plane, and will attempt to keep fixation. When tipped downwards the baby will respond by gazing upwards, and a little frown will appear above the eyebrows (Fig. 5.7).

At the age of about six to twelve months a baby will more readily follow stimuli such as a pen torch light (Fig. 5.8) or small toy, especially if the latter produces noises, although there will still be difficulties in restraining the patient's head during the procedure.

More sophisticated techniques for analysing ocular motility such as the Lees or Hess screens can be carried out from the age of about five years, and the test can take the form of a 'space invaders game' (Stidwill, 1990).

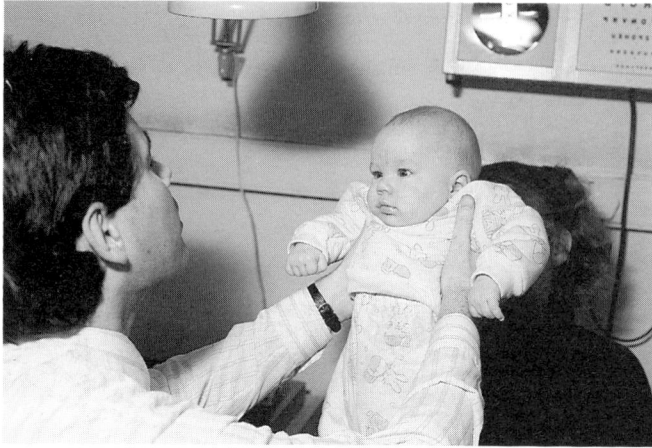

Fig. 5.5   Infant looking in the primary position at the practitioner's face.

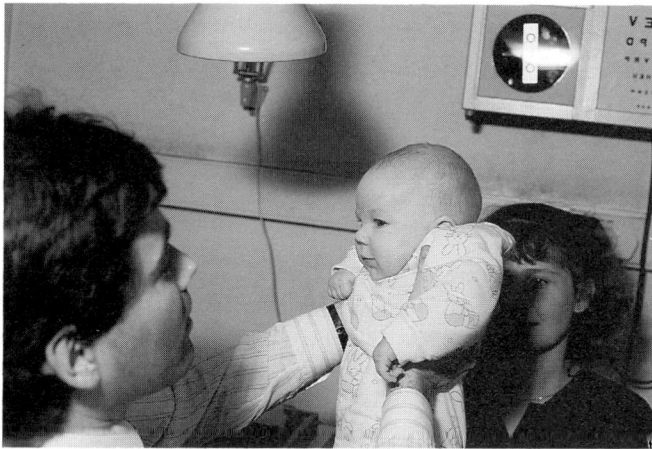

Fig. 5.6   The infant is slowly rotated to produce left horizontal gaze.

Bielshovsky's head tilt test

This may be used to differentiate a superior rectus palsy in one eye from a palsy of the superior oblique of the other eye. A patient with a right superior oblique palsy will normally have an habitual head tilt towards his left shoulder. In this test, if the head is tilted to the right and the eye moves upwards then this is indicative of a superior oblique palsy (see Mallett, 1988).

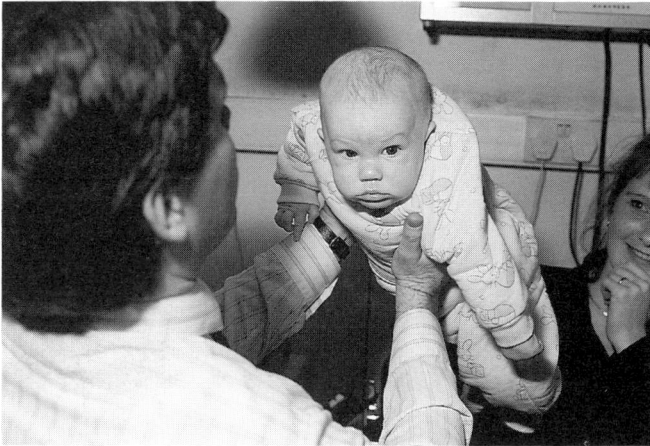

Fig. 5.7 Rotating an infant to produce vertical gaze.

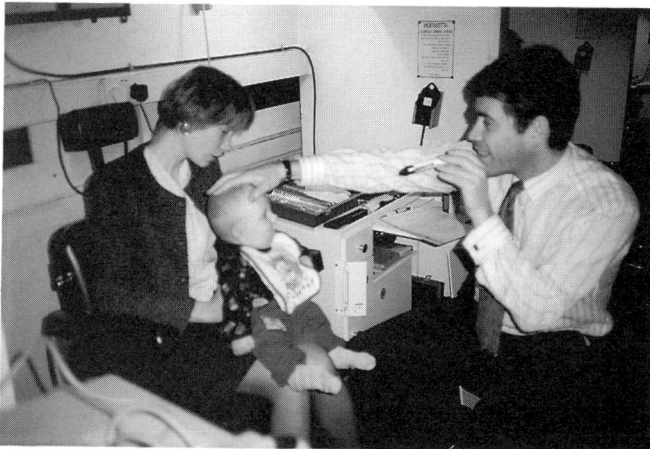

Fig. 5.8 Ocular motility using a pen torch.

5.13 Eye position and oculomotor balance

To assess the eye positions of an infant a two-step procedure may be used. First, the angle lambda can be measured (which, under clinical circumstances, is sometimes incorrectly termed angle kappa (Mallett, 1988)), and second the Hirschberg test may be performed.

5.13.1 Angle lambda

To measure angle lambda, defined as the angle between the line of sight and the pupillary axis, the first step is to occlude one of the patient's eyes. Direct the light from a pen torch, positioned immediately below the practitioner's sighting eye, into the patient's fixating eye from a distance of 50 cm. The practitioner then estimates, or measures, the distance in millimetres between the corneal reflex and the centre of the patient's pupil. If the corneal reflex is situated exactly in the centre of the pupil then angle lambda is zero. A nasally displaced reflex is denoted as a positive angle lambda, and a temporally displaced reflex as negative. Thus a 1 mm nasal displacement would be recorded as +1.0 angle lambda. This procedure is repeated for the other eye.

5.13.2 The Hirschberg test

Having estimated angle lambda for each eye, the Hirschberg test may be carried out by encouraging the patient to fixate binocularly the pen torch held just below the optometrist's sighting eye at a distance of 50 cm. The position of each corneal reflex is noted. They should be in the same position as when angle lambda was measured. If one of the reflexes is displaced with respect to the other and to its previous position, this suggests the presence of a squint. A 1 mm deviation is generally taken to be equivalent to approximately 22 Δ (Rosner & Rosner, 1990), though Eskridge *et al.* (1990) showed that for patients with corneal curvatures steeper than 46 D (=7.35 mm) and with deviations greater than about 30 Δ, then 1 mm = 27 Δ is more appropriate. This deviation can be estimated by the *Krimsky test*, in which prisms are interposed until the reflex of the deviating eye is positioned symmetrically with respect to the fellow eye (Krimsky, 1972). This technique will only detect relatively large angles of deviation, and is of limited value, but it can be of assistance in the presence of epicanthus.

5.13.3 The Bruckner test

The Bruckner test or 'transillumination test' (Bruckner, 1962) has been advocated as a useful technique to detect strabismus in young children. A bright light source is directed towards the patient's eyes from a distance of one metre. The practitioner compares the brightness of the right and left fundus reflexes. With an isometropic patient with both eyes aligned there will be no difference in brightness whereas if a squint is present the fixing eye may show a darker reflex than the deviating eye.

5.13.4   Cover test

The objective cover test is of great importance in investigating the oculomotor balance in children as subjective techniques cannot be relied upon. The cover test should be carried out at both distance and near using a fine target which should stimulate both fixation and accommodation. A spotlight should only be used in the case of infants or when the vision or visual acuity is less than 6/18 in either eye.

Conventional wisdom suggests covering each eye in turn for 2–3 seconds and assessing fixation and recovery movements or undertaking the 'alternate cover test' which tends to produce larger measurements of heterophoria as the slow fusional mechanism is broken down. However, in adult heterophoric subjects, Peli and McCormack (1983) found evidence that it may take up to eight seconds for the eye to reach full dissociation under the cover during a cover test.

It is probably important to cover the eye completely, to avoid any peripheral binocular lock which may prevent full dissociation, but this is not always possible with children and infants, particularly when using a thumb as the occluder.

The quality and speed of recovery of the occluded eye when the cover is removed may provide information of how well a heterophoria is compensated although there has been very little objective investigation carried out to confirm this relationship.

5.13.5   Assessment of associated (or uncompensated) heterophoria

The presence of associated heterophoria may be detected, and its size measured, on children from the age of about five years using a fixation disparity test. The method of choice is the Mallett unit (Mallett, 1964; 1983), which can be used for testing at both distance and near. Careful explanation of the task is required if the child is to respond adequately.

5.14   Recording eye movement

There are a number of systems available for recording and analysing eye movements. Infra-red limbal reflection systems are used by optometrists, particularly in the field of the visual assessment of children with learning difficulties, and can provide useful information concerning the version eye movements and tracking abilities of a patient. However, unless a head restraint and/or a dental bite is utilized to restrain head movements, the accuracy of the measurement of vergence eye movements can be limited.

Another use for eye movement recording is in the analysis of the characteristics of nystagmus. The technique may be used to determine the type of nystagmus, and to measure the amplitude, frequency and velocity of the various phases.

5.14.1   Fusional vergence

A fusional vergence response to the interposition of a base out prism in front of one eye will be found in the normal infant from between four-and-a-half and six months of age, and this test may be routinely carried out on infants and babies. Failure of one eye to move may indicate poor relative vergence or suppression. The measurement of fusional reserves is discussed in Chapter 8.

5.14.2   Stereopsis tests

The assessment of stereopsis is very important, because the presence of a reasonable stereoacuity suggests a good standard of binocularity and the absence of strabismus or amblyopia. Stereopsis can be present with deep harmonious abnormal retinal correspondence (HARC).

There are a variety of tests that are suitable for children. Some of the more commonly used tests are discussed below.

Lang test (Lang, 1988)

This is an excellent test for the gross screening of younger children, and some infants will even respond to the test. Infants responses are assessed with the practitioner observing if the infant preferentially fixates specific areas on the test card, or reaches out towards one of the targets.

The test is a combination of Julesz random dot stereograms and cylindrical gratings. The latter present disparate images to each eye which are fused by the patient with binocular vision to produce stereoscopic images. The images are either of a cat, car and star, or of an elephant, moon and van, and these represent stereoscopic disparities of between 1200″ and 550″ when the test is used at 40 cm.

These levels of stereopsis are gross, yet positive responses to the test probably rule out the presence of significant amblyopia, anisometropia in excess of 2 dioptres, suppression, squint, a central scotoma (such as that found in Stargardt's disease) and major deficits of accommodation and convergence (Lang, 1988). Stidwill (1990) suggests that conditions creating an intermittent squint are likely to cause a child to fail the test, even if the child eyes are not deviating during the test, and that such a failure is an indication for carrying out a cycloplegic refraction.

Titmus stereotest

The Titmus test (Fig. 5.9) utilizes a series of crossed polarized vectogram pairs, displaced to produce stereoscopic targets when viewed binocularly through polarized lenses (Levy & Glick, 1978). This test provides a variety of stereo patterns from the gross (3000″) fly, to 40″ on the circle test. A display of animals represents stereo thresholds of 400″, 200″ and 100″, and is useful for younger children. Older children usually respond to the nine sets of four circles. In this sequence one of the circles in each set is disparately imaged, producing stereo thresholds from 800–40″ when the test is shown at a distance of 40 cm. Children can be induced to respond to this test by encouraging them to 'push the button that sticks out'.

Simons & Reinecke (1974) reported that, with the exception of sets of circles 5 to 9, the Titmus test is not reliable for discriminating between normal patients and those with amblyopia or squint. Some stereo blind patients may receive monocular cues producing false positive results (von Noorden, 1990).

Random dot stereograms

Simons & Reinecke (1974) introduced the random dot E stereogram test used in conjunction with polarized lenses. The test was designed to screen at a distance of 50 cm, and to produce a pass or fail result, although performance could be graded by altering the working distance. The use of random dots removes the monocular cues encountered with the Titmus test.

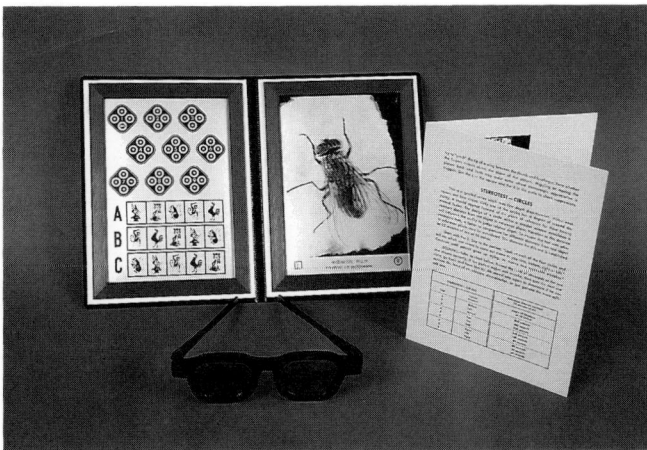

Fig. 5.9 Titmus stereotest.

The Randot test

Like the Titmus test, this employs polarized targets but also has four Julesz random dot patterns. The circles on this test give thresholds down to 20″.

TNO stereotest

This test utilizes random dot stereograms produced from superimposed red-green half images which are viewed through red-green goggles (Walraven, 1975). This test is graded to provide disparities ranging from 15–480″ of arc. This test compares favourably with the Titmus test (Okuda *et al.*, 1977).

Frisby test

This test provides 'real depth' by presenting random patterns printed on one side of three different transparent plates of varying thicknesses (Hinchcliffe, 1978). Each plate contains four squares, and within one of the squares some of the patterns are positioned on the opposite side of the plate. By using all three plates at different testing distances a range of disparities can be presented. At a 40 cm observation distance these three plates show a binocular disparity of approximately 340″, 170″ and 55″. With this test it is important to have the plate positioned in front of a white background positioned perpendicular to the patient's line of sight. Any movement of the patient's head will produce monocular cues which should be avoided. The test can be used from about the age of three years.

Super Stereoacuity Timed Tester (SSTT) (Super, 1991)

This stereo test contains three vectogram plates which may be viewed through either crossed or uncrossed polarized viewers from a distance of 40 cm. The SSTT allows the examiner to assess local, global, and combined local and global stereopsis, in front of, as well as behind, the plane of regard. In addition, Super (1991), found that the speed with which a person is able to process visual information accurately in a sequential order has been shown to be a developmental and learning related function. This test will be of interest to optometrists examining children with learning disorders.

Stereopsis at distance

The clinical measurement of stereopsis at distance may be obtained using vectographic stereotests in conjunction with a projector.

Table 5.5   A guide to examination procedures for different age groups of children in primary care optometric practice.

	Infants < 18 months	*18 months to 3 years*	*3 to 5 years*	*>5 years*
Vision	Preferential looking (forced choice or Visual Acuity Cards); Bock candy beads; Stycar graded-balls test, Cardiff Test; reponse to occlusion.	Visual acuity cards; Bock candy beads; Kay pictures; Cardiff; Sheridan-Gardiner; Sonksen-Silver.	Kay pictures; Cardiff; Sheridan-Gardiner; Cambridge crowding; Sonksen-Silver; Glasgow acuity cards.	Sheridan-Gardiner, Cambridge crowding, Sonksen-Silver; Glasgow acuity cards; Snellen.
External exam (incl. S/L)	✓	✓	✓	✓
Pupillary reflexes	✓	✓	✓	✓
Ophthalmoscopy	Attempt	Attempt	✓	✓
Ocular motility	*Binocular:* fixation on face, squeaky toy, pen torch.	*Binocular:* pen torch, toy.	*Binocular (& monocular):* pen torch.	*Binocular (& monocular):* pen torch, Hess or Lees screen.
Eye position/ oculomotor balance	Hirschberg/Krimsky/Bruckner; near cover test.	Hirschberg/Krimsky/Bruckner, near cover test, distance cover test sometimes possible.	Distance and near cover test.	Distance and near cover test, Maddox rod and wing, fixation disparity (Mallett).
Fusion	Gross convergence (light or toy); 5–10 Δ base out by six months.	Convergence (fine picture on fixation stick or toy); 10 Δ base out.	Convergence (fine picture on fixation stick or toy); >10 Δ base out.	Convergence (including subjective response).
Stereopsis	Lang	Lang, Titmus fly/animals, TNO butterfly.	Several stereo tests.	Several stereo tests.
Visual fields	–	Kinetic outline perimetry as young as 2½ years.	Kinetic outline perimetry.	Adult tests.
Colour vision	–	–	Ishihara (unlettered), Ishihara specific numbers, Fletcher-Hamblin.	As 3- to 5-year-olds plus other tests with increasing age.
Refraction	Retinoscopy (cycloplegia, Mohindra).	Retinoscopy (cycloplegia, Mohindra).	Distance fixation retinoscopy, cycloplegia.	Retinoscopy; attempt subjective.
Accommodation	Objective (retinoscopy).	Objective; picture recognition.	Objective; picture recognition; 'push-up subjective', accommodative facility; AC/A ratio.	Objective; picture recognition; 'push-up subjective'.

General comments
(1) Symptoms and history is required at all ages.
(2) Cycloplegic refraction is not always imperative. Indications for cycloplegia are listed in Chapter 7.
(3) Mydriasis using a cycloplegic drug is necessary for binocular indirect ophthalmoscopy.

5.14.3   The routine eye examination

For a routine eye examination the procedures that the practitioner may follow will vary depending on the age of the patient. Table 5.5 is a guide to the routines that a practitioner may wish to carry out at varying ages. The practitioner will obviously need to be flexible as infants and children develop at different rates.

5.15   The mentally and physically handicapped child

Apart from the visually impaired child who is discussed in Chapter 21, a busy pediatric practice is likely to attract children with other special needs including those with cerebral palsy, spina bifida, autism and attention deficit disorder. These conditions are discussed in Chapter 13, to which the reader may wish to refer, and will be further considered here along with the deaf child and Down's and Fragile X syndromes.

5.15.1   General considerations

It is important that the physically impaired child with, for example *cerebral palsy* or *spina bifida*, has easy access to the practice and consulting room. If the child is in a wheelchair this can be manoeuvred into the consulting room and then, if possible the patient can be physically assisted into the patient chair. Patients with cerebral palsy do tend to have difficulty in remaining sitting upright and keeping their limbs still (athetosis), and some surrounding support such as arm rests and cushions can be useful. If a child cannot be moved, or does not wish to be moved from the wheelchair the practitioner may adapt his examination technique to the situation.

When examining a *severely* mentally/physically impaired child the optometrist should welcome the assistance of the parent or helper (the latter sometimes known as the 'key worker'). The child may need to be supported and have his or her head restrained and the parent or helper may be the best person to do this. In such cases the optometrist needs to carry out any clinical tests as rapidly and efficiently as possible. Often, little more than retinoscopy and the Hirschberg test need be carried out, but the clinician may also wish to attempt other procedures including assessment of visual acuity (Gevene Hertz, 1988) depending on the individual characteristics of each patient. Assessment of ocular tensions with the Keeler Pulsair may be possible on some children.

Ametropia and squint is common amongst the multiply handicapped. Orel-Bixler *et al.* (1989) examined 59 patients with multiple neurological handicaps aged between 3–33 years, and found significant refractive error in 73% and strabismus in 71%. In 27 patients the refractive error was uncorrected and ranged from $-10\,D$ to $+20\,D$.

The practitioner will undoubtedly occasionally find a very large and previously undiagnosed refractive error and can be pleasantly surprised as to how the provision of such a spectacle prescription can make an apparent 'difference' to even the most severely neurologically impaired child.

5.15.2 Mental retardation

Mental retardation reportedly occurs in 3% of the population (Merck Manual, 1987) and *fragile X syndrome* is the most common form of familial retardation, being second only to Down's syndrome in prevalence among children with chromosomal abnormalities (Davies, 1989). It occurs in one in 1000 males and one in 2000 females. Maino *et al.* (1991) reviewed this condition and reported the ocular findings of 30 subjects with this genetic abnormality. They found that 30% of the subjects exhibited *strabismus* of whom 70% were esotropes; 59% of the eyes evaluated showed *hypermetropia* of $+1.00\,D$ or greater, 17% *myopia* of $-1.00\,D$ or greater, and 22% had at least $1.00\,D$ of *astigmatism*.

5.15.3 Down's syndrome

Langdon Down, in the mid-nineteenth century, was the first to describe the characteristics of this syndrome which is genetically determined and has an overall prevalence of one in 700 live births rising to one in 40 for mothers over the age of 40 years.

Down's syndrome people tend to be short in stature, have a small broad head and straight hair. They commonly have upward sloping eyes with epicanthal folds giving them an 'oriental' facial appearance. Other obvious signs may include an underdeveloped bridge to the nose, protruding tongue and short stubby hands. Heart disease occurs more frequently than in the normal population.

Connelly (1978) found that 60% of Down's syndrome people had an IQ of less than 50 and only 0.5% had an IQ of greater than 90.

Most Down's children go to special schools but the more intelligent, providing they have a good supportive home background, may benefit from attending normal schools.

Ocular anomalies

Epicanthus is very common in young Down's patients, persisting for longer than normal children but tending to disappear during puberty (Scully, 1973).

Blepharitis and *keratoconus* are more prevalent in Down's syndrome patients than in normal individuals (Shapiro & France, 1985).

The iris in Down's syndrome has been described as hypoplastic (Eissler & Longenecker, 1962) and up to 85% show a ring of yellow speckles concentric with the pupil on the iris. These are known as *Brushfield spots* and can occur in the normal population.

Cataract is commonly found in Down's syndrome patients with a reported prevalence of as high as 50% (Scully, 1973).

Williams *et al.* (1973) found a significant difference between the number and pattern of *retinal blood vessels* crossing the margin of the optic nerve head.

Strabismus appears to be common with a 34% prevalence being reported by Hiles *et al.* (1974) of which 81% were *esotropias*. Shapiro & France (1985) found 9% of their Down's patients to exhibit *nystagmus*.

The reported distribution of *refractive error* in the Down's population appears to vary considerably. Pesch *et al.* (1978) found 60% of their patients to be hypermetropic compared to 23% of the population found by Gaynon & Schimek (1977). Lyle *et al.* (1972) found the prevalence of myopia of 26% with 6% exhibiting myopia of 6 D or more. Both Pesch *et al.* (1978) and Shapiro & France (1985) found that 25% were astigmatic which perhaps should be expected considering the prevalence of keratoconus amongst Down's syndrome patients.

5.15.4   Optometric assessment of the Down's syndrome child

In view of the prevalence of ocular anomalies amongst the Down's population it is important that such patients have access to regular eye care. Generally, Down's children are very cooperative, pleasant and a delight to examine, though there are exceptions. The age, intelligence, behaviour and educational standard of the patient will determine which tests the practitioner will attempt and generally the optometrist will find himself using tests designed for children of a younger age. However, the optometrist should not be surprised if he finds that his patient is able to read and generally cooperate with a substantially normal routine.

When a refractive error requires correction, spectacles are normally tolerated very well and it may be possible to institute a course of orthoptic exercises or vision therapy with some Down's syndrome children. The use of cycloplegics in Down's Syndrome is contraindicated because of possible idiosyncratic cardio-accelerator response.

5.15.5   The optometric assessment of the autistic child

Autistic children are difficult to examine because of the child's inability to communicate or cooperate. These difficulties may vary considerably between patients depending on the severity of the handicap. The practitioner may need to follow the child around the room but a range of tests can often be carried out with some success. These include grating acuity using preferential looking, retinoscopy, Lang stereopsis test (by observing the patient's response), cover test during gaze episodes, pupillary reflexes, assessment of ocular motility by general observation or by attempting to elicit smooth pursuit movements, and an attempt at ophthalmoscopy. The practitioner should be ready to change to a different test and alternate between tests to take advantage of opportunities as they present themselves. The use of favourite toys or music may encourage some degree of concentration.

Scharre and Creedon (1992) assessed the visual function of 34 autistic children and found that refractive errors ranged from $-4.25\,D$ to $+3.25\,D$ using a near retinoscopy technique. Intermittent strabismus was reported present in 21% of the children. Rosenhall *et al.* (1988) investigated oculomotor function of 11 children who exhibited typical autistic features and found poor accuracy, reduced velocity of saccadic eye movements and difficulties in performing smooth pursuit movements in 55% of the children.

5.15.6 The optometric assessment of the child with attention deficit disorder (hyperactivity)

Hyperactive children are a challenge as the optometrist needs to work very efficiently while continually talking to and keeping the interest of the child. The practitioner may wish to try using two techniques in an attempt to complete a specific test without the child continually moving and fidgeting. The first is to make a 'bet' with the patient that he cannot keep his hands on his lap and keep absolutely still for thirty seconds. If the child remains still for half that time this may be long enough to complete a specific test. The second technique which works very well on some children entails the practitioner pretending to put some 'glue' on the back of the child's head and then gently 'sticking' the head back on the chair. Suggestion is a very powerful technique and can be very effective. It is important to inform the child that the 'glue' has been removed when the practitioner has finished his examination and this whole technique must be used light-heartedly.

5.15.7 The optometric assessment of the deaf child

For a deaf child vision is arguably even more important than in the child with normal hearing and yet visual impairment is more prevalent amongst the deaf.

The causes of deafness are varied and include congenital rubella, meningitis, various inherited conditions and syndromes, hypoxia at birth and Rh incompatibility of the parents.

Hearing loss is often associated with pigmentary retinopathy. Such syndromes include congenital rubella which may cause retinal pigment epithelial changes

(Boniuk & Zimmerman, 1967) and various subtypes of Usher's syndrome (an autosomal recessive condition), in which retinitis pigmentosa is a sign (Nicoll & House, 1988).

Woodruff (1986) examined 460 deaf children and reported that 55% had an ocular anomaly requiring professional care. Inherited deafness showed the fewest problems with respect to refractive errors. A high proportion of patients who were deaf due to Rh incompatibility were myopic, yet deafness due to meningitis or neonatal sepsis tended to be associated with hypermetropia. A wide variety of refractive error occurred amongst those with deafness caused by congenital rubella. Astigmatism greater than 1 D was common in patients whose cause of deafness was unknown or due to congenital rubella or meningitis.

The reported prevalence of strabismus amongst deaf patients varies from about 5% to 11% (Regenbogen & Godel, 1985; Alexander, 1973). Woodruff (1986) found the prevalence of strabismus and amblyopia in his population to be particularly high in children whose cause of deafness was Rh incompatibility, neonatal sepsis or congenital rubella.

The examination of a deaf child should not pose too many additional problems for the optometrist as the optometric investigation will rely on objective procedures. Obviously, a knowledge of sign language may be of great assistance in communicating with some profoundly deaf children though the patient may well be accompanied by a parent or teacher who will act as an interpreter. Many patients will have some residual hearing assisted by aids.

It is very important for the practitioner to gain a rapport with the child and this can be helped by using lots of smiles and eye contact particularly whilst the optometrist is speaking. For the older child, instructions can be written down and shown to the patient if necessary. The use of instruments, such as the phoropter, that remove the possibility of the child seeing the clinician's face and eyes should be avoided.

5.16   References

Alexander, J.C.C. (1973) 'Ocular abnormalities among congenitally deaf children'. *Canad J. Ophthalmol.*, 8, 428–33.

Barnard, N.A.S. (1989) 'Kinetic outline perimetry as a technique for examining the visual fields of young children'. *Ophthal. Physiol. Opt*, 9, 463–4.

Boniuk, M. and Zimmerman, L.E. (1967) 'Ocular pathology in the rubella syndrome'. *Arch. Ophthalmol.*, 77, 455–73.

Bruckner, R. (1962) 'Exacte strabismusdiagnostik bei $\frac{1}{2}$–3 jahrigen kindern mit einem ein-lached verlahren, dem "Durchleuchtunglest"'. *Ophthalmologica*, 144, 184–98.

Coleman, D.J., Lizzi, F.L. and Jack, R.I. (1977) *Ultrasonography of the Eye and Orbit.* Lea and Febiger, Philadelphia.

Connolly, J.A. (1978) 'Intelligence levels of Down's syndrome children. *Am. J. Ment. Defic.*, 83, No. 2, 193–6.

Cooper, J. (1987) 'Accommodative dysfunction', in *Diagnosis and management in vision care*. (J.F. Amos, ed.). Butterworth, London, 431–59.

Davies, K. (1989) *The Fragile X Syndrome*. Oxford University Press, Oxford.

Eissler, R. and Longenecker, L.P. (1962) 'The common eye findings in mongolism'. *Am. J. Ophthalmol.*, **54**, 398–406.

Elkins, L. (1991) 'Symptoms of children presenting for an eye examination'. Undergraduate thesis (unpublished), City University, London.

Eskridge, J.B. (1989) 'Clinical objective assessment of the accommodative response'. *J. Am. Optom. Assoc.*, **60**, No. 4, 272–5.

Eskridge, J.B., Perrigin, D.M. and Leach, N.E. (1990) 'The Hirschberg Test: Correlation with Corneal Radius and Axial Length'. *Optom. Vis. Sci.*, **67**, No. 4, 243–7.

Gaynon, M.W. and Schimek, R.A. (1977) 'Down's syndrome: a ten-year Group Study'. *Ann. Ophthal. (Chic)* **9**, 1493–7.

Gevene Hertz, B. (1988) 'Use of the acuity card method to test retarded children in special schools'. *Child: care, health and development*, **14**, 189–98.

Hiles, D.A., Hovme, S.H. and McFarlane, F. (1974) 'Down's syndrome and strabismus'. *Am. Orthoptic J.*, **24**, 63–8.

Hinchcliffe, H.A. (1978) 'Clinical evaluation of stereopsis'. *Brit. Orthopt J.*, **35**, 46–57.

Hoyt, C. and Lambert, S. (1990) 'Childhood glaucoma', in *Paediatric Ophthalmology*. (D. Taylor, ed.). Chapter 25, Blackwell Scientific Publications, Oxford.

Kasparek, G. (1981) 'Anforderungskriterien an Kinderbrillen'. *Deutsche Optikerzeitung*, **10**, 10–14.

Kestenbaum, A. (1925) 'Einfache Methode der Groben Gesichitsfeld-prufung'. *Wien Med. Wochenschnt.*, **46**, 2533.

Krimsky, E. (1972) *The corneal light reflex*. Thomas, Springfield, Illinois.

Levy, N.S. and Glick, E.B. (1974) 'Stereoscopic perception and Snellen visual acuity'. *Am. J. Ophthalmol.*, **78**, 722–4.

Lyle, W.H., Woodruff, M.E. and Zuccaro, V.S. (1972) 'A review of the literature on Down's syndrome and an optometric survey of 44 patients with the syndrome'. *Am. J. Optom. Arch. Am. Acad. Optom.*, **49**, No. 9, 715–27.

Maino, D.M., Wesson, M., Schlange D., Cibis, G. and Maino, J.H. (1991) 'Optometric findings in the Fragile X syndrome'. *Optom. Vis. Sci.*, **68**, No. 8, 634–40.

Mallett, R.F.J (1964) 'The investigation of heterophoria at near and a new fixation disparity technique'. *Optician*, **148**, 547–51.

Mallett, R.F.J. (1983) 'A new fixation disparity test and its applications'. *Optician*, **186**, 11–15.

Mallett, R.J. (1988) 'Techniques of investigation of binocular vision anomalies', Chapter 15, in *Optometry*. (Edwards & Llewellyn, eds). Butterworth, London.

Merck Manual of Diagnosis and Therapy (1987) 'Mental retardation', 1982, Merck & Co., Rahaway.

Mohn, G. and Von Hof-van Duin, J. (1986) 'Development of the binocular and monocular visual fields of human infants during the first year of life'. *Clin. Vision Sci.* **1**, 51–64.

Nicoll, A.M. and House, P. (1988) 'Ocular abnormalities in deaf children: a discussion of deafness and retinal pigment changes'. *Australian and New Zealand J. Ophthalmol.*, **16**, 205–208.

Okuda, F., Apt, L. and Wanter, B. (1977) 'Evaluation of the TNO random-dot stereogram test'. *Am. Orthopt. J.*, **27**, 124.

Orel-Bixler, D., Haegerstrom-Portnoy, G. and Hall, A. (1989) 'Visual assessment of the multiply handicapped patient'. *Optom Vis. Sci.*, **66**, No. 8, 530–6.

Ossoinig, K. (1977) 'Echography of the eye, orbit and periorbital region', in *Radiology of the Orbit*. (P.H. Arger, ed.). John Wiley, New York.

Peli, F. and McCormack, G. (1983) 'Dynamics of cover test eye movements'. *Am. J. Optom. and Phys. Opt.*, **60**, No. 8, 712–24.

Pesch, R.S., Nagy, D.K. and Caoen, B.W. (1978) 'A survey of the visual and developmental-perceptual abilities of the Down's syndrome child'. *Am. J. Optom. Assoc.*, **9**, 1031–7.

Pickwell, L.D. (1989) *Binocular Vision Anomalies*. Butterworth, London.

Regenbogen, L. and Godel, V. (1985) 'Ocular deficiencies in deaf children'. *J. Paed. Ophthalmol. and Strabismus.*, **22**, 231–3.

Rosenhall, U., Johansson, E. and Gillberg, C. (1988) 'Oculomotor findings in autistic children'. *J. Laryngol. Otol.*, **102**, 435–9.

Rosner, J. and Rosner, J. (1980) *Pediatric Optometry*. Butterworth, London.

Scharre, J.E. and Creedon, M.P. (1992) 'Assessment of visual function in autistic children'. *Optom. Vis. Sci.*, **69**, No. 6, 433–9.

Schwartz, T.L., Dobson, V., Sandstrom, D.J. and Van Hof-van Duin, J. (1987) 'Kinetic perimetry assessment of binocular visual field shape and size in young infants'. *Vis. Res.*, **27**, 2163–75.

Scully, C. (1973) 'Down's syndrome'. *Brit. J. Hosp. Med.*, **10**, 89 and 98.

Shapiro, M.B. and France, T.D. (1985) 'The ocular features of Down's syndrome'. *Am. J. Ophthalmol.*, **99**, 659–63.

Simons, K. and Reinecke, R.D. (1978) 'Amblyopia screening and stereopsis', in *Symposium on strabismus: Transactions of the New Orleans Academy of Ophthalmology*. C.V. Mosby, St Louis.

Stidwill, D. (1990) *Orthoptic Assessment and Management*. Blackwell Scientific Publications, Oxford.

Storey, J. (1988) 'Ultrasonography of the eye' (342–352), in *Optometry*. (K. Edwards & R. Llewellyn, eds). Butterworth, London.

Super, S. (1991) 'Stereopsis and its educational significance'. Doctoral Thesis, Rand Afrikaans University, Johannesburg, South Africa.

Taylor, D. (1990) 'Paediatric Ophthalmology' (702–707). Blackwell Scientific Publications, Oxford.

Walraven, J. (1975) 'Amblyopia screening with random-dot stereograms'. *Am. J. Ophthalmol.*, **80**, 893–900.

Wang, M. and Chryssanthou, G. (1988) 'Monocular eye closure in intermittent exotropia'. *Arch. Ophthalmol.*, **106**, 941–2.

Williams, E.J., McCormick, A.Q. and Tischler, B. (1973) 'Retinal vessels in Down's syndrome'. *Arch. Ophthalmol.*, **89**, 269–71.

Woodruff, M.E. (1986) 'Differential effects of various causes of deafness on the eyes, refractive errors, and vision of children'. *Am. J. Optom. and Physiol. Opt.*, **68**, 668–75.

CHAPTER 6

Clinical Measurement of Vision and Visual Acuity

David Edgar

Numerous clinical tests of children's visual acuity are available, which vary greatly in complexity. A selection of some of the more commonly used and innovative tests are described in this chapter. Most of these tests are suitable for children of a particular age-group, so they have been classified chronologically.

6.1 Infants of less than 18 months

6.1.1 Response to occluding one eye

Although a very gross and imprecise method, this is one of the few available for a very young infant, and may be attempted in infants from three months onwards. As the name suggests, the basis of the test is that the infant will react differently to monocular occlusion if there is a significant acuity difference between the two eyes. Each eye is occluded in turn, using either the parent's or practitioner's hand. If acuity is reduced significantly in one eye, the infant should object strenuously to occlusion of the dominant eye. However, if there is no acuity difference between the eyes, the infant should object equally whichever eye is occluded.

6.1.2 Bock candy beads ('hundreds and thousands')

These small, bright cake decorations can attract the interest of an infant, and may be used as a crude test of acuity for infants from 6 months onwards. At six months of age the infant should be interested in the decorations held in the palm of the mother's hand, and be equally interested when each eye is occluded in turn. Older infants may attempt to pick up the decorations. Again, the chief value of the test is not so much as an absolute measure of acuity, but as a means of checking for a gross difference between the eyes.

6.1.3   Forced-choice preferential looking (FPL)

Developed as a research tool, FPL requires sophisticated apparatus. In a typical set-up the infant is presented with two television monitors side by side. One monitor screen is uniform grey, and the other contains a pattern, usually a grating, of variable spatial frequency. Preferential looking is based on the phenomenon that, if he or she can discriminate between the two screens, an infant would prefer to look at the grating pattern, rather than the uniform field. In forced-choice preferential looking, the forced-choice is made by a trained observer who, without knowing on which screen the pattern is presented, has to make a decision about which screen the infant prefers to look at, based on observation of the infant's eye movements and general behaviour (Teller, 1979).

Three adults are required to conduct this test; the observer, someone to hold the infant (often a parent), and a scorer who monitors the observer's responses and directs the operation of the procedure. To ensure the results are statistically valid, a rather time-consuming method is adopted for determining acuity. Though useful for research, the time-consuming nature of this test, and the fact that it requires three adults and bulky, expensive equipment make it unsuitable for the optometrists' consulting room. Nevertheless, much of our current knowledge of the development of the visual system during the first 18 months of life has been obtained from studies using FPL. By simplifying the apparatus and speeding up the procedure, it has been possible to design tests, based on the same principle, which are suitable for the clinical environment.

6.1.4   Visual acuity cards

Although based on FPL, the acuity card procedure requires the presence of only two adults, one to hold the infant, while the other acts as examiner. Monitors are replaced by rectangular cards, used to present the grating on a grey background (Fig. 6.1). By rotating the card through 180 degrees, the examiner can present the grating on either the right or left of the card. Each card has a centrally positioned peephole, through which the examiner observes the infant. By combining the roles of observer and scorer into that of the examiner, some of the scientific rigour of FPL is lost, because the examiner usually selects which spatial frequencies to present to the infant, and may even know on which side of the card the grating is situated. However, it is a much more practicable and speedier test.

Two sets of cards are in widespread use, the Teller acuity cards and the Keeler acuity cards. The Teller cards have a high-contrast, black and white square grating patch, and the remainder of the card is a uniform grey, with a luminance equal to the mean luminance of the grating. One disadvantage of this arrangement is that the infant may be aware of an 'apparent edge' where the grating patch is delineated from the grey background (Robinson *et al.*, 1988). In cases where the infant is unable to resolve the grating, they may still prefer the grating side of the chart because they are aware of the edge, leading to an overestimate of acuity.

In the Keeler acuity cards the grating patch is circular, with a fine white border (see Fig. 6.1). A similar white border is placed symmetrically on the other half of the card, with the interior of the border the same uniform grey as the remainder of the background. The circular borders are an attempt to mask the visible edge apparent on the Teller cards. Two sets of cards are available, an infant assessment set of eight cards, and a children's additional set containing a further ten cards. With the additional set, the use of the cards can be extended beyond the first year of life, and they provide greater sensitivity when testing spatial frequencies below 12.5 c/deg. The test is designed for a working distance of 38 cm. A separate, free-standing puppet screen, similar to that used for a Punch and Judy show, can be purchased to reduce distractions. An aperture is cut in the centre of the screen, through which the cards can be presented. Bishop (1991), reports that the screen, which is a bulky and expensive item, does not seem to be essential.

The success of any test based on the preferential looking principle depends on the infant having complete freedom to move their eyes and head when the cards are presented. Any restrictions on movement will make the interpretation of the infant's responses more difficult. If occlusion is achieved by means of the parent's hand it is possible that the hand or arm may restrict the infant's range of movement. Such restrictions can be avoided if Opticlude eye patches are used for occlusion.

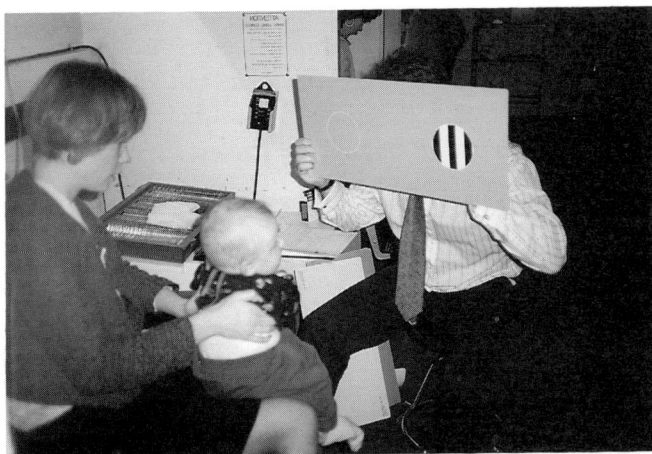

Fig. 6.1 The Keeler acuity card.

Many protocols have been proposed for use in the measurement of acuity with the Teller and Keeler acuity cards. One of the most widely used procedures is that recommended with the Teller cards, in which the examiner begins with a coarse grating patch (below the infant's expected acuity), in order to establish their behaviour with a target they can resolve. Further cards of increasing spatial frequency are presented, and the infant's looking responses are observed. The examiner should be unaware of the location of the grating patch, until after making his judgement based on the infant's looking responses.

The procedure is as follows: each card is presented twice; only if two consecutive correct judgements are made does the examiner present the next card of increasing spatial frequency. Once an incorrect judgement is made, the next larger grating card is presented. If correctly identified, this spatial frequency is taken as the acuity limit; if incorrect, it is assumed that the infant has lost interest in the test, and this spatial frequency is still taken to be the acuity limit, although the confidence level of the measurement is reduced. A procedure of this type enables acuity to be measured in approximately three minutes for each eye.

One alternative to this approach is the 'informed procedure', in which the examiner is aware of the spatial frequency and the location of the patch. The examiner is free to present the cards in any order, and to repeat cards as desired.

Acuity cards have proved effective in a variety of clinical settings (Chandna *et al.*, 1988; Mohn *et al.*, 1988), including vision screening of preschool children. Infants aged from a few weeks up to six months are the ideal patients to test using acuity cards. They are relatively passive, yet find the test interesting. Toddlers older than 12 months tend to get bored with this type of test, preferring something more interactive, and it may be difficult to keep their attention for the duration of the test (Atkinson & Braddick, 1982). Nevertheless, results can be obtained from infants of up to age three years. Lewis *et al.* (1993) found evidence to suggest that examiner bias can influence results, although McDonald *et al.* (1986) found no significant bias effects in their study.

Acuity cards are expensive to produce, and their high cost is a significant barrier to their routine use in optometric practice. Nevertheless, they enable acuity to be assessed quickly and with reasonable accuracy in an age group that are difficult to assess by any other means.

6.1.5 Stycar graded-balls vision test

A set of white polystyrene balls is used in this test, with sizes ranging from 3–61 mm in diameter. The spheres are rolled across a black cloth strip in front of the infant at a distance of 3 m, and the infant's responses observed. If the ball is seen, the infant should follow it with his eyes, and infants of crawling age may even attempt to pursue it. One weakness of this test is that it does not separate the infant's ability to detect motion from the infant's ability to resolve the sphere. To overcome this objection a static version of the test is available, in which the sphere remains stationary within the patient's field of view (Sheridan, 1973).

6.1.6 The Cardiff test

A preferential looking approach is combined with vanishing optotypes to produce this test, which is suitable for toddlers from 12 months of age up to $3\frac{1}{2}$ years, and for older children with either poor communication skills or delayed development (Adoh *et al.*, 1992). A single picture of a familiar object – such as a fish, a house, or a dog – is positioned either at the top or bottom of a rectangular card with a uniform grey background (Fig. 6.2). Each picture is composed of alternating black and white bands, with the width of the black band being one half of that of the white. Mean background luminance is equal to the average luminance of the black and white bands. Eleven spatial frequencies, equivalent to acuities from 6/6 to 6/60, can be tested by using cards with pictures made up

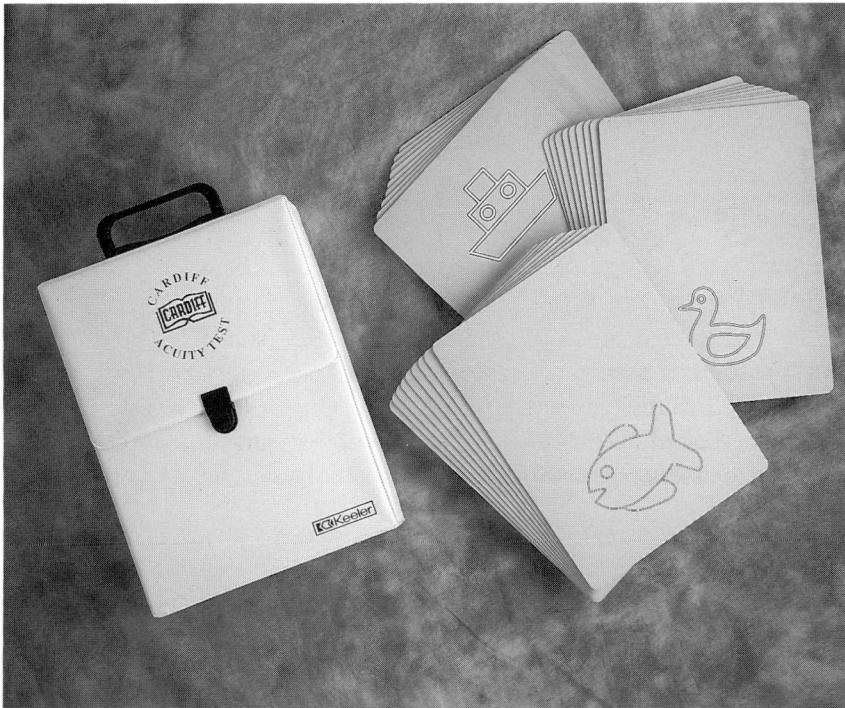

Fig. 6.2 The Cardiff test.

of lines of different band widths. Acuities progress in regular steps of 0.1 log units. Three cards are provided at each spatial frequency, giving a total of 33 cards. There is no peephole in the centre of each card, the designers regarding it as unnecessary and an additional distraction to the infant.

The procedure for the test, which is carried out at 1 metre from the subject, is as follows: beginning with the largest pictures, equivalent to 6/60, the examiner presents the first of two cards and observes the eye movements. Based on these movements he decides whether the picture is top or bottom, making a mental note of this position. The second card at that acuity level is presented, and the examiner again judges whether the picture is at the top or bottom of the card. The examiner then checks the cards to see if both estimations were correct. If they were correct the next set of cards is presented, and so on. If a wrong estimate of picture position is made, the examiner switches to the previous set of cards, and presents all three of them, and the end-point is reached when two of three cards are consistently seen correctly. By including three cards at each acuity level the order of presentation of the pictures can be varied, i.e. one top, one bottom; or two top; or two bottom. Compared with visual acuity cards, where only one card is provided at each acuity level, this helps to reduce the possibility of guessing by the child, and of bias by the examiner.

Preliminary studies show the Cardiff test to record acuities comparable with the Teller acuity card, but with considerably less variation between individuals. The Cardiff test is quicker to administer, and is well received by toddlers, who regard it as a game. Older children can point at or name the objects, giving information to support that obtained from observation of eye movements.

6.2   Children of 18 months to three years old

The following tests are also applicable to children of between 18 months and three years of age:

- visual acuity cards;
- the Cardiff test.

The visual acuity card test is covered above (see Section 6.1.4) as is the Cardiff test (Section 6.1.6).

6.2.1   Kay picture test

In this recognition test, pictures of familiar objects are presented singly to the child, who has to identify the object (Fig. 6.3). Pictures of various sizes are available to test a range of acuities at distances of up to 6 m, and the pictures

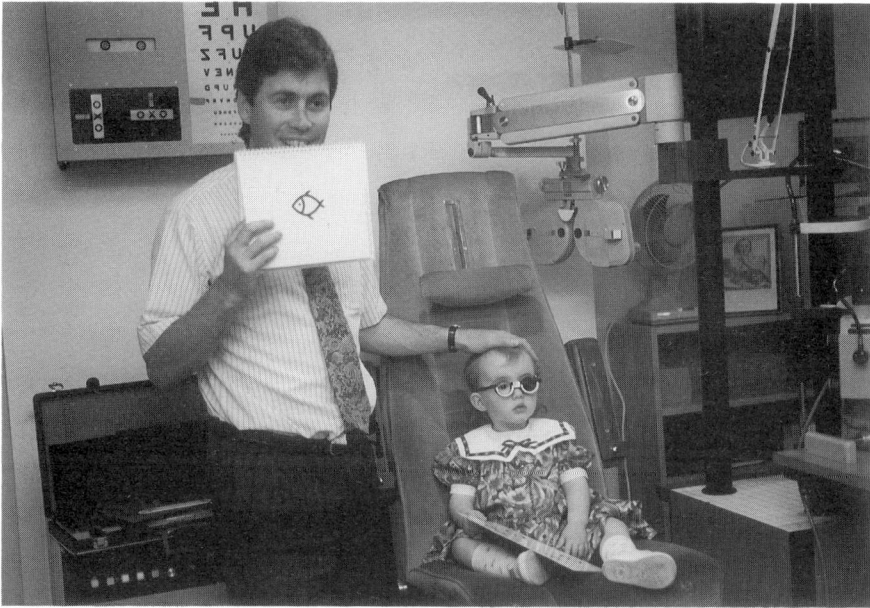

Fig. 6.3 The Kay picture test.

have been designed to conform to Snellen principles. Such tests can be criticized for having cultural limitations which may impair the test's validity. Also, they offer only a limited range of potential answers, and alert children quickly learn which objects are possible. Nevertheless, the test can be very useful with the 'terrible twos', and it is sensitive enough in practice to allow comparisons between the eyes to detect amblyopia.

6.2.2   Sheridan-Gardiner test

Seven Snellen letters are used in this matching test. They are presented at a distance of three or six metres. The mother, or child if old enough, holds a key card on which all seven letters are printed, and the child has to match the letter shown by the optometrist with one on the card (Fig. 6.4). By using letters that are identical when reversed, A, H, O, T, U, V, and X, the test can be used with or without a mirror. However, with young children it may be advisable to avoid the use of a mirror, because they can confuse children. This test is widely used in clinical practice, being cheap, portable, and simple to perform. It can be tried with children from about $2\frac{1}{2}$ years of age. One disadvantage of the test is that it only measures single letter or 'angular' acuity, which can lead to an overestimate of acuity (Fern *et al.*, 1986).

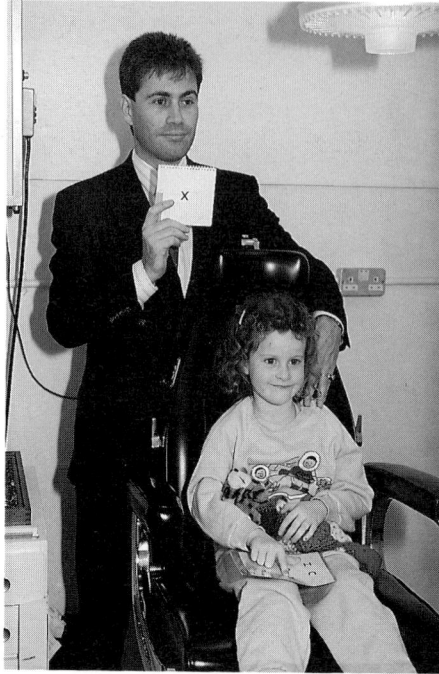

Fig. 6.4 The Sheridan-Gardiner test.

6.2.3   Sonksen-Silver acuity system

Using six of the seven letters in the Sheridan-Gardiner selection, the distance acuity test presents single lines of letters using two flipover booklets. The child views a key card on which all six letters are printed, and has to match the letter selected by the optometrist with one on the card (Fig. 6.5). Testing distances of 6 m or 3 m can be used as required, and the test is within the capabilities of above average $2\frac{1}{2}$ year olds. The system is packaged in two forms, the screening pack and the more comprehensive diagnostic pack. The screening pack contains the standard booklet with one line of letters on each page, and five letters on each line. Six letter sizes are available, namely 18, 12, 9, 6, 4.5, and 3 m. Two lines of letters are provided in the 6 m and 3 m sizes. Larger letter sizes of up to 60 m are provided in the second booklet, which is included together with the first in the more comprehensive diagnostic pack. A feature of the Sonksen-Silver test is the excellent test of near acuity, which is supplied in both packs, as is a pointer, used to select the letter to be matched when testing distance acuity. One objection raised to the use of a pointer is that it to some extent isolates the selected letter (Bishop, 1991).

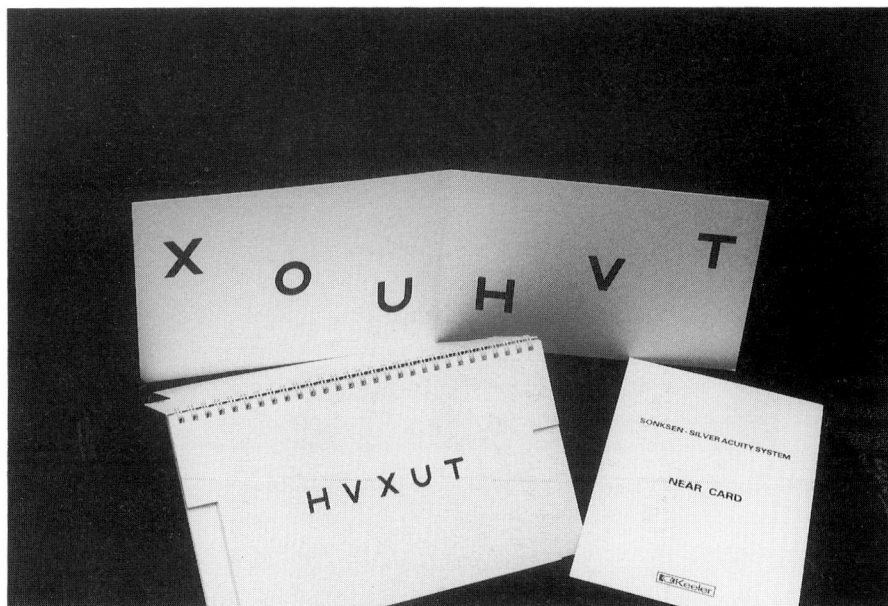

Fig. 6.5 The Sonksen–Silver test.

6.3 Children of three years to five years old

The following tests are suitable for the three- to five-year-old age-groups, as well as the 18-month to three-year-old group:

- the Kay picture test;
- the Sheridan-Gardiner test;
- the Sonksen-Silver acuity system.

These three tests are covered above, in Sections 6.2.1, 6.2.2 and 6.2.3 respectively.

6.3.1 Cambridge crowding cards

These cards provide a matching test, at a distance of 3 m, using two sets of cards. One set is designed to assess angular acuity using single letters, while the second tests 'crowded acuity' using a set of multiple or 'crowded' letters (Fig. 6.6). Each card in this set contains a central letter surrounded by four letters of the same size, and the child's task is to match the middle letter on the card with one from the key set. By making the five key letters moveable, they can be placed on a board in non-regular pattern which does not resemble the arrange-

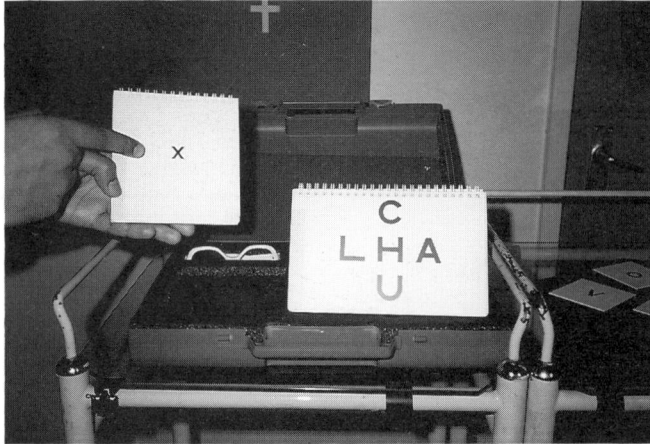

Fig. 6.6 The Cambridge crowding cards and single letter set.

ment on the crowded cards. It is stressed that pointing directly to the letters should be avoided, as this will introduce uncontrolled changes in the crowding effects. Both angular and crowded acuity should be tested on each child, and results can be compared with normal values which can be read from a simple table that comes with the test. A child who achieves normal acuities for single letters, but not for crowded acuity may have amblyopia (see Chapter 4).

6.3.2 Glasgow acuity cards

This matching test, suitable for three- to five-year-olds, uses lines of letters presented from a flip-book. The mother, or child if old enough, holds a key card on which all six letters used in the test are printed, and the child has to match each letter presented by the optometrist with one on the card (Fig. 6.7). Designed for use at 3 m, acuities from 3/19 to 3/1.5 (equivalent to 6/38 to 6/3) can be assessed. A regular progression of letter sizes is employed, in 0.1 log unit steps, as used in the Bailey-Lovie chart. Each line contains four letters to ensure a constant visual demand at each acuity level, allowing low levels of acuity to be measured with the same precision as higher acuity levels. Standardization for the crowding effect at each acuity level is controlled by using a crowding bar to surround the four letter array, the width of which is equal to the stroke width of a letter. To avoid children having to read too many letters, a screening set of three cards is provided which enables the practitioner to identify a starting point for the measurement of line acuity (McGraw & Winn, 1993). Reports of clinical investigations of this ingenious test are awaited.

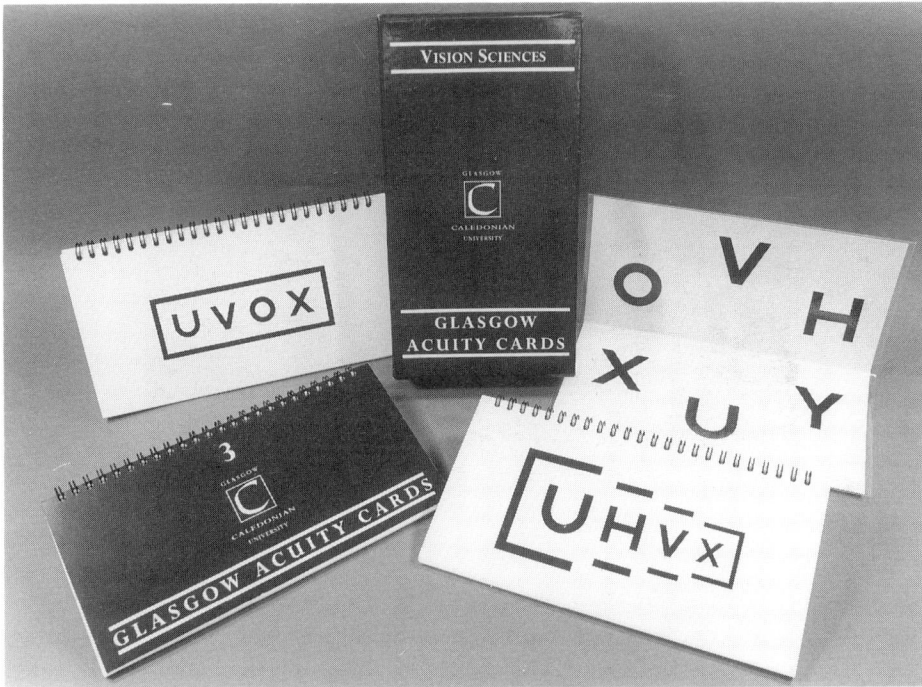

Fig. 6.7 The Glasgow acuity card test.

6.3.3 Stycar test

Snellen letters are used in this matching test, and are presented on a test chart of the conventional Snellen type. No line has more than three letters, and a key card is provided. When vision is tested in preschool screening by health visitors, it is likely they will use the Stycar test (Bishop, 1991).

6.4 Children of five years and older

Several of the tests appropriate for five-year-old and older children are also appropriate for younger children, and have been covered above:

- the Sheridan-Gardiner test (see Section 6.2.2);
- the Sonksen-Silver acuity system (see Section 6.2.3);
- the Cambridge crowding cards (see Section 6.3.1 above);
- the Glasgow acuity cards (see Section 6.3.2 above); and
- the Stycar test (see Section 6.3.3 above).

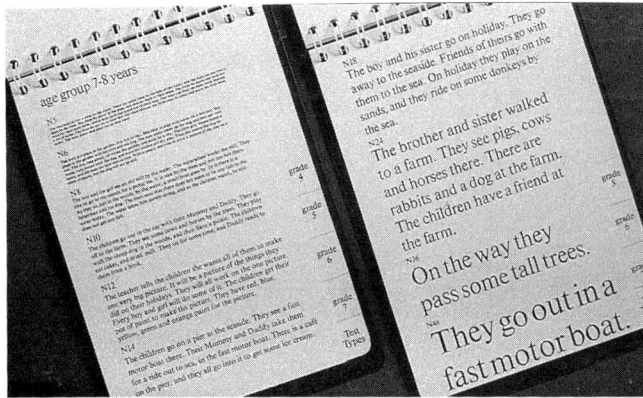

Fig. 6.8 Maclure test type.

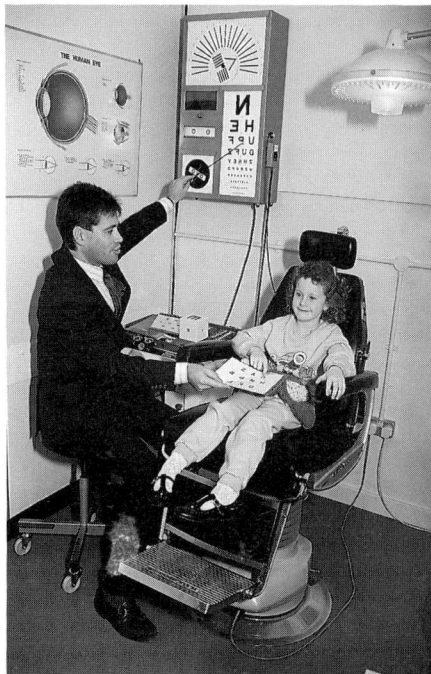

Fig. 6.9 The Snellen chart used with a key card.

6.4.1   Maclure test type

A test for near acuity which resembles the conventional near vision charts used with adults, and is used in a similar way. However, it is based upon the Ladybird Key words reading scheme, using school script, which is a simplified type without serifs (Fig. 6.8).

6.4.2   Snellen or LogMAR chart

By the age of about $6\frac{1}{2}$ years the average child should be able to cope with the standard Snellen or LogMAR chart without assistance. Bright, confident children may achieve the transfer to adult charts even earlier, especially with some assistance. This can take the form of the practitioner turning the test into a matching test by making up his own key card for use with his 6 m letter chart (Fig. 6.9). Further help can be given by pointing to a line of letters, or even pointing to individual letters, though this will cause some disturbance to the normal crowding characteristics of the chart, and could affect the acuity measurement.

6.5   References

Adoh, T.O., Woodhouse, J.M. and Oduwaiye, K.A. (1992) 'The Cardiff Test: A new visual acuity test for toddlers and children with intellectual impairment. A preliminary report'. *Optom. Vis. Sci.*, **69**, 427–32.

Atkinson, J. and Braddick, O. (1982) 'Assessment of visual acuity in infancy and early childhood'. *Acta. Ophthalmol. (Suppl.) (KBH)*, **157**, 18–26.

Bishop, A.M. (1991) '*Vision in childhood. Young children at visual risk*. The British College of Optometrists, London.

Chandna, A., Pearson, C.M. and Doran, R.M.L. (1988) 'Preferential looking in clinical practice: a years' experience'. *Eye*, **2**, 488–95.

Fern, K.D., Manny, R.E., Davis, J.R. and Gibson, R.R. (1986) 'Contour interaction in the pre-school child'. *Am. J. Optom. Physiol. Opt.*, **63**, 313–18.

Lewis, T.L., Reed, M.J., Maurer, D., Wyngaarden, P.A. and Brent, H.P. (1993) 'An evaluation of acuity card procedures'. *Clin. Vis. Sci.*, **8**, 591–602.

McDonald, M., Sebris, S.L., Mohn, G., Teller, D.Y. and Dobson, V. (1986) 'Monocular acuity in normal infants: the acuity card procedure'. *Am. J. Optom. Physiol. Opt.*, **63**, 127–34.

McGraw P.V. and Winn, B. (1993) 'Glasgow Acuity Cards: a new test for the measurement of letter acuity in children'. *Ophthal. Physiol. Opt.*, **13**, 400–405.

Mohn, G., van Hof-van Duin, J., Fetter, W.P.F., de Groot, L. and Hage, M. (1988) 'Acuity assessment of non-verbal infants and children: clinical experience with the acuity card procedure'. *Developmental Medicine and Child Neurology*, **30**, 232–44.

Robinson, J., Moseley, M.J. and Fielder, A.F. (1988) 'Grating acuity cards: spurious resolution and the "edge artifact"'. *Clin. Vis. Sci.*, **3**, 285–8.

Sheridan, M.D. (1973) 'The Stycar graded-balls vision test'. *Devel. Med. Child. Neurol.*, **15**, 423–32.
Teller, D.Y. (1979) 'The forced-choice preferential looking procedure: a psychophysical technique for use with human infants'. *Infant Behaviour and Development*, **2**, 135–53.

CHAPTER 7
Refraction
David Edgar & Simon Barnard

7.1   Introduction

The accurate refraction of infants and children is important not only for correcting ametropia – so that the child can develop or obtain optimum visual acuity – but also as the starting-point for the management of many anomalies of binocular vision.

7.2   Equipment

There is no doubt that the retinoscope is the most important instrument used for refracting infants and children. The techniques employed are discussed below.

A full-aperture trial set is preferred so that eye movements during, for example, the cover test can be observed. For younger children a small, light drop-cell trial frame is required. Pediatric trial cases with miniature lenses and trial frames are available (Fig. 7.1).

Some practitioners prefer to use the phoropter for refracting older children, and the phoropter can be used whenever a child is big enough to sit behind it, and still enough to remain in position. Most children enjoy 'looking through the space helmet', and the phoropter is also useful for measuring fusional reserves.

7.3   Retinoscopy

Retinoscopy is the most important technique used for obtaining the refractive error of a baby or child. Whilst children over the age of four can provide a subjective response the quality of this response cannot usually be relied upon until about the age of six years. The advantages of retinoscopy over other objective techniques are its speed, reliability and accuracy. Objective optometers, while quick and accurate in adults, are both expensive and generally poorly suited to young children and babies. Photorefractive techniques may have an important place in refractive screening, but are not likely to be found commonly in primary care optometric practice.

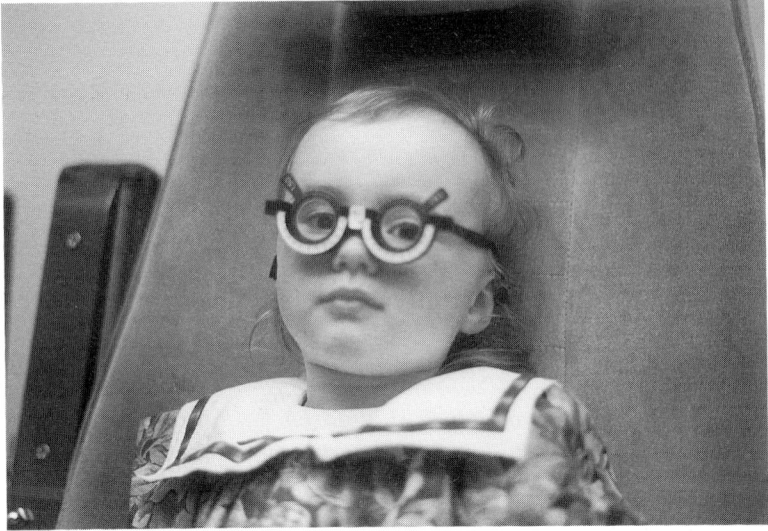

Fig. 7.1 A 20-month-old child wearing a pediatric trial frame secured with a velcro strap.

The only disadvantage of retinoscopy is that skill and therefore much practice is required to produce the rapid and accurate results required when refracting a child.

Retinoscopes may be either of spot or streak design. There has been much argument over the years as to the relative merits of the two designs, however, the authors believe that both can give precise results in expert hands. The authors prefer the *spot retinoscope* for pediatric work, because it lends itself both to dynamic and near retinoscopy, and can also be used for refining both power and axis if used in conjunction with a cross cylinder. The latter approach can prove very useful with children who cannot provide an adequate subjective refinement.

7.4   Static retinoscopy

Static retinoscopy is used to assess the refractive state of the eyes whilst efforts are made to relax the patient's accommodation. The optometrist generally uses a working distance of 67 cm in a dimmed or darkened room. With infants and babies, retinoscopy (and ophthalmoscopy), is usually more successful if the patient is sucking on a bottle, breast or dummy. In pediatric practice static retinoscopy is performed using one of the following methods:

Distance fixation retinoscopy

The patient is encouraged to fixate a target at least 6 m away. For a child it is important to present an interesting target such as a toy or a cartoon video. The latter is particularly useful as it can be remotely controlled. During the procedure the practitioner must keep up a steady banter to keep the child's attention on the target. For example, 'Can you see the teddy bear? Is he still there? What is he doing now?' and so on. The practitioner needs to work rapidly and efficiently. Distance fixation retinoscopy cannot easily be carried out on babies and infants because of the difficulty in attracting and maintaining attention on a distant fixation target. However, if a parent acts as a fixation target, a useful result can often be obtained using a binocular lens rack, with the practitioner estimating any cylinder power from the spherical lens powers required to achieve reversal in the principal meridians.

Under cycloplegia

Cycloplegic drugs need not be used on every patient in pediatric practice. However, there are some categories of patient who would benefit from the use of a cycloplegic (Taylor, 1988), including the following cases:

(1)   where a poor retinoscopy result is obtained due to, for example, poor fixation;
(2)   where a patient presents with a convergent squint;
(3)   where the child shows a significant or unstable esophoria;
(4)   where accommodation fluctuates during retinoscopy, or where a spasm is suspected;
(5)   where other anomalies of accommodation are present, these include insufficiencies such as reduced amplitudes or inertia of accommodation;
(6)   where a marked difference between retinoscopy and subjective findings is found in older children;
(7)   of newly diagnosed myopia, or of myopia apparently increasing more rapidly than expected;
(8)   where there is a poor response on the Lang (Stidwill, 1990) or other stereotest.

During a cycloplegic refraction the patient will be encouraged to, or will naturally fixate the retinoscope light itself, ensuring that the optometrist is refracting along the visual axis.

It is not essential for the child to wear a trial frame because, in the absence of significant accommodative ability, it is no longer necessary to fog the eye not under test. Some child patients refuse, or are most reluctant to wear a trial frame, but are more cooperative if trial lenses are hand held before their eyes. Wherever possible, results obtained from the principal meridians of the eye using hand-held spherical lenses should be confirmed with the full sphero/ cylindrical result placed in a trial frame.

Aberrations associated with the dilated pupil can confuse the interpretation of retinoscopy reflexes. The practitioner should concentrate on the centre of the pupil, and this can be achieved with the aid of an artificial pupil, consisting of a pinhole disc with an aperture of diameter between 3 mm and 4 mm, placed in a trial frame. Unfortunately, it is difficult to centre the aperture accurately, limiting the value of this approach.

It is conventional to record in red all results obtained under cycloplegia. This avoids possible confusion with the results of investigations performed before instillation of the cycloplegic or after the effects of the drug have worn off.

In the rare situation where a parent is concerned that the child may be allergic to the cycloplegic agent, referral to the general medical practitioner for a skin patch test is most useful.

During sleep

A baby can occasionally be refracted whilst asleep by gently lifting the lids. The practitioner must get as close to the visual axis as possible, and this can prove difficult when Bell's phenomenon occurs. Whilst the exact state of accommodation is unknown, at worst a useful comparison between the two eyes is obtained.

7.4.1   Near fixation retinoscopy

There are a number of methods of obtaining the 'static' refraction by *near fixation retinoscopy*. Many optometrists use the Barrett method, which is suitable for adults and children in whom accommodation is not too active, and is carried out as follows:

(1)   The trial frame (or refractor head) is adjusted and centred on (or before) the face and the room lights are dimmed as for static retinoscopy.

(2)   The retinoscopist places himself or herself along the midline of the patient's head, and at a convenient working distance (usually 67 cm). A lens of dioptric power equivalent to the working distance may be placed before each eye, according to the practitioner's preference.

(3)   If the patient has no manifest ocular deviation, he or she views a target in the plane of the retinoscope and usually below the sighthole position, with both eyes. The target should not contain any fine detail that could stimulate accommodation. If he or she has a manifest deviation of greater

than a few prism dioptres, the need to work on axis may require occlusion of the fixing eye when performing retinoscopy on the squinting eye.

(4) The eye not under examination should be fogged, as in conventional retinoscopy. When performing retinoscopy on medium and high hyperopes it is wise to check from time to time, as increasing positive power is added to the eye under test, that fogging is maintained.

(5) Reversal is obtained for both eyes.

(6) The patient is then directed to observe a distance target, and the retinoscopist checks whether an adjustment of the spherical element of the correction is required to maintain reversal. The retinoscopist should be careful to position himself or herself on the visual axis of the eye being measured – observation of the corneal reflex with respect to the pupil will help with this. It is usually sufficient to check the spherical element in one eye only, and to make equal changes to the spheres before both eyes to maintain reversal.

(7) An adjustment for the working distance is made to the spherical element to obtain a 'static refraction'.

One advantage associated with the use of the Barrett method in children is that they often find it easier to maintain fixation at the retinoscopy working distance than at 6 m. Also, fixation in the plane of the retinoscope guarantees that retinosocopy is performed along the visual axis in a non-squinting child. Off-axis errors can occur with distance fixation retinoscopy, and these are more serious in children in whom there is unlikely to be any subjective refinement of the cylinder. One disadvantage of this technique, when used with children, is that fixation at the working distance may induce significant accommodation, which may not always fully relax when fixation is switched to 6 m for final sphere checking.

7.4.2 The Mohindra technique

This useful modification to the near fixation technique, first described by Mohindra (1975), may be used to refract children of all ages, but is most useful as a routine method for examining babies and infants.

Method

(1) The infant is placed on the mother's lap, facing the practitioner.

(2) The consulting room is made completely *dark*.

(3) If possible, one of the patient's eyes is occluded, preferably by the parent.

(4) Retinoscopy is then carried out rapidly at a working distance of 50 cm,

with the optometrist encouraging the baby to fixate the *retinoscope light*, both naturally by its very movement, and also by continually whistling, clucking or calling to the baby. Reversal is achieved using a lens rack or trial case lenses. Mohindra advocates the use of monocular lens racks for infant patients. Lens racks containing spherical lenses allow the rapid examination of the principal meridians of the eye, thus avoiding the use of cylindrical lenses.

(5) Add −1.25 DS to the result obtained, rather than the −2.00 DS required by the 50 cm working distance. Owens *et al.* (1980) suggest that this 0.75 D discrepancy is the result of a form of inadequate stimulus myopia caused by the absence of any visual detail in the darkened consulting room.

High correlations have been reported between results obtained with this technique and (a) subjective refraction in young adults (Mohindra, 1977); and (b) cycloplegic refraction in children aged five to seven years (Mohindra & Molinari, 1979). However, Maino *et al.* (1984) found little agreement between the Mohindra technique and cycloplegic retinoscopy in a large sample of children aged between 18 and 48 months. Rosner & Rosner (1990) suggest that the Mohindra technique, while reasonably accurate for non-hypermetropic patients, performs poorly for young hypermetropes.

7.5   Dynamic retinoscopy

Unlike static retinoscopy, the aim of dynamic retinoscopy is to evaluate the accommodative state of the eye when viewing targets at near or intermediate distances. Dynamic retinoscopy is a most useful technique in pediatric practice (see Chapter 9), and the description that follows should serve as a brief introduction to the technique.

A young patient with full normal accommodation, wearing their distance correction, *critically* fixates a fine target placed at their reading or working distance. If retinoscopy is undertaken with the retinoscope placed close to, and in the same plane as the target, a with movement is observed in the patient's pupil. This is termed the *objective* (or *dynamic*) *lag*. It may be measured in terms of dioptric value by moving the retinoscope away from the subject (whilst maintaining the target at the original distance) until reversal is obtained. The objective lag in normal, young emmetropic eyes may vary between +0.25 D and +1.00 D with a mean of approximately +0.50 D. For example, in a typical case in which the fixation target is placed at 33 cm from the patient's eyes, reversal is obtained with the retinoscope at 40 cm, a distance equivalent in dioptric terms to +0.50 D (+3.00 D −2.50 D).

There are a number of explanations to account for this objective lag. At least part of it is likely to be due to a true lag of accommodation or laxity of focusing.

The *low neutral point* is equivalent to the objective lag but measured in a different fashion. If pairs of lenses of *rapidly escalating*, equal positive power are placed before the patient's eyes whilst he fixates *fine detail* in the plane of the retinoscope, a point is quickly reached at which the retinoscopist observes reversal. If the patient is emmetropic or wearing his distance correction, then the amount of positive power added to reach this point is called the *low neutral*. As speed is of the essence a binocular lens rack is very useful.

If, following the low neutral being reached, the retinoscopist continues binocularly to increase the positive spherical power before the patient's eyes, reversal is maintained up to a point. Beyond this point the addition of a further pair of +0.25 D spheres gives an against movement. The strongest reversing lens is known as the *high neutral*. If the patient is maintaining binocular fixation, then the difference between the low and high neutrals is likely to represent the true flexibility between accommodation and convergence, and is probably a true measure of *negative relative accommodation*.

For further information, the reader is directed to Taylor (1988), who presents a table (after Swann, 1939), showing the differential diagnoses afforded by dynamic retinoscopy.

7.6 MEM retinoscopy

A variation of dynamic retinoscopy is the *monocular estimation method* (MEM), which was developed by Haynes (1960). In this variation the fixation distance is equal to the distance from the child's elbow to his knuckle (*Harmon distance*). The practitioner *estimates* the power of the low neutral, and quickly and briefly inserts a lens equal to this power before one eye to assess the accuracy of the estimate. The aim of this technique is to determine the low neutral without disrupting the accommodative state.

7.7 Prescribing from the retinoscopic findings

The practitioner needs to take into account a number of factors when using static retinoscopy findings to prescribe spectacles. These include the effect of refractive intervention on oculomotor balance, and the strong body of evidence which suggests that, particularly in the young eye, the effective reflective layer for retinoscopy is situated some 0.18 mm anterior to the receptive layer of the retina. This may produce a retinoscopy result which contains up to approximately 0.50 DS of pseudo-hypermetropia (Glickstein & Millodot, 1970). Such a discrepancy would usually be corrected during the subjective examination of an adult, but in the absence of reliable subjective responses in a child, allowance may have to be made when prescribing.

7.8   Subjective refraction

Generally, very little can be done in the way of a meaningful subjective refraction on a child until the age of about five or six years. When a subjective routine is attempted on children of this age, it must be kept as simple as possible, with careful explanations that avoid complex terminology. Children respond well to encouragement and praise, but are quick to detect, and react negatively to, impatience or annoyance on the part of the practitioner. A pointer is an invaluable tool when attempting a subjective test using a Snellen or LogMAR chart. It can be used to direct the child's attention to a particular line of letters, or to individual letters on a line.

A rough subjective check of the sphere found by retinoscopy is often possible, although it is usually unwise to place much reliance on a child's judgement of clarity, because children are prone to guesswork and to suggestion. Instead the optometrist, having established the smallest letters that can be read, can ask the child to read this line again following the addition of positive power. This process can be repeated until a reduction in acuity occurs.

When attempting a subjective routine on a child many practitioners adopt what is known as a 'bracketing' technique, in which large dioptric intervals are used initially. This approach helps to ensure that the differences in clarity produced by lenses placed in front of the eye are appreciated by the child, and allows him to gain in confidence. With some children it may be best to begin with $\pm 1.00\,D$ spheres, or even stronger in certain circumstances. Once the refraction has been determined to the nearest dioptre, the practitioner can refine his result with $\pm 0.50\,D$ spheres, using $0.25\,D$ spheres last of all, and only if the child is capable of appreciating the changes in clarity produced by 0.25 steps. If the initial positive power is rejected, the addition of negative power can be tried. In this case the optometrist should direct the child to the next smallest line of letters, and only give extra negative power if it enables the child to read more letters.

The attention span of a child is so short that there is an onus on the optometrist to work quickly before cooperation is lost. With this in mind, a child who successfully reads two letters on a line without error or hesitation can be considered to have successfully resolved the line.

It is difficult to state with any certainty the age at which more complex tests can be attempted, since so much depends on the intelligence and cooperation of the child. Often the astigmatic correction can be checked with cross cylinders. A trial run can quickly establish if the child understands what is required. One approach is to rotate the cylinder away from the axis found by retinoscopy until there is no doubt as to which position of the cross cylinder should be preferred. Both sides of the cross cylinder are presented, and the patient's performance can be assessed. The bracketing technique can also be applied to the determination of astigmatism, with a ±0.50 cross cylinder used initially, with refinements to follow if the changes in clarity produced by a ±0.25 cross cylinder are appreciated by the patient.

7.9 The use of cycloplegic drugs

It is always desirable to perform a precycloplegic examination on a child patient, as it enables the optometrist to assess the eyes' refractive state under normal accommodative conditions. In the course of this examination the optometrist often identifies the patient as one for whom a cycloplegic refraction is required. Perhaps the most obvious candidate for a cycloplegic is the child with unstable accommodation during retinoscopy. This instability may simply be the sign of an uncooperative child, or it may be unstable accommodation in an otherwise cooperative child. In either case, an accurate determination of the refractive error is impossible without the use of a cycloplegic.

Another indicator for cyloplegia is a precycloplegic examination which suggests that there could be a latent component to the child's refractive error. A relatively common indication of a latent error in a hypermetrope is the presence of asthenopic symptoms, especially those associated with close work, in a patient with a low refractive error. Further signs of latent hypermetropia are an amplitude of accommodation that is low for the patient's age, and the presence of marked esophoria. If either or both of these signs is found in a previously uncorrected myope, the practitioner should be alert to the possibility of pseudo-myopia (spasm of accommodation), another indication for a cycloplegic refraction.

A third indication for cycloplegia is the presence of a squint, whether constant or intermittent. Accommodation plays a role in the development of many squints, and a cycloplegic refraction is required in a squinting child to identify the extent of any accommodative component.

It has been argued that a cycloplegic examination should always be performed on a child's first examination, because it allows the determination of a baseline refraction with the accommodation relaxed. However, while such information is always useful, its value must be weighed against the disadvantages of cycloplegic refraction. These include the risk of upsetting the child due to initial stinging produced on instillation of the cycloplegic, the possible inconvenience resulting from difficulty with close work, photophobia from the prolonged pupillary dilation, and the slight risk of adverse systemic reactions to the drug. One of the virtues of the precycloplegic examination is that it allows identification of those patients for whom a cycloplegic examination is unnecessary. A cooperative child with no symptoms, good visual acuities, stable accommodation that permits an accurate retinoscopy, and no binocular vision anomaly is unlikely to benefit from cycloplegia.

Prior to instillation of any ophthalmic drug the practitioner must take a careful history to ensure that he is aware of any previous drug allergies. Details of general health and other medications are also relevant. Many drugs taken for a wide range of systemic disorders have antimuscarinic effects, and the addition of a further antimuscarinic, in the form of a cycloplegic, increases the risk of adverse reactions. Patients with Down's syndrome have an increased susceptibility to antimuscarinic drugs.

7.9.1   Cyclopentolate

In current optometric practice, cyclopentolate is overwhelmingly the cycloplegic of choice. It is available in the UK in both 0.5% and 1% concentrations in either single-dose Minim form, or in a multidose container. The choice of concentration and number of instillations is influenced by the age of the child and the degree of pigmentation of the irides. As a rule, the 1% solution is used in children under 12 years of age, and 0.5% in those over 12. In a black or oriental child over the age of 12 years, 0.5% may be insufficient, and it may be wiser to use the 1% concentration. Similarly, a very fair-skinned child under the age of 12 may only require the 0.5% solution. Individual responses to drugs vary enormously, and it must be emphasized that only general guidelines can be given. It should be the practitioner's aim to use the lowest concentration possible, and the smallest number of drops to achieve the desired effect. Optometrists should not instil cyclopentolate in a child under three months of age, primarily owing to the increased risk of systemic reactions in neonates.

Atropine, the most potent cycloplegic available to optometrists, is even more strongly contra-indicated in children under the age of three months, when in addition to the risk of adverse reactions there is the danger of deprivation amblyopia as a result of the prolonged paralysis of accommodation. Faced with a neonate in whom it is essential to produce cycloplegia, cyclopentolate is the drug of choice, but ophthalmological advice should be sought prior to its use.

Cyclopentolate produces a rapid onset of cycloplegia. An excellent review of the findings of clinical trials investigating the time course of action of cyclopentolate has been made by Manny *et al.* (1993). Standard clinical routines for the use of cyclopentolate have been based on these findings, and a typical approach would be that recommended in O'Connor Davies *et al.* (1989). One drop of either 0.5% or 1% cyclopentolate is instilled, followed by a second drop if little effect on accommodation is measurable after about 15 minutes.

Retinoscopy can be carried out at 40 to 60 minutes, or sooner if adequate cycloplegia is obtained earlier than this. Residual accommodation can be measured objectively by dynamic retinoscopy, or subjectively with a child capable of reliable subjective responses. A modified form of the push-up method can be used, in which an auxiliary pair of positive lenses, typically of power +2.50 D, is placed in a trial frame. The measurement is taken as described in Chapter 5, and residual accommodation calculated by subtracting 2.50 D from the 'amplitude' as recorded on the rule. An alternative is the 'distance accommodation ability' test recommended by Rosenfield & Linfield (1986). With the child wearing their distance correction and fixating a distance target, which is typically the lowest line that can be read on a letter chart, negative spherical lenses are added until the letters can no longer be read. This technique is considered to be an easier test to perform than the push-up method, when measuring residual accommodation in young children.

Cycloplegia is usually taken to be adequate for retinoscopy when less than 2 D of residual accommodation is measured by the push-up method. There is evidence to suggest that this method gives an inflated estimate of residual accommodation. On theoretical grounds this can be expected, because the retinal image size of the target increases as it approaches the eye, making it easier to resolve. A clinical comparison between residual accommodation measured by the push-up method, and by the distance accommodation ability test supports this theoretical argument (Rosenfield & Linfield, 1986). Mean residual accommodation measured after instillation of 10 µl of 0.5% cyclopentolate was 0.55 D with the distance method, compared to 1.17 D with the push-up approach. Similar conclusions emerge when the push-up method is compared with objective measures of accommodation using dynamic retinoscopy (Rasgorshek & McIntyre, 1955) or optometers (Mordi *et al.*, 1986; Manny *et al.*, 1993). These findings suggest that clinicians can feel confident that when push-up accommodation is measured to be less than 2 D, the true value is almost certainly lower still. Furthermore, the accuracy of all the methods of measurement of accommodation depends upon the patient attempting to exert maximum accommodative effort, yet this is actively discouraged during retinoscopy. As a result, a child can be expected to exert less accommodation during the retinoscopy routine than when accommodation is being measured.

Although many authorities recommend waiting a minimum of 40 minutes after instillation of the drug before beginning retinoscopy, clinical experience has encouraged a number of practitioners to commence retinoscopy before 40 minutes has elapsed. Recent scientific evidence supports this view, at least for children with lightly pigmented eyes. In young adults and children, all of whom had light coloured irides, Manny *et al.* (1993) found maximum cycloplegia to occur 10 minutes after instillation of 1% cyclopentolate. Similar results were obtained by Rosenfield & Linfield (1993), who investigated a young adult population of mixed iris colour. In this sample the mean time to reach maximum cycloplegia was 12 minutes. Clearly, a 40-minute delay prior to refraction is unnecessary in practice for children with light coloured irides.

Patients with dark coloured irides are known to respond more slowly to cycloplegic drugs. This slow response occurs because during the initial period following instillation a proportion of the drug binds with melanin in the eye, preventing it reaching the receptor. Gradually, the melanin releases the drug, which eventually arrives at the receptor site. The more melanin present in a patient's eye, the longer it takes for the drug to produce its maximum effect. Although the maximum effect is delayed in dark coloured irides, it appears to be just as profound as in light coloured eyes when assessed in terms of the residual accommodation (Manny *et al.*, 1993), and the final effect on refractive error (Chan & Edwards, 1994). In patients with dark irides, maximum cycloplegic effect is reached 40 minutes after instillation (Manny *et al.*, 1993). In clinical terms this means that the widely recommended minimum 40-minute waiting period seems appropriate for those with dark coloured irides. However, it must be emphasized that, wherever possible, the practitioner should measure the residual accommodation, because this is invariably the best indicator of the correct time to begin retinoscopy.

There have been several reports of central nervous system adverse reactions to cyclopentolate. These include hallucinations, ataxia, incoherent speech, confusion and drowsiness. Fortunately, most are associated with the 2% solution, not available to the optometrist in the UK. Nevertheless, there have been reports of mild, adverse reactions with 0.5% and 1% solutions (Khurana *et al.*, 1988), and the practitioner should follow the sound advice, issued in O'Connor Davies *et al.* (1989), to use 0.5% cyclopentolate whenever possible, and to use 1% cyclopentolate sparingly. Peripheral adverse reactions of the type associated with atropine, such as dryness of the skin and mouth, and flushing of the skin around the face, have not been reported with cyclopentolate, and allergic reactions are rare.

7.9.2 Atropine

The use of atropine as a cycloplegic has declined steeply in recent years, although this decline in no way reflects its efficacy, for atropine is by far the most potent cycloplegic available to optometrists. However, it is slow acting, its effects are long-lasting, and it causes more adverse systemic reactions than any other cycloplegic used in optometric practice. Atropine is available as atropine sulphate in 0.5% and 1% solutions, and as ointment in a 1% concentration. For cycloplegic refraction ointment is generally used, and should be instilled in both eyes, twice a day, for three days prior to the examination. Ointment should not be instilled on the day of the examination because any ointment remaining in the eye may confuse the retinoscopy reflex. Optometrists favour the ointment form, because the drug is released more slowly from ointment, reducing the risk of a toxic reaction. It is also argued that, as the drug is usually instilled by the parents at home, ointment is to be preferred because in unskilled hands successful instillation may be more likely with ointment than with drops.

Complete atropine cycloplegia leaves no residual accommodation, and recovery may take from seven to ten days, although accommodation may be adequate for close work after four to five days. Mydriasis may last for 10–14 days, and this must be particularly distressing to an infant during long summer days. The use of atropine is controversial in children without a constant squint, because the long-term disruption to the normal relationship between accommodation and convergence can result in a phoria becoming a squint, or an intermittent squint becoming constant. Optometrists increasingly reserve the use of atropine for those children in whom adequate cycloplegia cannot be produced using cyclopentolate, and very few children seen in optometric practice fall into this category. Even in hospitals, where the use of atropine was once widespread, cyclopentolate has become the drug of choice. A typical hospital attitude to the use of atropine would be (a) to avoid it in children under the age of three months, (b) to use cyclopentolate 1% for the first refraction of a child aged from three months upwards. If adequate cycloplegia is produced by cyclopentolate, it would be used for subsequent cycloplegic examinations, and (c) to use atropine only if cyclopentolate fails to produce adequate cycloplegia on the first visit.

Atropine cycloplegia, when complete, totally abolishes the dependent tone of the ciliary muscle. No other cycloplegic abolishes this ciliary muscle tone. Consequently, complete atropine cycloplegia will, in theory, produce a greater positive refractive error than that produced by complete cycloplegia with cyclopentolate. To compensate, an allowance, the 'tonus allowance', is made to the retinoscopy result obtained under atropine cycloplegia, in anticipation of the return of ciliary muscle tone following recovery. The amount of tonus allowance given is of the order of 1 D to hypermetropic and low myopic children. In higher degrees of myopia the ciliary muscle tone is less, and a reduced allowance is given, with no allowance at all for myopes greater than about 3 D. However, these somewhat vague rules are not always followed. For example, in esotropic hypermetropes, the tonus allowance is frequently reduced, and in many hospitals no tonus allowance is given whatever the refractive error. In optometric practice, where cyclopentolate is the drug of choice and atropine is rarely used, all this is fortunately rather academic, because no tonus allowance is ever required with cyclopentolate.

Adverse reactions are more common with atropine than cyclopentolate, and can occur after topical instillation or after accidental ingestion of the drug. Reactions include peripheral effects such as dryness of the skin, mouth and throat, flushed skin of the face and neck, a rapid heart rate, restlessness, and irritability or delirium due to stimulation of the central nervous system. More severe cases may result in ataxia, insomnia, convulsions, drowsiness and coma. Death has occurred following the use of atropine, but is rare, as atropine is rapidly excreted from the body. Vale & Cox (1978) point out that it is a 'sobering thought' that as little as 10 mg of atropine can be a lethal dose in a child, and that a standard 3 gram tube of ointment contains 30 mg of atropine sulphate. This potential lethal dose of 10 mg is also equivalent to about 20 drops of the 1% solution, so vigilance is required to ensure the child does not accidentally ingest the contents of a bottle or tube. In cases of overdose or ingestion, the patient should be rushed to a casualty department. Allergic reactions to atropine are more common than with other cycloplegics. Contact dermatitis and allergic conjunctivitis can occur. For a thorough review of the adverse ocular effects of atropine the reader is referred to North & Kelly (1987).

7.9.3 Tropicamide

Tropicamide is a less effective cycloplegic than cyclopentolate, and is generally regarded as an unreliable cycloplegic in children. It is available in 0.5% and 1% solutions in both Minim form and in multidose containers. In 1993 it was introduced in the form of NODS (novel ophthalmic delivery system) 125 mcg, on an applicator strip with the drug contained in a detachable water-soluble membrane. In its 0.5% concentration, tropicamide is used solely as a mydriatic. The great advantage of tropicamide is its short duration of action, which makes the 1% concentration an attractive cycloplegic to use in patients in their late teens or older. It is associated with very few cases of adverse systemic effects. For cycloplegia one drop of 1% solution repeated after 5 minutes is usually sufficient, although a third drop may be used if required. Retinoscopy can commence 30 minutes after instillation.

Egashira *et al.* (1993) confirmed that cyclopentolate reduced accommodation to a greater extent than tropicamide. However, their well-designed study revealed no difference between the refractive errors obtained by retinoscopy with either cyclopentolate or tropicamide. Their subjects were hypermetropic children between six and twelve years of age. Both drugs were used in 1% concentration, and two drops of each were instilled into one eye only at each visit. Prior to instillation, one drop of the local anaesthetic proxymetacaine was instilled to decrease lacrimation, and to increase the corneal penetration of the cycloplegic agent. If these results can be confirmed in other studies, and with other patient populations, the current restriction of tropicamide to older age-groups may be worthy of reappraisal.

7.9.4 Drug installation

Eyedrops

The standard method for instillation of eyedrops may work perfectly well with many children. The patient's head should be tilted backwards, with their eyes looking back over the patient's head. The lower lid is gently pulled down and away from the eye. One drop is instilled from the Minim or multidose container, which is held close to the eye but avoiding contact with the lashes. It is advisable to keep the part of the hand holding the container in contact with the child's forehead, in an effort to minimize the risk of a sudden forward movement by the child bringing the container into contact with the cornea. With infants and young children it can be easier if the child is lying face upwards on the parent's lap, looking at the corner of the ceiling. The lower lid is pulled down to expose the lower bulbar conjunctiva and the eye drop instilled. In an uncooperative child, who refuses to open their eyes, the drug may be instilled onto the everted lower palpebral conjunctiva, or a drop may be placed at the inner canthus where it forms a pool, some of which will enter the eye when it is eventually opened. Some authorities recommend that routine canalicular occlusion is highly desirable to reduce the risk of systemic absorption (O'Connor Davies *et al.*, 1989), while others question the value of this manoeuvre (Havener, 1983).

Eye ointment

When instilling ointment in the practice, the optometrist transfers a grape-pip size amount from the tube to the end of a clean glass rod. The child adopts an upright head position, looking in a slightly upward direction, and the lower lid is pulled down and away from the eye. With the glass rod held horizontal, the end of the rod is placed gently into the sac. The lower lid is released, and the child asked to close their eyes. Keeping the rod as horizontal as possible it is removed from the sac, leaving the ointment behind. By adding a gentle rotational movement of the rod as it is removed the efficiency of the procedure can be improved. Excess ointment should be carefully removed from the lids and eye surrounds with a soft tissue or cotton wool.

Atropine is frequently instilled by parents at home, and the practitioner can demonstrate the method by making the first instillation himself in the practice. For demonstration purposes it may be more convenient to instil simple eye ointment, which contains no active agent. Parents can be given a rod, or rods, to use at home, or alternatively can instil the ointment direct from the tube. The procedure is similar to that followed with a rod. Parents should be advised to observe good standards of hygiene, and of the risks of overdose and ingestion. It is often possible to instil the ointment while the child is asleep. By pulling the lower lid down and away, the parent can insert a $\frac{1}{4}$ inch ribbon of atropine into the sac.

Spray application

Spray application of cyclopentolate may become a possible alternative to traditional eyedrop instillation. The spray can be applied to the lashes of the upper lid while the child lightly closes their eyes. Preliminary clinical studies report a significant preference among children for the spray application as compared with conventional eyedrop instillation. Adequate cycloplegia is produced, and there have not been any reports of contact dermatitis or allergic conjunctivitis (Ismail *et al.*, 1994).

7.10 Photorefraction

The technique was introduced by Howland & Howland in 1974, and a version of the procedure for clinical use is commercially available as the Clement Clarke videorefractor. The basic principle of the test is to use a flash source on a camera to produce a series of in-focus, and out-of-focus, images of the child's illuminated pupil. By controlling the amount of defocus, the flash pictures produced by this method produce blur circles, the size of which are proportional to the child's ametropia. In hypermetropia the far point is closer to the picture taken when the camera is focused behind the eye, and the blur circles so caused are relatively bright and well defined. In myopia the reverse applies. Elliptical blur circles are produced in astigmatism. Hodi & Wood (1994), have assessed the videorefractor in the clinical situation, and for astigmatic errors found very poor correlation between the retinoscopy findings and those obtained with the videorefractor. This may be because changes of gaze alter the measured refraction. The videorefractor can be used to identify those with large refractive errors, but other methods should be used to determine the exact magnitude of the error.

7.11 Optometers

Edwards (1988) observed that autorefractors have no role to play in the examination of young children, because they are intimidating, impractical and unlikely to yield accurate results, owing to poor control of accommodation. While accommodation is better controlled in modern autorefractors, they can still scare children, and infants can be extremely difficult to position at the instrument. Good results have been obtained by Zadnik *et al.* (1992) using the Canon R-1 autorefractor, which permits the child to view a target in reasonably natural conditions.

7.12 References

Chan, O.Y.C. and Edwards, M. (1994) 'Comparison of cycloplegic and noncycloplegic retinoscopy in Chinese preschool children'. *Optom. Vis. Sci.*, **71**, 312–18.

Egashira, S.M., Kish, L.L., Twelker, J.D., Mutti, D.O., Zadnik, K. and Adams, A.J. (1993) 'Comparison of cyclopentolate versus tropicamide in children'. *Optom. Vis. Sci.*, **70**, 1019–26.

Glickstein, M. and Millodot, M. (1970) 'Retinoscopy and eye size'. *Science*, **168**, 605–606.

Havener, W.H. (1983) *Ocular Pharmacology*, 5th edn. CV Mosby, St Louis.

Haynes, H. (1960) 'Clinical observations with dynamic retinoscopy'. *Opt. Wkly*, October 27(2243) and November 3(2306).

Hodi, S. and Wood, I.C.J. (1994) 'Comparison of the techniques of videorefraction and static retinoscopy in the measurement of refractive error in infant'. *Opthal. Physiol. Opt.* **14**, 20–24.

Howland, H.C. and Howland, B. (1974) 'Photorefraction: a technique for study of refractive state at a distance'. *J. Opt. Soc. Am.*, **64**, 240–49.

Ismail, E.E., Rouse, M.W., De Land, P.N.A. (1994) 'Comparison of drop instillation and spray application of 1% cyclopentolate hydrochloride'. *Optom. Vis. Sci.*, **71**, 235–41.

Khurana, A.K., Ahluwalia, B.K., Rajan, C. and Vohra, A.K. (1988) 'Acute psychosis associated with topical cyclopentolate hydrochloride'. *Am. J. Ophthalmol.*, **105**, 91.

Maino, J.H., Cibis, G.W., Cress, P., Spellman, C.R. and Shores, R.E. (1984) 'Noncycloplegic versus cycloplegic retinoscopy in pre-school children'. *Annals Ophthalmol.*, **16**, No. 9, 880–82.

Manny, R.E., Fern, K.D., Zervas, H.J., Cline, G.E., Scott, S.K., White, J.M. and Pass, A.F. (1993) '1% cyclopentolate hydrochloride: another look at the time course of cycloplegia using an objective measure of the accommodative response'. *Optom. Vis. Sci.*, **70**, 651–65.

Mohindra, I. (1975) 'A technique for infant vision examination'. *Am. J. Optom. Physiol. Opt.*, **52**, 867–70.

Mohindra, I. (1977) 'Comparison of near retinoscopy and subjective refraction in adults'. *Am. J. Optom. Physiol. Opt.*, **54**, 319–22.

Mohindra, I., Molinari, J.F. (1979) 'Near retinoscopy and cycloplegic refraction in early primary grade school children'. *Am. J. Optom. Physiol. Opt.*, **56**, 34–8.

Mordi, J., Tucker, J. and Charman, W.N. (1986) 'Effects of 0.1% cyclopentolate or 10% phenylephrine on pupil diameter and accommodation'. *Ophthal. Physiol. Opt.*, **6**, 221–7.

North, R.V. and Kelly, M.E. (1987) 'A review of the uses and adverse effects of topical administration of atropine'. *Ophthal. Physiol. Opt.*, **7**, 109–14.

O'Connor Davies, P.H., Hopkins, G.A. and Pearson, R.M. (1989) *The Actions and Uses of Ophthalmic Drugs*, 3rd edn. Butterworth, London.

Owens, D., Mohindra, I., Held, R. (1980) 'The effectiveness of a retinoscope beam as an accommodative stimulus'. *Inv. Ophthal. Vis. Sci.*, **19**, 942–9.

Rasgorshek, R.H., McIntyre, W.C. (1955) 'Cyclogyl®: re-evaluation and further studies'. *Am. J. Ophthalmol.*, **40**, 34–7.

Rosenfield, M. and Linfield, P.B. (1986) 'A comparison of the effects of cycloplegics on accommodation ability for distance vision and on the apparent near point'. *Ophthal. Physiol. Opt.*, **6**, 317–20.

Rosner, J. and Rosner, J. (1990) *Pediatric Optometry* (157). Butterworth, London.

Stidwill, D. (1990) *Orthoptic Assessment and Management*. Blackwell Scientific Publications, Oxford.

Swann, L.A. (1939) *Recent advances in objective refraction*. Raphaels, London.

Taylor, S. (1988) 'Retinoscopy' (81–91), in *Optometry*. (Edwards and Llewellyn, eds). Butterworth, Oxford.

Vale, J. and Cox, B. (1985) *Drugs and the eye*, 2nd edn. Butterworth, London.

Zadnik, K., Mutti, D.O., Friedman, N.E. and Adams, A.J. (1993) 'Initial cross-sectional results from the Orinda longitudinal study of myopia'. *Optom. Vis. Sci.*, **70**, 750–8.

CHAPTER 8
Investigation of Binocular Vision in the Child

Adrian Jennings

8.1   Introduction

Chapters 5, 6 and 7 discussed the various techniques and equipment required to undertake the routine examination of the young patient. Some of these tests appertain to binocular vision and may be carried out on patients with normal as well as abnormal binocular vision. This chapter will consider further investigative techniques that may be particularly useful in the assessment of children with binocular vision anomalies. The examination routines for patients of different age-groups will also be considered.

Failure of binocular vision may have little effect on everyday behaviour and, unless accompanied by a large squint, it is unlikely to be noticed by either the parent or the child. The practitioner should be aware that various binocular anomalies have been correlated with some types of educational difficulties in children (see Chapter 9). In the absence of overt symptoms a diagnosis of abnormal binocular vision is based on assessment of the motor status, the refractive error and the sensory performance.

With young children subjective data are sparse and unreliable. The diagnosis has to be made on the objective formation gleaned in brief periods of cooperation. As discussed in Chapter 5, it is wise to collect the most critical data first in case the child's interest is lost. For example, an initial stereopsis measurement can exclude the possibility of squint or gross amblyopia (Reinecke & Simons, 1974; Levy & Glick, 1974; Cooper & Feldman, 1978, 1981; Dobson & Sebris, 1989).

It is hoped to collect the following essential data for all ages:

(a)   an estimate of the vision and visual acuities;
(b)   the motor status as deduced from the cover test;
(c)   an indication of normal ocular motility;
(d)   the refractive error and ability to accommodate;
(e)   the state of the media and fundus on ophthalmoscopy.

When the patient reaches an age where he or she is able to give some subjective reponses, various other assessments can be carried out, for example tests to determine the sensory status.

8.2 Facilities required

The practice facilities have been discussed in Chapter 5. With respect to the consulting room it is worth mentioning again that a room length of about 5 m or more avoids the needs for a mirror which can be confusing for the child (see Chapter 5). It will also make divergent excess deviations less susceptible to voluntary control.

Sound-proofing is useful as noisy children in the waiting room can be a great distraction for the patient and, conversely, any sounds of protest against the instillation of cyclopentolate spreads apprehension in the waiting area.

Table 8.1 lists the basic equipment required for the assessment of the binocular vision in the child. Each practitioner will have his own preferences and the optometrist specializing in children will certainly require additional equipment.

8.3 Appointments and timing

If appointment times are scrupulously observed it is usually possible to avoid keeping children waiting. Any delay makes the child more apprehensive and probably less cooperative.

Ideally, cyclopentolate refractions are best done in the late afternoon so that the binocularly stressful period of increased AC/A ratio (Burian & von Noorden, 1974) occurs overnight while the child sleeps.

Table 8.1 Basic equipment and uses.

Equipment	Uses
Full aperture trial case	Simplifies retinoscopy and cover test
Lightweight child's trial frame	Essential for children with astigmatism
Cyclopentolate hydrochloride 0.5% and 1%	Cycloplegic refraction and ophthalmoscopy
Opticlude eye patches	Occlusion during the preferential looking test
Fixation bar	Near cover test, NPC, near acuity, accommodation
Pen torch	Near cover test, motility, pupils, NPC
Various pediatric acuity tests	Visual acuity
Stereopsis tests	To establish the presence of binocular vision or probable absence of amblyopia
Bagolini glasses	Investigation of sensory status
Large aperture 10 Δ prism	Fusional eye movements in infants

8.4   Further investigative techniques

As well as various tests discussed in Chapter 5, the following tests or investigations may be additionally required as part of the assessment of a child with a binocular vision anomaly.

8.4.1   AC/A ratio

The gradient test attempts to measure AC/A ratio by assessing the change in vergence for each supposed change in accommodation. Inaccuracies occur because, whilst convergence needs to be precise (within the limits of Panum's fusional areas), accommodation frequently lags by 0.50 D or more. As spheres are introduced binocularly, the change in phoria is measured using the Maddox rod, Mills test or Maddox Wing. Another method is to introduce spheres binoculary, increasing their power until a retinal slip is noted on the Mallett unit, then repeat with prisms instead of spherical lenses until the slip reappears. Both negative spheres/base out prism and positive spheres/base in prism can be used. Most of these techniques (apart from the cover test) are generally limited to children of about five years and older, because of the subjective responses required.

8.4.2   Fusional reserves

Fusional reserves are also termed prism vergences (Pickwell, 1989) and relative vergences (Stidwill, 1990), and refer to motor fusion ability. Measurement of horizontal fusional reserves is made by asking the patient to fixate a vertical line of letters. Horizontal prism is gradually increased until the patient reports that the target blurs, and further increased until the target 'breaks' to give diplopia. The prism is then reduced until the patient reports recovery of single vision. These three measures are known as 'blur, break and recovery' and may be measured for distance and near vision. Negative and positive fusional reserves may be measured by using base-in and base-out prisms respectively, with base in being measured first. A Risley rotary prism gives the smoothest change in prism power, and is preferable to a prism bar. The rotary prism system is found in a phoropter, and in the variable-prism stereoscope. Alternatively a loose Risley prism can be positioned in a trial frame. A further method utilizes the synoptophore. Fusional reserves vary not only between patients but also according to which technique and target is used. For example, stereoscopic targets tend to produce greater ranges, the synoptophore results are affected by proximal convergence, and increasing the rate of change of prism power will reduce the measured ranges. A rate of change of approximately 1 Δ per second is often recommended when using a Risley rotary prism.

Table 8.2 Vergence ranges in a large group of non-presbyopic patients (adapted from Morgan, 1960).

	Positive fusional vergences (Δ) *(measured with base out prism)*	*Negative fusional reserves (Δ)* *(measured with base in prism)*
6 m		
Blur	7–11	–
Break	15–23	5–9
Recovery	8–12	3–5
40 cm		
Blur	14–20	11–15
Break	18–24	19–23
Recovery	7–15	10–16

N.B. Vertical reserves are usually of the order of 3 prism dioptres for right and left supra and infra vergences.

Convergence normally is greater than divergence, and horizontal vergences measured in distance fixation are smaller than those obtained in near fixation (von Noorden, 1990). Table 8.2 shows examples of normal ranges.

The practitioner should become familiar with the technique of his choice and with the normal ranges obtained using this technique. Measurement of fusional reserves is useful when diagnosing oculomotor anomalies, and for monitoring the progress of treatment. There is evidence that poor fusional reserves may be a correlate of some types of learning under achievement (see Chapter 9).

8.4.3   Detection of foveal suppression

One reason why a poorly compensated heterophoria might not produce symptoms is the presence of foveal suppression. Any test to detect this small area (5'– 15' arc) must not introduce retinal rivalry or other artefacts. A test for foveal suppression is incorporated in the near Mallett Unit (Mallett, 1964), which is used in conjunction with polarized spectacles. If the child is unsure of the letters then the practitioner should ask him to count the number of letters on each line. A note should be made of which eye is suppressing, and at what angular subtense. These tests cannot generally be used before the age of about four years.

Other more crude tests can be employed, for example the Javal FL card in a plano prism stereoscope, the Worth four dot test and the synoptophore. Some stereopsis tests include targets designed specifically to detect suppression.

8.4.4   Assessment of sensory status in strabismus

Tests for abnormal retinal correspondence (ARC) or suppression in a squinting child can be carried out from the age of about three to five years. Non-dissociating tests are much preferred, as these do little to disrupt the natural sensory status of the patient. The methods of choice are the Bagolini striated glasses, and the modified Mallett unit.

Bagolini glasses

Bagolini glasses consist of plano lenses with very fine lines etched into the surface. When a spot light is viewed through the lens, a thin streak of light is produced at right angles to the striations. Bagolini No. 4 glass produces a brighter streak than No. 2. The Bagolini glasses are placed in a trial frame with one positioned at 45° and the other at 135°. If the patient reports only seeing one streak then suppression is present, and its depth can be investigated using a graded neutral density filter bar over the non-squinting eye. If the patient reports seeing two spotlights, each with a streak passing through, then either normal retinal correspondence with diplopia is present, or the patient has unharmonius ARC, which is likely to be accompanied by diplopia. If the patient reports, in the presence of a manifest squint, one spot light with both streaks passing through it then harmonious ARC (HARC) is present. Its depth can be assessed by slowly increasing the strength of neutral density filters in front of the squinting eye until suppression is reported. The patient will often report that a small central portion of the streak seen by the squinting eye is missing. This is due to a small area of central suppression at the zero point measure (Mallett, 1988).

Modified Mallett test (Mallett, 1983)

The distance fixation disparity test is viewed at 1.5 m (or alternatively the enlarged fixation disparity test on the newer version of the near unit is viewed at 25 cm) through polarized filters, with additional compensatory ambient illumination. A larger angular subtense for the target is required to avoid the retinal image falling into the 1° suppression area at the zero point measure. HARC is present if both strips are seen simultaneously, and the depth of HARC can be investigated with filters, as with the Bagolini glasses.

8.4.5   Assessment of fixation

Fixation is invariably eccentric in patients whose amblyopia is purely strabismic and there is a fairly linear relationship between the visual acuity and the degree of eccentricity with 15′ arc of eccentric fixation for every line of morphoscopic acuity below the norm of 6/5 or 6/6 (Mallett, 1988). Assessment of the degree of eccentric fixation may be used to aid differential diagnosis from other types of amblyopia, and it is particularly useful in diagnosing a microtropia with deep HARC and in which the objective angle of strabismus is equal to the degree of eccentric fixation. In such a case the strabismic eye will be amblyopic but there will be no movement during the cover test. Apart from the reduced acuity the only other clue may be the presence of eccentric fixation.

For children the method of choice is to use a direct ophthalmoscope containing a graticule. The Visuscope is designed for this purpose and has a graticule consisting of a central fixation star surrounded by a series of fine concentric circles which can be focused on the retina. Children of all ages will usually fixate the star and the position of the fovea within the graticule pattern can be recorded. In convergent squint eccentric fixation is normally nasal and thus the clinician observes the fovea temporal to the star. If the concentric rings are removed most infants will fixate a Visuscope star and central fixation could be taken as being a reliable indication that no *strabismic amblyopia* is present (Mallett, 1988)

Subjective methods of measurement such as the Hadinger brush and 'after image transfer' (AIT) are generally unsuitable for younger children because the phenomena can be difficult the child to appreciate but both these techniques can be used for active amblyopia therapy for the older child.

8.5 The examination

On a general note, with infants and younger children the practitioner can sometimes feel that the investigation is not proceeding with the accuracy that is normally thought to be essential. Many refractions will be just a retinoscopy based on a few seconds' observation of each eye. This approximation can be refined, if necessary, at the next appointment, by which time the child will have become accustomed to wearing spectacles, the whole experience will be less intimidating and the prescription can be fine tuned.

8.6 Examination of infants of less than eighteen months

Blindness at birth is fortunately rare. When it does occur it is almost always accompanied by abnormal eye movements and other congenital anomalies. The parents may notice a lack of eye contact and that the infant's head posture relates more to sound than to visual stimuli (Tallents, 1987; Fulton, 1989).

Very low birth weight children (<1500 g) are particularly at risk for visual disorders such as strabismus and amblyopia (Van Hof-van Duin et al., 1989; Pott & Van Hof-van Duin, 1989; Lennerstrand & Gallo, 1989).

Infants under the age of eighteen months are uncommon as patients in most optometric practices because once early onset anomalies have been detected they are often treated in hospital. The exception is the infant presenting to an optometrist because he is the sibling of an older patient or who has been previously designated as normal but is now thought to have recently developed a visual problem.

8.6.1 History and symptoms

The optometrist needs to enquire about a number of general factors. Was the birth full-term or premature? What was the birth weight? Were there any complications, any subsequent illness or trauma or any additional investigations or treatment required? Useful information can be obtained by enquiring of the general and ocular health of the siblings. Binocular anomalies in the immediate family may suggest a hereditary influence (Cantolino & von Noorden, 1969; Jay & Elston, 1987). A very high prevalence of strabismus (40%) has been found in the children of treated amblyopes (Sarniguet-Bardouche & Pincon, 1982), though excess hypermetropia rather than squint *per se* is the more critical hereditary factor (Wattam-Bell *et al.*, 1987; Dobson & Sebris, 1989). The parents should be asked for their impressions of the infant's visual attention, face recognition and fixation ability.

8.6.2 Motor assessment

Ocular motility in the younger infant can be assessed by holding and rotating the infant, with the practitioner's face acting as the fixation stimulus (see Chapter 5). The infant will briefly fix a pen torch or small 'squeaky toy' held in the diagnostic directions of gaze. A tendency to move the head to keep fixation in the field of one particular eye suggests possible amblyopia or restricted motility (Sarniguet-Bardouche & Pincon, 1982). Early onset esotropes often cross fixate so that on motility testing they change the fixing eye soon after the target crosses the midline.

Monocular motility is tested to exclude pareses and congenital anomalies such as Duane's syndrome. In infants any incomitance will quickly acquire more symmetrical characteristics making diagnosis difficult (Mallett, 1969). If any oculomotor restriction is found immediate referral is appropriate. Pupil reactions should be checked. Latencies are slightly longer than in the adult (Shea *et al.*, 1985) and are indicative of a functioning retina (Fulton, 1989).

8.6.3 Eye position

When fixing a pen torch the corneal reflexes (Figure 8.1) are normally nasally displaced in the pupil because of the large angle lambda of the infant, $\cong 9°$

(Slater & Findlay, 1972). This gives an appearance of exotropia which is counteracted by the epicanthal folds commonly seen at this age. This makes the assessment of strabismus by eye position and corneal reflex very complicated (Paliaga, 1989; Quick & Boothe, 1989; Brodie, 1987). It has been suggested that neonates tend to be exotropic and become more orthotropic at three months (Archer *et al.*, 1989). Esotropia at birth is very unusual ($\cong 0.1\%$), the incidence starting to increase after three months (Nixon *et al.*, 1985; von Noorden, 1988). Small unilateral squints are unusual (Lennerstrand & Gallo, 1989). Infantile esotropia is usually of a large angle, e.g. $\cong 30\,\Delta$. The ill-defined fovea at birth (Yuodelis & Hendrickson, 1986) makes it doubtful if precise fixation is possible. In these circumstances the designation of esotropia and exotropia is perhaps not appropriate.

8.6.4   Cover test

The cover test at this age is not easy. Keeping the infant's attention on a distance target is rarely successful and the introduction of the cover causes further distraction. Covering with the thumb while resting the fingers on the head is sometimes more successful. Any difference in tolerance of one eye being covered as opposed to the other, should be considered suspicious. If covering an eye is made difficult by the child repeatedly grasping for or pushing away the occluder, it can be useful to get the mother to occlude the eye with her hand. After the infant becomes used to this situation, the practitioner can gain the

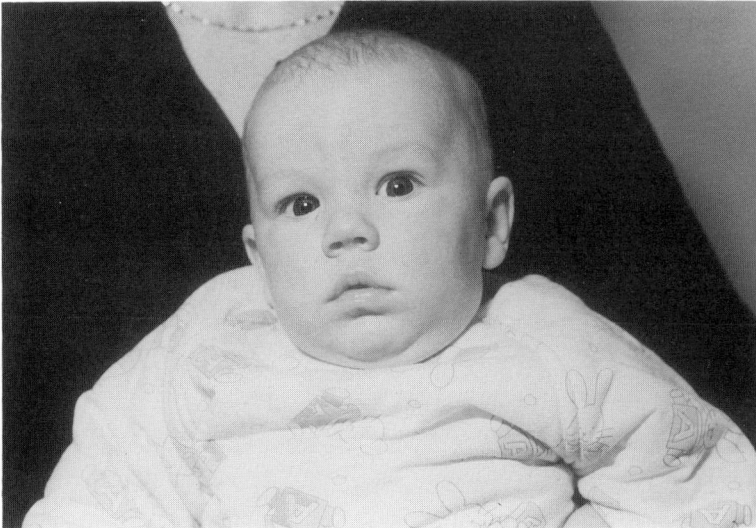

Fig. 8.1 Infant showing corneal reflexes.

attention of the unoccluded eye and observe its movement when the mother's hand is removed from the fellow eye.

Significant heterophoria is unusual in the infant though the accommodation convergence relationship is functional by about three months (Aslin & Jackson, 1979).

8.6.5   Motor fusion

Motor fusion can be demonstrated by holding a large aperture prism in front of one eye and observing if a fusional movement occurs to restore binocular vision (Fig. 8.2). A 5 or 10Δ base out is normally overcome by the cooperative infant of six months, but the reflex is not established until about four-and-a-half months (Aslin, 1977; Archer *et al.*, 1989).

8.6.6   Stereopsis

Stereopsis can be assessed in the infant by evoked potentials (Petrig *et al.*, 1981), preferential looking (Birch *et al.*, 1985) or by observation of the eye movements precipitated by a moving random dot stimulus (Fox *et al.*, 1980). Despite the clear experimental demonstration of stereopsis in the infant there is at present no reliable clinical method of measurement in the very young child though operant preferential looking shows promise (Ciner *et al.*, 1989). In the consulting room, the Lang stereo test can be used with occasional success to show the

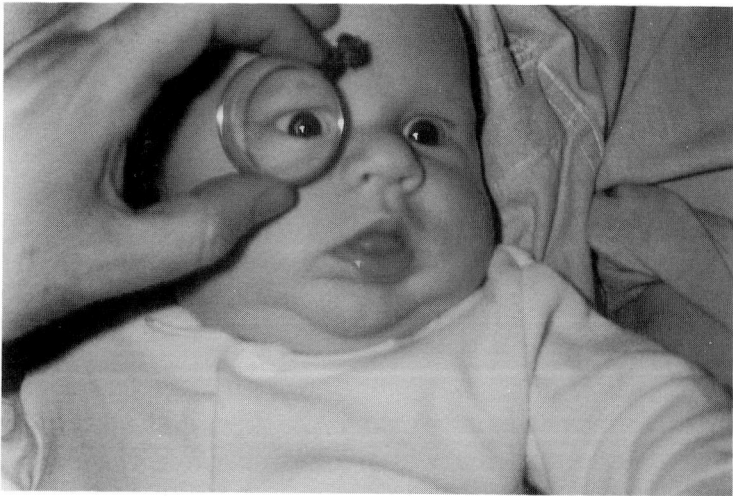

Fig. 8.2 10Δ prism over one eye.

presence of stereopsis in infants from the age of about six months (Stidwill, 1990).

Stereo acuity is at least 45 minutes of arc by about four months and increases to about 100 seconds by three years (Ciner *et al.*, 1989). Clinical measures of stereopsis show increases up to the early teens, probably as a result of the younger children's lack of attention (Romano *et al.*, 1975; Heron *et al.*, 1985). Under ideal conditions and high motivation the stereoscopic acuity of children (three- to five-year-olds) is similar to that of adults (Fox *et al.*, 1986).

8.6.7   Refraction

Retinoscopy is the method of choice for refraction because it is accurate over the whole range of refractive error and is tolerant of considerable movement of the infant.

Alternative methods of measuring refractive error have been developed based on video or photographic recording of the coaxially illuminated pupil (Howland & Howland, 1974; Howland *et al.*, 1983; Howland, 1985; Bobier, 1988; Crewther *et al.*, 1988; Wagner & Wearn, 1988; Hsu-Winges *et al.*, 1989). Typically, the accuracy of these methods is not high and the refractive range can be limited (Howland *et al.*, 1983; Braddick & Atkinson, 1984; Crewther *et al.*, 1988). However these newer methods hold promise in the refractive screening of large numbers of children (Atkinson *et al.*, 1987). These techniques are discussed in Chapter 7.

Infants are best held firmly on the parent's knee. They tend to close their eyes and turn their head away from any threatening approach so that attempts to use a trial frame are usually counterproductive. A pair of hand held lenses is easier to keep in position and the refraction of both eyes can be estimated at the same time (Fig. 8.3). If the trial lenses are grasped for or pushed away, a lens vertex of 10 or 15 cm may be the closest that can be managed and this must be allowed for in the final prescription.

Cycloplegia is required for reliable results and this subject, as well as other non-cycloplegic retinoscopy techniques, is discussed in Chapter 7.

8.6.8   Refractive error

Retinoscopy should be done as accurately as possible. Assessing both eyes at the same time by quickly alternating between the two eyes helps to reveal any anisometropia. Astigmatism can be estimated or measured in each meridian with spheres and then the full sphero/cylindrical result put up in a trial frame for as long as possible to verify power and axes.

All measures of refraction based on light reflection from the fundus suffer from a systematic error caused by the difference between the perceptual layer of

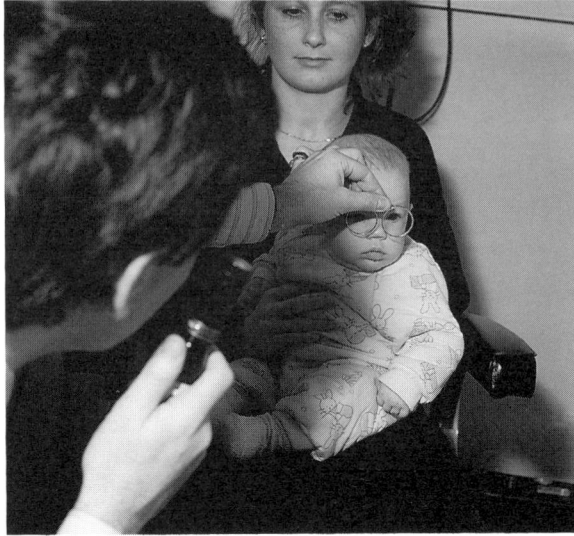

Fig. 8.3 Infant held by mother whilst refraction proceeds through a hand held pair of full aperture lenses.

the retina and the reflecting surface (Glickstein & Millidot, 1970; Howland, 1982). This error varies inversely with the square of the focal length of the eye and could amount to about 0.50 D of hypermetropia in the infant.

In the newborn, refractive error is widely distributed with a mean of $+2.00$ D ± 2 D. The spread diminishes over the first year under the influence of emmetropization to produce a typical refractive error at one year of approximately $+1.00$ D. Amblyopic eyes emmetropize less effectively and remain more hypermetropic (Lepard, 1975; Nastri *et al.*, 1984). Premature infants can be myopic (Banks, 1980; Keith & Kitchen, 1983) but otherwise normal, low birth weight infants (<2000 g) develop unremarkable refractive errors (Shapiro *et al.*, 1980).

Large refractive errors are unusual, only about 5% of six- to nine-month-olds have hypermetropia $>+3.50$ D and only about 0.5% have myopia >-3.00 D (Atkinson *et al.*, 1984). Astigmatism of $1-2$ D is common and it regresses spontaneously over the first twelve months (Mohindra *et al.*, 1978; Howland *et al.*, 1978; Atkinson *et al.*, 1980) as the cornea becomes more spherical (Howland & Sayles, 1985) without causing any permanent meridional amblyopia (Gwiazda *et al.*, 1985a, 1985b) though there may be some effect on meridional vernier acuity (Gwiazda *et al.*, 1986). Remaining astigmatism diminishes over the next year or two (Abrahamson *et al.*, 1988) towards the typical adult prevalence of $<30\%$ of eyes having more than 1 D of astigmatism (Satterfield, 1989).

The minority of children whose astigmatism persists or even increase

(Abrahamson *et al.*, 1988) are likely to get meridional amblyopia (Mitchell *et al.*, 1973; Mitchell & Wilkinson, 1974) if left uncorrected. This is a permanent, cortical, loss in contrast sensitivity for gratings of the habitually most defocused orientation, despite optimum refractive correction of the astigmatism (Thibos & Levick, 1982). The Snellen chart is not very sensitive at detecting meridional defects (Atkinson *et al.*, 1987).

Further discussion on refractive development and amblyopia may be found in Chapters 3 and 4.

8.6.9   Assessing visual acuity

Parents have the opportunity of observing the development of their children and can be very astute observers of visual anomalies. Their opinion should be sought of the infant's visual ability, for example in recognizing faces and finding toys.

At birth, acuity is limited by the immaturity and wide spacing of the foveal cones (Banks *et al.*, 1989) and is about 6/240 regardless of the method of measurement (Fulton *et al.*, 1981; Banks & Dannemiler, 1987; von Noorden, 1988; Thomson & Drasdo, 1988). The evoked potential indicates that acuity increases rapidly to approach adult levels in the first year (Marg *et al.*, 1976; Norcia & Tyler, 1985) whereas preferential looking indicates a slower development, taking at least two years to reach adult levels (Mayer & Dobson, 1982). Optokinetic nystagmus methods can give similar acuities to preferential looking but the results are heavily influenced by field size (Schor & Narayan, 1981). There is a monocular asymmetry of optokinetic nystagmus in normal infants (Naegel & Held, 1982b) which persists in amblyopes (Westall *et al.*, 1989) and the extent to which the technique assesses midbrain as opposed to cortical function is not known (Naegel & Held, 1982a; Tallents, 1987). These considerations make optokinetic nystagmus a dubious measure of developing acuity.

Preferential-looking is the method of choice and this is discussed in Chapter 6.

In the absence of apparatus for preferential-looking a crude impression of the acuities can be gained by observing the facility with which small sweets (e.g. hundreds and thousands) spread out before the infant can be located and retrieved (Gruber, 1984). This is sometimes known as the Bock candy bead test.

Also, poor fixation, failure to follow a target with one eye, impaired pupil reaction, marked difference in the reaction to covering one eye compared to the other are all suggestive of poor acuity but all are unreliable and can be very misleading.

8.6.10   Ophthalmoscopy

This is best carried out under mydriasis.

8.7   Examination of children of eighteen months to three years

This can be the most difficult age group to cope with. The child is mobile and is continually being distracted by novel objects. Unless the parent is firm and supportive there can be great difficulties in conducting an adequate examination. Ideally, the mother keeps the child on her knee the right way round and the right way up!

8.7.1   History and symptoms

The parents will have an opinion as to the adequacy of the child's visual acuity to the extent that people and objects can be recognized at the appropriate distances and that samll objects can be manipulated under visual control. The child will have established head postures and patterns of visually guided behaviour. The parent's descriptions of eye movements and deviations should be noted and given credence. For example, they may report that an intermittent deviation may only be present when the child is tired. Any childhood illnesses, for example measles or chicken pox, or any trauma should be related to the onset of visual problems.

8.7.2   Motor assessment

It should be possible to attract fixation into the diagnostic directions but there is rarely sufficient cooperation to do a monocular motility test. Pupil reactions should be normal.

8.7.3   Cover test

A pen torch at about 30 cm can hold the child's attention for several seconds if he or she is encouraged to 'blow it out' and is rewarded by switching it off after a concerted effort. The practitioner should note the corneal reflexes and do the cover test with a thumb or cover as appropriate. If the cover is such a distraction that the child always looks around, it can be helpful to cover the putative 'good' eye and establish fixation by the suspect eye as suggested above. In unilateral squint, removal of the cover gives an unambiguous saccadic movement as fixation is taken up by the good eye.

Heterophoria may be present, particularly esophoria associated with hypermetropia.

8.7.4   Motor fusion

The $10\,\Delta$ base out test can be attempted with a cooperative child.

The amplitude of convergence can be tested using an interesting target to attract the child's attention.

8.7.5   Stereopsis

Clinical stereo tests are extremely useful. Examples are the Lang test (Lang, 1984), TNO test (Walraven, 1975), Titmus test (Levy & Glick, 1974), Frisby test (Hinchcliffe, 1978). There are substantial differences between the design and sensitivity of these tests (Frisby *et al.*, 1981; Heron *et al.*, 1985) and it is prudent to use more than one test. Low-grade stereopsis may be found with the Titmus test but not with the TNO. This is probably caused by monocular detection of asymmetry within the Titmus test figures (Cooper & Warshowsky, 1977; Simons & Reinecke, 1974).

The Lang stereo test is the most appropriate for this age group and successful results have been obtained on surprisingly young children (Stidwill, 1985). A reaction to the Titmus fly and reaching above the page for its wings suggests the presence of stereopsis. At about two years, children will often be able to point to which animal is 'coming out to say hello' on the Titmus test. If goggles are tolerated for the Titmus then it is worth trying the less ambiguous TNO test.

8.7.6   Refraction

If cycloplegic retinoscopy proves difficult because the child is uncooperative and dislikes lenses being held near his or her eyes photorefraction may be a useful alternative. The child may be happier at a distance from the apparatus and the video technique only requires a few seconds of attention. Significant spherical and astigmatic errors present at this age are unlikely to emmetropize and must be fully corrected.

8.7.7   Visual acuity

Children of this age are poor subjects for preferential looking because of their short attention span and insatiable curiosity. Kay pictures or the Cardiff test can be attempted, often with some success at as young as twenty months.

8.7.8   Ophthalmoscopy

Indirect ophthalmoscopy may be more acceptable to the child than direct ophthalmoscopy but a satisfactory result must be obtained by whatever method.

8.8   Examination of children of three to five years of age

8.8.1   History and symptoms

The history should allow a distinction to be made between those congenital or early onset binocular anomalies which have been untreated and those acquired under normal development. There is general agreement that the more long standing a condition the worse the prognosis though the significance of 'age of onset' and 'time since onset' on the effectiveness of amblyopia treatment is debatable (Ingram *et al.*, 1977, 1990). The onset of accommodative squints is most common at this age. These often present initially as an intermittent deviation occurring when the child is tired.

8.8.2   Motor assessment

It should be possible to encourage or cajole the child into an acceptable motility and cover test. Compensation may be inferred from the quality of cover test recovery movements. A comparison of distance and near cover tests shows the effect of accommodation and the AC/A relationship.

8.8.3   Stereopsis

Every effort should be made to get a quantitative measure of stereopsis from several stereo tests. Unfortunately, failure to demonstrate stereopsis only indicates either lack of stereopsis or a lack of cooperation. If stereopsis is doubtful the cover test remains the final arbiter, although with a microtropia there may not be a movement. For a discussion on microtropia the reader is referred to von Noorden (1990).

8.8.4   Refraction

If the history suggests an intermittent deviation it is essential to use a short acting cycloplegic, such as cyclopentolate hydrochloride 0.5% or 1%, rather than the longer acting atropine. During the several days of partial cycloplegia which follows the use of atropine the AC/A ratio is greatly increased putting additional stress on an already vulnerable vergence system. After cycloplegic retinoscopy, a crude subjective may be possible, at least to the extent of reassessing the acuity with the cycloplegic results in place.

8.8.5   Visual acuity

Most children of this age have some ability for matching shapes. Repeatable results can usually be gained with the Sheridan–Gardner or Kay picture test

(Fern & Manny, 1986). These tests consist of isolated single symbols which are not affected by 'crowding' (Flom *et al.*, 1963; Fern *et al.*, 1986) giving an overestimate of the acuity in an amblyopic eye. Any consistent difference in acuity, however small, should be considered suspicious. Multiple character tests (Rodier *et al.*, 1985; Elliott, 1985; Atkinson *et al.*, 1988) have the test letter surrounded by other letters to give a 'crowding effect' and make the test more sensitive to amblyopia. These tests are discussed in Chapter 6.

8.8.6   Ophthalmoscopy

The opportunity should be taken to check for eccentric fixation in an amblyopic child. There needs to be a systematic difference in the pattern of fixation in the good and amblyopic eyes for a diagnosis of eccentric fixation to be made with certainty. This can be crudely assessed with the cross target of, for example, the Keeler specialist ophthalmoscope or measured using a Visuscope.

8.9   Examination of children of five years and older

Children of seven or eight years old are often more forthcoming when seen alone, uninhibited by parental presence. It can be difficult to know that a child is old enough to be seen without the parents, but this possibility should be considered at the second or third visit. A discussion with the parents is obviously necessary after the examination.

Children of this age can confirm or deny the presence of symptoms and a subjective verification of the prescription is usually possible. The reduction in acuity caused by rotating large cylinders 10° or 15° each side of the axis helps to confirm the astigmatic correction. The effect of a +1.00 DS addition will adequately check the sphere.

8.9.1   Motor assessment

Patients who have undergone previous surgery may have secondary motility anomalies and these can be assessed with the patient following a pen torch in the diagnostic positions of gaze. A Hess screen plot is of great assistance in the recording of oculomotor anomalies and can be undertaken by quite young children. A permanent record of ocular motility is a useful aid to initial diagnosis, assessment of sequelae and to assist in monitoring subsequent change (Lyle & Wybar, 1967; Mallett, 1969; Duke-Elder, 1973).

8.9.2   Video recording

A video recording of ocular motor anomalies has the great advantage of allowing a leisurely study of repeated playbacks. This can be very helpful in complex cases and allows a more considered diagnosis than may otherwise be possible.

Nystagmus investigation generally requires quantitative data on the eye movement speed and amplitude. Simple observation is not adequate and quantitative eye movement recording apparatus is needed.

8.9.3   Cover test

The distance and near cover test should present no special difficulty.

8.9.4   Fixation disparity tests

Whilst fixation disparity tests are not easy for children, the task can be understood at this age if carefully explained. The Mallett unit is the technique of choice and this may be used for both distance and near. The amount of prism or sphere to correct a retinal slip (associated heterophoria) can be measured and this gives guidance as to the optimum over-minus or near addition required for any treatment regime. It is the non-dominant eye that usually shows the slip. Any sensory suppression can also be noted with the Mallett unit.

8.9.5   Amplitude of convergence

Convergence may be assessed at this age using conventional techniques, and at also this age the practitioner should assess the ability to maintain convergence. Both the near-point and jump convergence can be assessed.

8.9.6   AC/A ratio

The AC/A ratio is apparent from the effects of cycloplegia and the change in deviation at distance compared to near. It may be also be specifically measured using other techniques (see Chapter 5).

8.9.7   Fusional reserves

Fusional reserves can be measured from about six years of age using either a variable prism stereoscope or a phoropter.

8.9.8   Stereopsis

Adult levels of stereo acuity should be expected and the TNO, Frisby or Titmus tests may be used.

8.9.9　Sensory status

At this age further tests of binocularity and sensory status can be carried out. In the case of squint, Bagolini glasses or the Mallett unit can be used to investigate the presence of suppression or abnormal retinal correspondence. The use of a filter bar may be used to assess the depth of either. In the case of heterophoria, suppression at near can be investigated using the Mallett unit binocularity test and asking the child to read the letters or, failing that, count the number of letters on each line.

8.9.10　Refraction

If a previous refraction has been done under cycloplegia and the management is proceeding satisfactorily then further cycloplegia is not usually necessary on routine rechecks.

8.9.11　Refractive error

The normal refraction at this age is approximately emmetropic. Some children will start to develop myopia and for several years the refractive error may increase. Oculomotor balance needs to be reviewed at each subsequent recheck which might be required every six months or less.

8.9.12　Visual acuity

The Snellen chart, perhaps with a matching card, can be used to confirm the results of Sheridan–Gardiner, Cambridge crowding cards or other pediatric tests of visual acuity. Acuity should normally be 6/6 with each eye.

8.9.13　Ophthalmoscopy

A full ophthalmoscopic examination of the media and fundus should be possible.

8.10　References

Abrahamson, M., Fabian, G. and Sjöstrand, J. (1988) 'Changes in astigmatism between the ages of 1 and 4 years: a longitudinal study'. *Brit. J. Ophthalmol.*, **72**, 145–9.

Archer, S.M., Sondhi, N., and Helveston, E.M. (1989) 'Strabismus in infancy'. *Ophthalmology*, **96**, 133–7.

Aslin, R.N. (1977) 'Development of binocular fixation in human infants'. *J. Exptl. Child Psychol.*, **23**, 133–50

Aslin, R.N. and Jackson, R.W. (1979) 'Accommodative-convergence in young infants: Development of a synergistic sensory-motor system'. *Canad. J. Psychol.*, **33**, 222–31.

Atkinson, J., Anker, S., Evans, C., Hall, R. and Pimm-Smith, E. (1988) 'Visual acuity testing of young children with the Cambridge Crowding Cards at 3 m and 6 m'. *Acta Ophthalmologica*, **66**, 505–508.

Atkinson, J., Braddick, O., Durden, K., Watson, P.G. and Atkinson, S. (1984) 'Screening for refractive errors in 6–9 month old infants by photorefraction'. *Brit. J. Ophthalmol.*, **68**, 105–12.

Atkinson, J., Braddick, O. and French, J. (1980) 'Infant astigmatism: its disappearance with age'. *Vis. Res.*, **20**, 891–3.

Atkinson, J., Braddick, O., Wattam-Bell, J., Durden, K., Bobier, W., Pointer J. and Atkinson, S. (1987) 'Photorefractive screening of infants and effects of refractive correction'. *Invest. Ophthalmol. Vis. Sci. Suppl.*, **28**, 399.

Banks, M.S. (1980) 'Infant refraction and accommodation. Electrophysiology and psychophysics: their use in ophthalmic diagnosis'. *International Ophthalmology Clinics Vol. 20, No. 1*. (S. Sokol, ed.). Little Brown & Co., Boston.

Banks, M.S., Bennett, P.J. and Schefrin, B. (1989) 'Foveal cones and spatial vision in human neonates'. *Invest. Ophthalmol. Vis. Sci. Suppl.*, **30**, 4.

Banks, M.S. and Dannemiller, J.L. (1987) *Infant visual psychophysics. Handbook of infant perception Vol. I*. (P. Salapatek & L. Cohen, eds). Academic Press, New York.

Birch, E.E., Shimojo, S. and Held, R. (1985) 'Preferential-looking assessment of fusion and stereopsis in infants aged 1–6 months'. *Invest. Ophthalmol. Vis. Sci.*, **26**, 366–70.

Bobier, W.R. (1988) 'Quantitative photorefraction using an off centre flash source'. *Am. J. Optom. Physiol. Opt.*, **65**, 962–71.

Braddick, O. and Atkinson, J. (1984) 'Photorefractive techniques: applications in testing infants and young children'. *1st Int. Cong. Brit. Coll. Ophthal. Opticians Part II*, (Charman, ed.). WN, London (25–34).

Brodie, S.E. (1987) 'Photographic calibration of the Hirschberg test'. *Invest. Ophthalmol. Vis. Sci.*, **28**, 736–42.

Burian, H.M. and von Noorden, G.K. (1974) *Binocular Vision and Ocular Motility*. CV Mosby, St Louis.

Cantolino, S.J. and von Noorden, G.K. (1969) 'Heredity in microtropia'. *Arch. Ophthalmol.*, **81**, 753–7.

Ciner, E.B., Scheiman, M.M. and Schanel-Klitsch, E. (1989) 'Stereopsis testing in 18 to 35 month-old children using operant preferential looking'. *Optom. Vis. Sci.*, **66**, 782–7.

Cooper, J. and Feldman, J. (1978) 'Random-dot stereogram performance by strabismic, amblyopic and ocular-pathology patients in an operant-discrimination task'. *Amer. J. Optom. Physiol. Opt.*, **55**, 599–609.

Cooper, J. and Feldman, J. (1981) Depth perception in strabismus. *Brit. J. Ophthalmol.*, **65**, 510.

Cooper, J. and Warshovsky, J. (1977) 'Lateral displacement as a response cue in the Titmus stereo test'. *Am. J. Optom. Physiol. Opt.*, **54**, 537–41.

Crewther, D.P., Kelly, P.M., McCarthy, A. and Crewther, S.G. (1988) 'Evaluation of paraxial photorefraction in screening a population of monkeys for refractive error'. *Clin. Vision. Sci.*, **3**, 213–20.

Dobson, V. and Sebris, S.L. (1989) 'Longitudinal study of acuity and stereopsis in infants with or at-risk for esotropia'. *Invest. Ophthalmol. Vis. Sci.*, **30**, 1146–58.

Duke-Elder, S. (1973) *Ocular motility and Strabismus. System of Ophthalmology, Vol. VI*. Henry Kimpton, London.

Elliott, R. (1985) 'A new linear picture test'. *Brit. Orthopt. J.*, **42**, 54–7.

Fern, K.D. and Manny, R.E. (1986) 'Visual acuity of the pre-school child: a review'. *Amer.*

J. Optom. Physiol. Opt., **63**, 319–45.

Fern, K.D., Manny, R.E., Davis, J.R. and Gibson, R.R. (1986) 'Contour interaction in the per-school child'. *Amer. J. Optom. Physiol. Opt.*, **63**, 313–18.

Flom, M.C., Weymouth, F.W. and Kahneman, D. (1963) 'Visual resolution and contour interaction'. *J. Opt. Soc. Amer.*, **53**, 1026–32.

Fox, R., Aslin, R.N., Shea, S.L. and Dumais, S.T. (1980) 'Stereopsis in human infants'. *Science*, **207**, 323–4.

Fox, R., Patterson, R. and Francis, E.L. (1986) 'Stereoacuity in young children'. *Invest. Ophthalmol. Vis. Sci.*, **27**, 598–600.

Frisby, J.P., Nielsen, P. and Parker, J. (1981) 'Clinical tests of stereoacuity: do they measure the same thing?', in *Orthoptics: Research and Practice. Trans. 4th Int. Orthopt. Cong.* (J. Mein. & S. Moore, eds). Kimpton, London.

Fulton, A.B. (1989) 'Testing the possibly blind child', in *The Eye in Infancy* (S.J. Isenberg, ed.). Year Book Medical Publishers, London.

Fulton, A.B., Hanson, R.M. and Manning, K.A. (1981) 'Measuring visual acuity in infants'. *Survey Ophthalmol.*, **25**, 325–32.

Glickstein, M. and Millidot, M. (1970) 'Retinoscopy and eye size'. *Science*, **168**, 605–606.

Gruber, J. (1984) 'Examination of the young child (in 6 parts)'. *Optician*, **187**, 4949 June 22, 26–7; 4950 June 29, 14–17; 4958 Aug 24, 18–20; **188**, 4959 Aug 31, 12–14; 4962 Sept 21, 11–14; 4956 Oct 12, 10–12.

Gwiazda, J., Bauer, J., Thorn, F. and Held, R. (1986) 'Meridional amblyopia does result from astigmatism in early childhood'. *Clin. Vis. Sci.*, **1**, 145–52.

Gwiazda, J., Mohindra, I., Brill, S. and Held, R. (1985a) 'Infant astigmatism and meridional amblyopia'. *Vis. Res.*, **25**, 1269–76.

Gwiazda, J., Mohindra, I., Brill, S. and Held, R. (1985b) 'The development of visual acuity in infant astigmats'. *Invest. Ophthalmol. Vis. Sci.*, **26**, 1717–23.

Heron, G., Dholakia, S., Collins, D.E. and McLaughlin, H. (1985) 'Stereoscopic threshold in children and adults'. *Amer. J. Optom. Physiol. Opt.*, **62**, 505–15.

Hinchcliffe, H.A. (1978) 'Clinical evaluation of stereopsis'. *Brit. Orthopt. J.*, **35**, 46–7.

Howland, H.C. (1982) 'Optical techniques for detecting and improving deficient vision', in *Optics in Biomedical Sciences.* (G. von Bally & P. Greguss, eds). Springer-Verlag, Berlin.

Howland, H.C. (1985) 'Optics of photoretinoscopy: results from ray tracing'. *Amer. J. Optom. Physiol. Opt.*, **62**, 621–5.

Howland, H.C., Atkinson, J., Braddick, O. and French, J. (1978) 'Infant astigmatism measured by photorefraction'. *Science*, **202**, 331–3.

Howland, H.C., Braddick, O., Atkinson, J. and Howland, B. (1983) 'Optics of photorefraction: orthogonal and isotropic methods'. *J. Opt. Soc. Am.*, **73**, 1701–1708.

Howland, H.C. and Howland, B. (1974) 'Photorefraction: a technique for study of refractive state at a distance'. *J. Opt. Soc. Am.*, **64**, 240–49.

Howland, H.C. and Sayles, N. (1985) 'Photokeratometric and photorefractive measurements of astigmatism in infants and young children'. *Vis. Res.*, **25**, 73–81.

Hsu-Winges, C., Hamer, R.D., Norcia, A.M., Wesemann, H. and Chan, C. (1989) 'Polaroid photorefractive screening of infants'. *J. Paed. Ophthalmol. Strab.*, **26**, 254–60.

Ingram, R.M., Rogers, S. and Walker, C. (1977) 'Occlusion and amblyopia'. *Brit. Orthop. J.*, **34**, 11–22.

Ingram, R.M, Walker, C., Billingham, B., Lucas, J. and Dally, S. (1990) 'Factors relating to visual acuity in children who have been treated for convergent squint'. *Brit. J. Ophthalmol.*, **74**, 82–3.

Jay, B. and Elston, J. (1987) 'Genetic aspects of strabismus'. *Orthoptic horizons*, 11–14', in *Trans 6th Int. Orthopt. Cong.* (M. Lenk-Schafer, ed.), Harrogate.

Keith, C.G. and Kitchen, W.H. (1983) 'Ocular morbidity in infants of very low birth weight'. *Brit. J. Ophthalmol.*, **67**, 302–305.

Lang, J. (1984) 'The two-pencil test and the new Lang stereotest'. *Brit. Orthopt. J.*, **41**, 15–21.

Lennerstrand, G. and Gallo, J.E. (1989) 'Prevalence of refractive errors and ocular motility disorders in 5 to 10 year-old Swedish children born prematurely or at full-term'. *Acta Ophthalmol.*, **67**, 717–18.

Lepard, C.W. (1975) 'Comparative changes in error of refraction between fixing and amblyopic eyes during growth and development'. *Am. J. Ophthalmol.*, **80**, 485–90.

Levy, N.S. and Glick E.B. (1974) 'Stereoscopic perception and Snellen visual acuity'. *Am. J. Ophthalmol.*, **78**, 722–4.

Lyle, T.K. and Wybar, K.C. (1967) *Lyle and Jackson's practical orthoptics in the treatment of squint*, 5th edn. HK Lewis & Co. Ltd, London.

Mallett, R.F.J. (1964) 'The investigation of heterophoria at near and a new fixation disparity technique'. *Optician*, **148**, 547–51; 574–81.

Mallett, R.F.J. (1969) 'The sequelae of ocular muscle palsy'. *Ophthalmic Optician*, **9**, 920–3.

Mallett, R.F.J. (1983) 'A new fixation disparity test and its applications'. *Optician*, **186**, 11–15.

Mallett, R.F.J. (1988) 'Techniques of investigation of binocular vision anomalies'. Chapter 15, in *Optometry*. (Edwards & Llewellyn, eds). Butterworth, London.

Marg, E., Freeman, D.N., Peltzman, P. and Goldstein, P.J. (1976) 'Visual acuity development in human infants: evoked potential measurements'. *Invest. Ophthalmol. Vis. Sci.*, **15**, 150–3.

Mayer, D.L. and Dobson, V. (1982) 'Visual acuity development in infants and young children as assessed by operant preferential looking'. *Vis. Res.*, **22**, 1141–51.

Mitchell, D.E., Freeman, R.D., Millidot, M. and Haegerstrom, G. (1973) 'Meridional amblyopia: evidence for modification of the human visual system by early visual experience'. *Vis. Res.*, **13**, 535–58.

Mitchell, D.E. and Wilkinson, F. (1974) 'The effect of early astigmatism on the visual resolution of gratings'. *J. Physiol.*, **243**, 739–56.

Mohindra, I., Held, R., Gwiazda, J. and Brill, S. (1978) 'Astigmatism in infants'. *Science*, **202**, 329–31.

Morgan, M.W. (1960) 'Anomalies of the neuromuscular system of the ageing patient and their correction', in *Vision of the Ageing Patient*. Chilton Co., Philadelphia.

Naegle, J.R. and Held, R. (1982a) Development of optokinetic nystagmus and effects of abnormal visual experience during infancy. Spatially Orientated Behaviour (155–74). (Jeannerod & Hein, eds). Springer, New York.

Naegle, J.R. and Held, R. (1982b) 'The postnatal development of monocular optickinetic nystagmus in infants'. *Vis. Res.*, **22**, 341–6.

Nastri, G., Caccia Perugini, G., Savastano, S., Polzella, A. and Sborbone, G. (1984) 'The evolution of refraction in the fixing and the amblyopic eye'. *Doc. Ophthalmol.*, **56**, 265–74.

Nixon, R.B., Helveston, E.M., Miller, K., Archer, S.M. and Ellis, F.D. (1985) 'Incidence of strabismus in neonates'. *Am. J. Ophthalmol.*, **100**, 798–801.

Norcia, A.M. and Tyler, C.W. (1985) 'Spatial frequency sweep VEP: visual acuity during the first year of life'. *Vis. Res.*, **25**, 1339–408.

Paliaga, G.P. (1989) 'Validity, sensitivity and specificity of the (Hirschberg) corneal light reflection test in 390 patients'. *Binocular Vision*, **4**, 59–62.

Petrig, B., Julesz, B., Kropfl, W., Baumgartner, G. and Anliker, M. (1981) 'Development of stereopsis and cortical binocularity in human infants: electrophysiological evidence'. *Science*, **213**, 1402–1405.

Pott, J.W.R. and Van Hof-Van Duin, J. (1989) 'Visual function in very low birth weight children at 5 years of age'. *Ophthal. Physiol. Optics.*, **9**, 473.

Quick, M.W. and Boothe, R.G. (1989) 'Measurement of binocular alignment in normal monkeys and in monkeys with strabismus'. *Invest. Ophthalmol. Vis. Sci.*, **30**, 1159–68.

Reinecke, R.D. and Simons, K. (1974) 'A new stereoscopic test for amblyopia screening'. *Am. J. Ophthalmol.*, **78**, 714–21.

Rodier, D.W., Mayer, D.L. and Fulto, A.B. (1985) 'Assessment of young amblyopes – arrays vs single picture acuities'. *Ophthalmology*, **92**, 1197–202.

Romano, P.E., Romano, J.A. and Puklin, J.E. (1975) 'Stereoacuity development in children with normal binocular single vision'. *Am. J. Ophthalmol.*, **79**, 966–71.

Sarniguet-Bardouche, J.M. and Pincon, F. (1982) 'The prevalence of strabismus in children born of squinters', in *Paediatric Ophthalmology*. (J. Francois & M. Maione, eds). J. Wiley & Sons, Chichester (375–7).

Satterfield, D.S. (1989) 'Prevalence and variation of astigmatism in a military population'. *J. Amer. Optom. Assoc.*, **60**, 14–18.

Schor, C. and Narayan, V. (1981) 'The influence of field size upon the spatial frequency response of optokinetic nystagmus'. *Vis. Res.*, **21**, 985–94.

Shapiro, A., Yanko, L., Nawratski, I. and Merin, S. (1980) 'Refractive power of premature children at infancy and early childhood'. *Am. J. Ophthalmol.*, **90**, 234–8.

Shea, S.L., Doussard-Roosevelt, J.A. and Aslin, R.N. (1985) 'Pupillary measures of binocular luminance summation in infants and stereoblind adults'. *Invest. Ophthalmol. Vis. Sci.*, **26**, 1064–70.

Simons, K. and Reinecke, R.D. (1974) 'A reconsideration of amblyopia screening and stereopsis'. *Am. J. Ophthalmol.*, **78**, 707–13.

Slater, A.M. and Findlay, J.M. (1972) 'The measurement of fixation position in the newborn baby'. *J. Exptl. Child Psychol.*, **14**, 349–64.

Stidwill, D. (1985) 'The Lang stereopsis test'. *Optician*, **190**, 11 (No. 5009, Aug 23).

Stidwill, D. (1990) *Orthoptic Assessment and Management*. Blackwell Scientific Publications, Oxford.

Tallents, C.J. (1987) 'The child who appears not to see'. *Research and Clinical Forums*, 9, (**I**); *New Perspectives in Ophthalmology* (**V**), 7–13.

Thibos, L.N. and Levick, W.R. (1982) 'Astigmatic visual deprivation in cats: behavioural, optical and retinophysiological consequences'. *Vis. Res.*, **22**, 43–53.

Thomson, C. and Drasdo, N. (1988) 'Neonatal vision: changes in refraction and grating acuity in the first post natal week'. *Invest. Ophthalmol. Vis. Sci. Suppl.*, **29**, 138.

Van Hof-van Duin, J., Heerseman, D.J., Groenendaal, F., Baerts, W. and Fetter, W.P.F. (1989) 'Visual impairments in very low birth weight (VLBW) infants during the first year after term'. *Ophthal. Physiol. Opt.*, **9**, 468.

von Noorden, G.K. (1988) 'A reassessment of infantile esotropia. XLIV Edward Jackson Memorial Lecture'. *Am. J. Ophthalmol.*, **105**, 1–10.

Wagner, P. and Wearn, G. (1988) 'Instant photographic refractometry in children'. *Acta Ophthalmologica*, **66**, 165–9.

Walraven, J. (1975) 'Amblyopia screening with random-dot stereograms'. *Am. J. Ophthalmol.*, **80**, 893–900.

Wattam-Bell, J., Braddick, O., Atkinson, J. and Day, J. (1987) 'Measures of infant binocularity in a group at risk for strabismus'. *Clin. Vis. Sci.*, **1**, 327–36.

Westall, C.A., Woodhouse, J.M. and Brown, V.A. (1989) 'OKN asymmetries and binocular function in amblyopia'. *Ophthal. Physiol. Opt.*, **9**, 269–76.

Youdelis, C. and Hendrickson, A. (1986) 'A qualitative and quantitative analysis of the human fovea during development'. *Vis. Res.*, **26**, 847–55.

CHAPTER 9

The Optometric Investigation of Children with Dyslexia

Bruce Evans

9.1   Introduction

9.1.1   Definition

The World Federation of Neurology defined dyslexia (Critchley, 1970) as:

> A disorder manifested by difficulty in learning to read despite conventional instruction, adequate intelligence, and socio-cultural opportunity. It is dependent upon fundamental cognitive disabilities which are frequently of constitutional origin.

A good popular definition of specific reading difficulties or dyslexia is:

> . . . an unexpected problem in learning to read in children who seem otherwise capable and intelligent.

9.1.2   Terminology

The phrase specific learning difficulty is normally used as a generic term for those children who have specific difficulties in certain academic activities (i.e. their performance in these areas is not commensurate with their intelligence). Specific reading difficulty (dyslexia) is the most common type of specific learning difficulty (Helveston, 1987). Specific spelling difficulty is almost invariably associated with specific reading difficulty. This chapter will concentrate on dyslexia, although the conclusions might also apply to other forms of specific learning difficulty. A source of some confusion is that the term 'learning disabilities' is increasingly used, without the prefix 'specific', to describe individuals who might previously have been described as 'mentally retarded'.

There are many synonyms of dyslexia and these include specific reading disability, specific reading retardation, developmental dyslexia, specific developmental dyslexia, and strephosymbolia. These terms are normally only used when there is a fairly severe degree of reading difficulty. A criterion that is often adopted is that the child should be behind in reading by 18 months or more. Less intelligent children would generally not be expected to read as well as the more intelligent. Hence, any quantification of reading difficulty usually takes account of the child's IQ (intelligence quotient), or of some other measure of performance (such as listening comprehension). Although this method of diagnosing dyslexia as a discrepancy between aptitude and achievement has been questioned (Stanovich, 1991), there is considerable evidence supporting this method and it is still widely used in the clinical field. It should be stressed that children do not need to have a high IQ to be dyslexic: they simply need to be worse at reading than one would expect from their general performance at tasks which are independent of reading skill.

Some authorities disapprove of the label 'dyslexic', preferring the terms specific reading difficulty or specific learning difficulty; others feel equally strongly that the term dyslexia is most appropriate for this condition. It is sometimes wrongly claimed that children are dyslexic when they are poor achievers across the board, possibly owing to low intelligence. However, optometrists can be reasonably sure of a diagnosis if they find that a psychologist has described the child as having dyslexia (or a synonym of this condition).

9.1.3 Prevalence of dyslexia

Many estimates suggest that dyslexia occurs in 4–10% of all children (Rutter, 1978; Yule, 1988). The prevalence of dyslexia amongst children consulting an optometrist is probably higher than this, since dyslexic children may be more likely to seek primary eye care. Hence, optometrists would be well advised to enquire about the reading performance of all children they see. Estimates for the prevalence of a visual component of the dyslexia vary enormously from zero (Brown, 1988) to 60–70% (Stein & Fowler, 1985).

More boys than girls suffer from dyslexia. This implies that there may be a genetic component to dyslexia and there is some evidence to support this notion (Pennington & Smith, 1983). Some recent research has argued that dyslexia is equally common in the two genders and has suggested that dyslexia is not a specific condition but simply represents the tail-end of a normal distribution of reading performance (Shaywitz *et al.*, 1992). However, this finding has itself been questioned (Miles *et al.*, 1994).

9.1.4 Correlates of dyslexia

It has been known for some time that there are factors or problems that are more likely to be present in a dyslexic population than in a non-dyslexic (control) population. In other words, these factors are correlates of dyslexia. This does not imply that they will always be present in a dyslexic person and does not necessarily mean that these factors are a cause of the reading difficulty.

Most of the correlates of dyslexia do not relate to vision but are psychometric correlates that are best measured by a psychologist. These include poor short-term memory, difficulty with decoding, poor rhyming skills, defective planning skills, confused or mixed laterality, and difficulties with sequential tasks (Miles & Miles, 1990). Some of these psychological correlates represent skills that are important components of the reading process (e.g. short-term memory and decoding) and are likely to be causally related to the reading difficulty. In addition to these psychometric correlates there are a few optometric correlates of dyslexia. These will be described in more detail below, but it should be noted that most authorities think these are of less causal significance than the psychological correlates (Critchley, 1981; Hulme, 1988).

9.1.5   Etiology of dyslexia

There are many theories concerning the cause of dyslexia and it is likely that this condition is heterogeneous. Recent anatomical and electrophysiological research has addressed the structure and function of the brain in dyslexia (Hynd & Semrud-Clikeman, 1989). This suggests that there may be very slight abnormalities of cerebral organization in dyslexia and there may be subtle lesions at several focal sites, mainly in the left cerebral cortex. Not all of these sites are affected in all dyslexic people and the pattern of lesions varies greatly from one individual to another.

Possibly the functions that are sometimes abnormal in dyslexia may be associated with the cortical areas where subtle focal lesions have been found. Hence, recent research could provide a model with an anatomical basis for dyslexia being a 'syndrome of difficulties', most of which contribute to poor reading and only some of which are present in a given dyslexic individual.

One such hypothesis suggests that these lesions might occur during fetal development and it could just be coincidence that many of these lesions impair functions that are important for reading. If this model is correct, then not all of the correlates of dyslexia need necessarily be a cause of the poor reading. A child who had been diagnosed as dyslexic might be expected to have several of the psychometric problems that can contribute to poor reading, and treatment of a visual problem should not be expected, therefore, to cure their reading difficulty. It should also be stressed that the anatomical findings described above are extremely subtle and that ascribing a functional corollary to them is speculative.

9.1.6   The Education Acts (England and Wales)

It is generally recognized that the most important therapy for dyslexia is individualized, structured teaching appropriate to the child's needs (Miles &

Miles, 1991). The Education Act 1981 set about integrating most children with special educational needs into the ordinary classroom. Dyslexia is generally accepted to represent a special educational need (SEN). The Education Act 1988 placed an obligation on Local Education Authorities to secure that adequate provision is made for all children with SEN.

The Education Act 1993 set time-scales for a staged procedure starting with the identification of a problem by teachers (Stage 1), and progressing through degrees of increasing support by teaching staff from inside (Stage 2) and outside (Stage 3) the school. If the Local Education Authority considers it appropriate, it may arrange for a multidisciplinary assessment (Stage 4). It seems unfortunate that this assessment does not usually, at present, include the opinion of an optometrist. The assessment may culminate in a Statement (Stage 5) of the child's strengths and weaknesses which makes recommendations for the child's future education. Parents have the right of appeal to a SEN tribunal if they have trouble obtaining or maintaining an assessment or statement, or if they are unhappy with the choice of school in a statement.

Unfortunately, this system rarely seems to work as well as it ought to. In many areas the authorities seem very reluctant to recognize specific learning difficulties, possibly to avoid extra demands on limited resources. This means that sometimes only those dyslexic children with articulate and persistent parents receive the extra help that they are entitled to. Parents can obtain information on their rights, and support, from the British Dyslexia Association and from the Dyslexia Institute whose addresses can be found at the end of this chapter. Information on the Education Acts in Scotland can also be obtained from the Dyslexia Institute.

Professional investigation and remediation of dyslexic individuals is also available through the Dyslexia Institute. This organization has local institutes throughout the country where appropriately qualified psychologists carry out private assessments. These assessments are very thorough and usually result in a report, suggesting appropriate action (normally extra teaching, but sometimes also suggesting an eye examination). Specialist teaching is also available at the dyslexia institutes. The investigation and remediation of dyslexia is time-consuming and this approach can, therefore, be expensive. If appropriate, an educational or child psychologist can recommend that a child is allowed extra time in examinations.

9.2   Optometric correlates of dyslexia

9.2.1   Introduction

In addition to the psychometric correlates of dyslexia, the research literature suggests that there may also be optometric correlates of dyslexia. However, for most of these visual factors, any causal relationship with the dyslexia is unclear. Furthermore, many dyslexic people do not have such visual problems and many people with the same visual problems are not dyslexic. There is little reason to believe that special criteria should be applied in deciding whether or not to treat visual problems in dyslexic people.

The following review of these optometric correlates is a brief summary of the considerable literature on this subject. The literature is reviewed in more detail by Evans and Drasdo (1990, 1991), Grisham and Simons (1990) and in depth by Evans (1991). Only references that are particularly pertinent, or do not appear in the preceding reviews, will be cited here.

The optometric correlates of dyslexia form a problematical area to research and the literature can be difficult to interpret for several reasons. First, the correlates of dyslexia are numerous: 'it would be difficult to find a task on which reading-disabled children have not been reported to be deficient' (Benton, 1978). This must diminish the significance of each correlate when taken individually. Second, the diagnosis of dyslexia should be made carefully, preferably by a psychologist. Third, research looking for correlates, or at the effect of treatment, must include adequate controls. Usually, this necessitates a control group which is matched for age (or reading age), sex, socio-cultural background, educational opportunity, and intelligence. Finally, any results must be supported by appropriate statistical analysis.

9.2.2 Refractive errors and accommodative dysfunction in dyslexia

Refractive errors

Although distance visual acuity does not appear to be highly correlated with dyslexia, there is some evidence suggesting a slightly increased prevalence of hypermetropia in the reading disabled. Normal clinical criteria should be applied in deciding whether to carry out a cycloplegic refraction and in deciding whether to correct a hyperopic refractive error.

Accommodation

A reduced amplitude of accommodation seems to be unusually common in dyslexic children (Evans *et al.*, 1994a); this can be detected by conventional techniques. As with all tests of ocular motor performance, it may be most appropriate to make this measurement when the child is fatigued. For example, this test could be repeated at the end of the examination, after a day at school, or after the child has been reading for some time in the waiting room.

The accommodative lag can be measured by retinoscopy using the monocular estimate method (Cooper, 1987). The subject binocularly fixates a detailed target on the retinoscope and is asked to keep this clear. Retinoscopy is carried out along the horizontal meridian and lenses are very briefly held in front of each eye to neutralize the retinoscope reflex. Each lens should only be present for a split second so as not to disrupt the status of the patient's accommodative and binocular response. The accommodative lag is usually about $+0.75\,\text{D}$ and values greater than $+1.25\,\text{D}$ may represent accommodative insufficiency. If a negative lens is required to neutralize the reflex this suggests that accommodative spasm is occurring. This test may give useful additional information when there is a low amplitude of accommodation, and with uncooperative patients.

A third aspect of accommodative function that can be assessed clinically (Cooper, 1987) is the accommodative facility (the rate at which the accommodation can be changed). A binocular twirl ('flipper') is used comprising two pairs of lenses (usually $+2.00\,\text{DS}$ and $-2.00\,\text{DS}$). (These are available from Paul Adler Optometry, 50 High Street, Stotfold, Herts., SG5 4LL.) The patient fixates a near target and his stimulus to accommodate is varied by twirling the lenses. After each change of the stimulus the patient reports as soon as the target becomes clear, when the stimulus is immediately changed again; the number of cycles that can be achieved in a given time is recorded. The literature on the relationship between accommodative facility and asthenopic symptoms is equivocal.

9.2.3   Binocular vision dysfunction and dyslexia

Amplitude of convergence

A reduced amplitude of convergence is frequently associated with dyslexia and some dyslexic children demonstrate poor convergence of a degree that would be expected to cause symptoms.

Usually, a near point of convergence (NPC) that is more remote than $6-10\,\text{cm}$ (Lyle & Wybar, 1979) would be considered for treatment, and such patients should be questioned carefully about any asthenopia during near visual tasks. If this is present, then convergence exercises should be prescribed. Most dyslexic children are intelligent and highly motivated, and respond well to orthoptic therapy.

The type of convergence exercises that are prescribed are very much a matter of personal preference. Some authorities prefer ramp (push-up) methods where a near target is gradually brought closer (Stidwill, 1990); others favour step (jump) techniques where the patient alternately fixates a distant and near (just outside the NPC) target. Alternatively, exercises based on physiological diplopia can be used (Pickwell, 1989). It is important to choose exercises that the child can understand and about which the practitioner is enthusiastic.

Heterophoria

Heterophorias of all types at near have been reported as correlates of dyslexia. These conditions can be treated with exercises or by prismatic therapy. It is only necessary to treat a heterophoria if it is likely to break down into a strabismus or if it is producing symptoms. In dyslexia, the situation is complicated because the children often report symptoms that may or may not result from a heterophoria. It is unlikely that any one clinical test can diagnose a symptomatic heterophoria in all cases (Sheedy & Saladin, 1983). A fixation disparity test with a good fusional lock may be the best diagnostic tool (Mallett, 1983; Jenkins *et al.*, 1989; Yekta *et al.*, 1989) and an assessment of vergence reserves can also be useful (Pickwell, 1989). Synonyms for vergence reserves (Stidwill, 1990) include: relative vergences, although this phrase is sometimes used to refer to the blur point only; fusional reserves, an undesirable term owing to ambiguity over motor or sensory fusion; fusion amplitudes, also potentially confusing since amplitudes are sometimes used to refer to the difference between positive and negative break points; and binocular ductions (Solomons, 1978), although this term no longer seems to be in common use. Pickwell (1989) preferred the term prism vergences, although this may be criticized since the measurement can be made without varying the prism (e.g. with a synoptophore).

Foveal suppression may develop as a compensatory mechanism to minimize symptoms from a decompensated heterophoria (Pickwell, 1989; Sucher, 1991). This can be detected using the polarized latters on a near Mallett Unit (Mallett, 1988). Stereopsis tests may be useful in identifying accommodative and binocular vision dysfunction, but these should be very sensitive, preferably measuring to 20″. Conventional clinical stereopsis tests may not detect transient or dynamic ocular motor anomalies.

Heterotropia

Stable uni-ocular strabismus is not especially likely to occur in dyslexia, although an alternating deviation may be particularly common. An alternating strabismus could result in unstable perception of print, and can sometimes be treated with eye exercises or by occlusion (Fowler & Stein, 1983). Care should be taken in giving occlusion therapy to a young person with an alternating strabismus, since this could lead to a permanent strabismus in one eye with associated amblyopia.

Binocular instability

Binocular instability is a term that conventionally has been used to describe an unstable heterophoria and reduced vergence reserves resulting in difficulty compensating for a heterophoria (Gibson, 1955; Giles, 1960). Both base in and base out vergence reserves are often reduced in dyslexia (Evans *et al.*, 1994a), as is the vergence amplitude (the difference between the convergent and divergent break-points). A low vergence amplitude represents a reduced ability to converge or diverge the eyes away from their natural resting point. This may explain why various authors have held contradictory views on the type of heterophoria which is important in dyslexia. The vergence reserves opposing a heterophoria are an important factor in determining a person's ability to compensate for a heterophoria. Hence, it may not be the heterophoria that is unusual in dyslexia but rather the reduced vergence reserves (Evans *et al.*, 1994a).

Therefore, it is useful to measure vergence reserves at near in dyslexic children. These can be measured using binocular rotary prisms (on a refractor head or in a trial frame) while the patient fixates fine print at near. The reserve opposing the heterophoria should be measured first (Rosenfield *et al.*, 1995). The prisms should be altered smoothly at the rate of about 1Δ per second. Divergent reserves to diplopia (the break point) should be at least 12Δ and convergent reserves 14Δ. In particular, the vergence reserve opposing the heterophoria should be at least twice the heterophoria. Low reserves should be treated if they occur together with asthenopic symptoms or if the heterophoria is likely to break down to a strabismus. Inadequate vergence reserves usually respond well to vergence exercises (described above). A prism bar can be used to measure vergence reserves, although the norms for this technique may be different from those with rotary prisms.

Another sign of binocular instability that can often be seen in dyslexia is an unstable heterophoria, signifying that the control of the binocular alignment of the eyes may be unstable. This can be detected by excessive movement of the arrow in the Maddox wing test or as an unstable exo- and/or eso-slip on the Mallett unit. If an underlying binocular vision problem can be detected (e.g. fixation disparity or low vergence reserves) treatment of this may render any binocular instability subclinical.

Binocular vision problems are sometimes associated with asthenopia (Yekta *et al.*, 1989) and may, therefore, discourage a child from reading and thus *indirectly* contribute to a reading problem. However, there is very little evidence to suggest that binocular anomalies are major *direct* causes of dyslexia by resulting in an unstable perception of print; many people with severe binocular anomalies read quite normally. Although it is good clinical practice to treat a binocular vision problem when it is associated with symptoms, or is likely to break down into a strabismus, the treatment of subtle binocular anomalies in other cases is hard to justify from the research literature.

9.2.4   Ocular dominance and the Dunlop test

Historically, there have been many theories concerning crossed dominance or unstable ocular dominance in dyslexia, and this area has attracted considerable controversy. One reason may be that various tests of ocular dominance measure different functions. There are three basic categories of ocular dominance: sighting, sensory, and motor. Even within each of these categories, different tests of ocular dominance are likely to produce different results in a given person. Most authorities now agree that atypical sighting dominance is not a factor in dyslexia (Evans, 1991).

The Dunlop test

Interest in this area has been revived in recent years by a new test of ocular dominance called the Dunlop test. Research using the Dunlop test has been extensively published (e.g. Stein & Fowler, 1985) and optometrists in the UK are often asked about this test.

In the Dunlop test the eyes are diverged to induce a fixation disparity, and the eye in which the fixation disparity occurs is said to be the non-dominant or non-referent eye. In theory, this is a sensitive test of motor ocular dominance that may be more relevant to dyslexia than sighting tests of ocular dominance. Importance is not attached to which eye is the referent eye, but rather to the stability of the dominance. The Dunlop test is usually repeated 10 times, and if the same eye is the referent eye 8 or more times out of 10 then the dominance is said to be 'stable'. Any other result is described as 'an unstable reference eye', with the worst result occurring when each eye is the referent one 5 times out of 10. A synoptophore is usually used for the Dunlop test, but Evans *et al.* (1992) found that a modified procedure employing a near Mallett unit can be employed.

It has been claimed that an unstable referent eye is a sign of 'poor visuomotor control' and that this is a cause of the reading problem in two-thirds of dyslexic children and can be treated by occluding one eye for up to 6 months for all reading and writing. Some research has shown that this treatment establishes the uncovered eye as the referent eye and that this leads to a scholastic improvement. However, there is considerable debate over the validity and significance of these results (Bishop, 1989). The Dunlop test is a difficult test, and the results are likely to be influenced more by the child's intelligence and responsiveness than by any visual parameter (Bishop *et al.*, 1979; Evans *et al.*, 1994a). Hence, it may be unwise to base a treatment on this controversial test.

9.2.5   The use of tinted lenses in dyslexia

The Irlen therapy

It has been stated that 50% of dyslexic individuals have a visual perceptual dysfunction that can be treated with tinted lenses (Irlen & Lass, 1989). The second person to describe this condition in detail Helen Irlen, and she called it 'scotopic sensitivity syndrome'. The meaning of this description is unclear and 'Meares-Irlen syndrome' may be a better term. People who suffer from this syndrome are said to report a range of anomalous visual effects when they view text, such as illusions of shape, motion, and colour. Irlen has claimed that these effects can be ameliorated with tinted lenses that have been individually pre-scribed, manufactured, and supplied through her organization. The literature reveals considerable controversy over this therapy and this has been fuelled by a lack of rigorously controlled scientific studies (Evans & Drasdo, 1991).

It seems likely that in some cases these tinted lenses merely act as a placebo. However, some children and adults continue using tinted lenses for many years and certain cases seem to derive a considerable benefit from this therapy. This has led many to believe that individually prescribed tinted lenses represent a breakthrough in the treatment of specific learning difficulties.

Potential mechanisms for a benefit from coloured filters when reading

There are several potential theoretical explanations for a benefit from tinted lenses (Evans & Drasdo, 1991). Some authorities have suggested that this therapy helps reduce asthenopia associated with binocular anomalies, although this would not account for the highly specific nature of the optimal tint. A more feasible explanation may relate to 'pattern glare' (Wilkins et al., 1984). If the striped pattern in Fig. 9.1 is viewed (in focus) at a distance of about 23 cm the observer may experience asthenopia or may see illusions of shape, motion, and colour; this is pattern glare. Lines of text can have spatial properties that might cause pattern glare and this could account for a benefit from tinted lenses (this potential mechanism is described in detail by Wilkins, 1995).

Optometric management

Wilkins has developed an 'intuitive colorimeter' (Wilkins et al., 1992) and technique of 'precision tinting' (Wilkins et al., 1992) which allows the precise prescription of person's preferred tinted lens to be accurately specified and reliably reproduced. (This system is available from Cerium Visual Technologies, Cerium Technology Park, Appledore Road, Tenterden, Kent, TN30 7DE.)

A double-masked placebo-controlled trial has shown that some children who

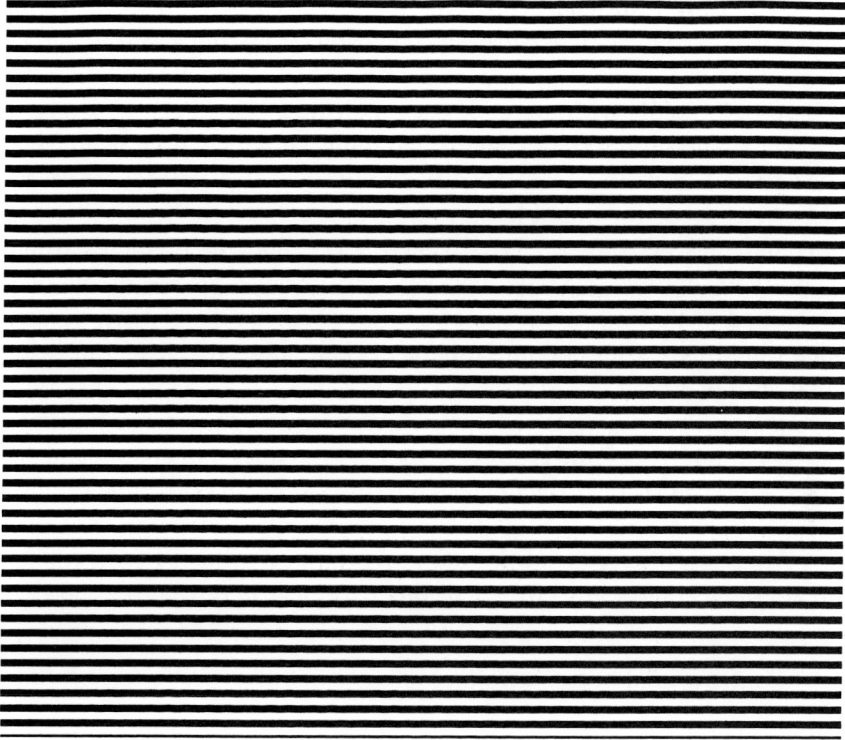

Fig. 9.1 A grating which may cause pattern glare when viewed from about 23 cm.
DO NOT STARE AT THIS FIGURE IF YOU SUFFER FROM EPILEPSY OR MIGRAINE.

report anomalous visual effects and asthnopia during reading do experience a reduction of asthenopic symptoms with a tinted lens of their preferred colour. This benefit reduced significantly if they were given a colour that was very slightly different from their optimal one, even if they did not know which was their preferred colour. Hence, the benefit from tinted lenses in this study was not solely attributable to a placebo effect (Wilkins *et al.*, 1994). The children who request tinted lenses tend to manifest the optometric correlates of dyslexia outlined above (Evans *et al.*, 1995a); but these optometric factors do not appear to be the reason for the benefit from coloured lenses. There may be a common underlying mechanism which accounts for both the ocular motor factors and for the benefit from coloured lenses (Wilkins, 1995).

One potential problem is that many dyslexic children may choose to try tinted lenses simply as a placebo. This may be why the British College of Optometrists has advised that children with the symptoms of Meares-Irlen syndrome, once any clinically significant conventional optometric anomalies have been treated, should be screened with coloured overlays. A representative range of coloured overlays can be obtained inexpensively (available from IOO Marketing Ltd., 56–62 Newington Causeway, London, SE1 6DS; 0171 378 0330) and patients can be screened rapidly with these. Those reporting a benefit can be issued with an overlay of their preferred colour, and only those children who show a sustained benefit from this (continued voluntary use after about a school term) should be considered for tinted lenses.

The colour of a person's preferred tinted lens cannot be predicted from the colour of their optimal overlay; nor can the optimal colour of an overlay be determined with the intuitive colorimeter. With adults it may be safe to prescribe tinted lenses simply on the basis of their subjective response, without screening with overlays.

Tinte lenses, like any other optometric intervention, should not be expected to 'cure' a reading problem. However, they may reduce asthenopia and hence encourage a person to read for longer (Wilkins *et al.*, 1994). It should also be noted that there is only one double-masked placebo-controlled trial of this therapy. Although the results of this are positive, they will need to be replicated by similar studies before the efficacy of this treatment is proven beyond doubt.

9.2.6   Controversial optometric therapies

In recent years some optometrists (mainly in the USA) have become involved in a series of controversial optometric therapies, sometimes described as develop-mental vision therapy. This seems to be based on a philosophy of 'behavioural optometry' which postulates that training can improve visual information pro-cessing in individuals who do not appear to have a specific (conventional) ocular or vision defect (Gilman, 1990).

Although there has been some support in the literature for these therapies (Cohen *et al.*, 1988), many authorities have criticized them and the lack of rigorous research to support the protagonists' claims (Keogh, 1974; Pierce, 1977; Beauchamp, 1986). One recent review concluded that 'the results of the preponderance of controlled studies in the research literature have been negative or inconclusive' (Grisham & Simons, 1990). The placebo effect can be very large (Evans, 1992) and, as with the Irlen therapy, practitioners have a professional obligation to counsel their patients on the basis of the results of controlled scientific investigations rather than anecdotal observations.

9.2.7   Eye movements and dyslexia

During reading the eyes proceed along a line in a series of step-like saccades, which are separated by 'fixation pauses' (Fig. 9.2). During the fixation pauses, information is acquired from the relevant section of text; the width of this

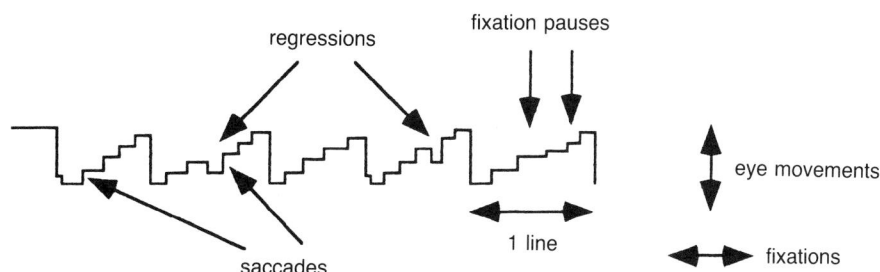

Fig. 9.2 Schematic illustration of eye movements during reading. Further details are given in the text.

section, normally measured in the number of letters, is termed the perceptual span. At the end of a line the eyes make a large saccade, or return sweep. Most of the other saccades are in a left-to-right direction, but occasionally one is made in the opposite direction to return to previously read text, usually for cognitive reasons; these latter are called regressions. Reading of more complicated, less comprehensible, text is normally associated with an increase in the number of regressions and fixations and a decrease in the perceptual span and speed of reading.

Research suggests that dyslexic children make an increased number of fixations, particularly regressions, when reading. These findings may be linked to the reading difficulty in three ways: they could be the cause of the dyslexia; they may be caused by the reading problem; or they could be the result of a higher-level problem that also, through another mechanism, causes the reading difficulty (e.g. a sequencing problem). These questions can, to some extent, be investigated by studying the eye movements during simple, non-verbal, tasks. Although the results of studies using this paradigm are equivocal, most workers have not found abnormal non-reading saccadic eye movement in dyslexia (Evans & Drasdo, 1990). The evidence, therefore, supports the tentative conclusion that abnormal reading eye movements in dyslexia are usually the result of cognitive difficulties with text.

Attempts have been made to develop simple subjective tests of saccadic function; one of these is the developmental eye movement test. This test seems to be based on the questionable assumption that saccadic dysfunction would interfere with horizontal but not vertical eye movements. The test results also seem to be confounded by the effects of intelligence (Garzia *et al.*, 1990).

Eye movements and binocular instability

It is sometimes difficult to decide whether binocular vision problems are linked to symptoms in dyslexia. Further, it has been noted that the presence of normal binocular vision during static viewing (e.g. when looking at a fixation disparity unit) does not necessarily mean that binocular function is normal under dynamic conditions (e.g. as the eyes are moving when reading). Methods are available for objectively recording eye movements whilst reading and it has been suggested that these techniques could be used clinically to look for vergence drifts during reading. This information might help in deciding whether to treat a subtle binocular anomaly.

Whilst this may prove to be a useful investigative tool, there are some limitations that should be borne in mind. Eye movement apparatus that is affordable usually uses infra-red light and a photocell to detect changes in reflectivity from the movement of the limbus (or sometimes one or more Purkinje images). To assess subtle binocular anomalies the apparatus should be able to reliably and repeatably detect vergence drifts of less than 5 minutes of arc (Mallett, 1988). Although manufacturers of eye movement equipment sometimes claim this order of sensitivity under ideal test conditions, this may not be achievable with a child in a clinical environment. Additional errors may result from difficulties of calibration and from translation of the globe during eye movements.

More research is needed to validate these clinical tools. In the meantime, it may be unwise to diagnose a binocular anomaly on the basis of clinical eye movement recording. However, eye movement analysis may be able to play a useful role in the further investigation of a binocular anomaly that has been detected by more conventional means.

9.2.8　　A defect of the transient visual subsystem in dyslexia

Parallel visual processing

Visual perception (in photopic conditions) is believed to operate through two visual subsystems, the transient and sustained systems. The sustained subsystem is relatively slow, does not respond well to moving or flickering stimuli, but does respond well to stationary fine detail, particularly in the central visual field. The transient subsystem responds optimally to flickering or moving stimuli, does not respond well to fine detail, and tends to relate more to peripheral vision. These subsystems are not completely separate since they interact with one another; they are also able to suppress (inhibit) one another. Recent research suggests that up to 70% of dyslexic individuals have a defect of the transient visual system (Lovegrove *et al.*, 1986).

The reading process

During reading each fixation pause lasts for about a quarter of a second, which is long enough for the information from a perceptual span of about 6 letters to be assimilated. The eyes then make a saccade to the next group of letters.

The image formation during a fixation is thought to be mediated via the sustained visual pathway. The characteristics of this system mean that the image will only fade slowly after the fixation has ended, so that the image could persist into the next fixation. This might be expected to cause a superimposition of subsequent images. This undesirable consequence is thought to be prevented by inhibition from the transient visual system. During a saccade the transient system is stimulated (by movement of the visual image across the retina), and this is thought to inhibit the sustained image (see Fig. 9.3).

In other words, during a fixation an image is formed by the sustained system, rather like writing on a slate; during the following saccade the transient system wipes this slate clean so that a new sustained image can be formed at the next fixation. It has been suggested, therefore, that a transient system deficit in dyslexia may result in visual confusion from a superimposition of subsequent sustained images during reading. It should be noted, however, that the preceding explanation is a theoretical model that awaits experimental validation.

Although it is unclear whether the transient deficit could be detected or

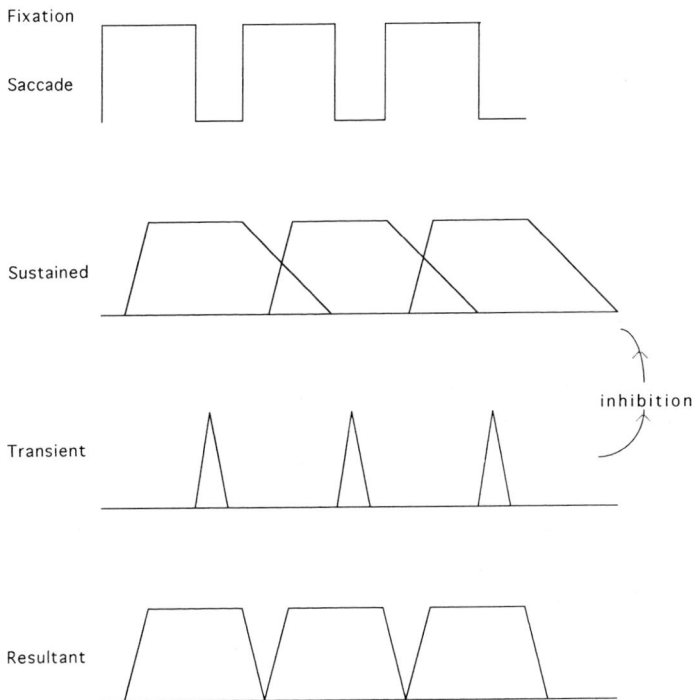

Fig. 9.3 The hypothetical response of the transient and sustained subsystems for three consecutive fixations and saccades during reading (modified with permission from Breitmeyer, 1980).

treated by the optometrist, recent research has suggested that it may be linked to binocular and accommodative dysfunction in dyslexia (Evans *et al.*, 1994a, 1994b, and 1995b). It is possible that the research on the transient system deficit may provide a unifying explanation of the visual correlates of dyslexia.

9.3   Conclusions

Dyslexia is an unexpected problem with reading and, although its causes are not fully known, visual problems are unlikely to be the main cause. However, several optometric problems are more likely to be present in dyslexia and these include poor accommodation and binocular instability (low vergence reserves and an unstable heterophoria), and possibly hypermetropia, poor convergence, and exophoria at near. Normal clinical criteria should be applied in deciding whether to treat these problems. It has been claimed that a test of motor ocular dominance (the Dunlop test) detects binocular instability in dyslexia. This assertion is controversial and the Dunlop test has been found to be unreliable.

It has been claimed that some dyslexic children may benefit from the use of tinted lenses and a recent double-masked placebo-controlled trial supports this claim. Replication and further research is required to study the mechanism for this benefit and the proportion of individuals who can be helped in this way. More research is also needed on controversial optometric therapies and to investigate the role of binocular eye movement recording in dyslexia.

There is considerable evidence for a sensory visual correlate of dyslexia in the form of a deficit of the transient visual subsystem. There are no clinical tests or treatment regimens based on this, but recent research suggests that this is linked to the binocular dysfunction in dyslexia.

People with specific learning difficulties are best helped a multidisciplinary team. Ideally this team should be headed by a child or educational psychologist, but the optometrist should be an important member of the team. Written reports describing optometric findings, even when no abnormalities are detected, will aid the patient, will lead to more referrals, and will help to increase awareness of the role of the optometrist in the community.

9.4   References and bibliography

Beauchamp, G.R. (1986) 'Optometric vision training'. *Pediat.*, **77**, 121–4.

Benton A. (1978) 'Some conclusions about dyslexia', in *Dyslexia, an Appraisal of Current Knowledge*. (A.L. Benton & D. Pearl eds). Oxford University Press, New York (453–476).

Bishop, D.V.M. (1989) 'Unfixed reference, monocular occlusion, and developmental dyslexia – a critique'. *Brit. J. Ophthalmology.*, **73**, 209–15.

Bishop, D.V.M., Jancey, C. and Mc P. Steel, A. (1979) 'Orthoptic status and reading disability'. *Cortex*, **15**, 659–66.

Borish, I.M. (1975) *Clinical Refraction*. The Professional Press Inc., Chicago.

Breitmeyer, B.G. (1980) 'Unmasking visual masking: a look at the "why" behind the veil of "how"'. *Psychological Review*, **87**, 52–69.

Brown, G.D.A. (1988) 'Cognitive analysis of dyslexia'. *Perception*, **17**, 695–8.

Buzzelli, A.R. (1991) 'Stereopsis, accommodative and vergence facility: do they relate to dyslexia?'. *Optom. Vis. Sci.*, **68**, No. 11, 842–6.

Cohen, A.H., Lowe, S.E., Steele, G.T., Suchoff, I.B., Gottlieb, D.D. and Trevorrow, T.L. (1988) 'The efficacy of optometric vision training'. *J. Am. Optom. Assoc.*, **59**, 95–105.

Cooper, J. (1987) 'Accommodative dysfunction', in *Diagnosis and management in vision care*. (J.F. Amos, ed.). Butterworth, London, 431–59.

Critchley, M. (1970) *The Dyslexic Child*. Thomas, Springfield, Illinois.

Critchley, M. (1981) 'Dyslexia: an overview', in *Dyslexia Research and its Application to Education*. (G. Th. Pavlidis & T.H. Miles, eds). Wiley & Sons, Chichester, 1–12.

Evans, B.J.W. (1991) 'Ophthalmic Factors in Dyslexia'. PhD Thesis, Aston University, Birmingham, U.K., pp. 110–50 (Available from the British College of Optometrists Library).

Evans, B.J.W. (1992) 'Academy Europe conference report'. *Optician*, 28 August.

Evans, B.J.W., Busby, A., Jeanes, R., Wilkins, A.J. (1995a) 'Optometric correlates of Meares-Irlen syndrome: a matched group study'. *Ophthal. Physiol. Opt.* **15** (in press).

Evans, B.J.W. and Drasdo, N. (1990) 'Review of ophthalmic factors in dyslexia'. *Ophthal. Physiol. Opt.*, **10**, 123–32.

Evans, B.J.W. and Drasdo, N. (1991) 'Tinted lenses and related therapies for learning disabilities – a review'. *Ophthal. Physiol. Opt.*, **11**, 206–17.

Evans, B.J.W., Drasdo, N. and Richards, I.L. (1992) 'An investigation of the optometric correlates of reading disability'. *Clin. Exper. Optom.*, **75**, No. 5, 15–23.

Evans, B.J.W., Drasdo, N. and Richards, I.L. (1994a) 'Investigation of accommodative and binocular function in dyslexia'. *Ophthal. Physiol. Opt.* **14**, No. 1, 5–19.

Evans, B.J.W., Drasdo, N. and Richards, I.L. (1994b) 'An investigation of some sensory and refractive visual factors in dyslexia'. *Vis. Res.*, **34**, No. 14, 1913–26.

Evans, B.J.W., Drasdo, N. and Richards, I.L. (1995b) 'Dyslexia: the link with visual deficits'. *Ophthal. Physiol. Opt.*

Fowler, M.S. and Stein, J.F. (1983) 'Consideration of ocular motor dominance as an aetiological factor in some orthoptic problems'. *Brit. Orth. J.*, **40**, 43–5.

Galaburda, A.M. (1990) 'The testosterone hypothesis: assessment since Geschwind and Behan, 1982'. *Annals Dyslexia*, **40**, 18–36.

Garzia, R.P., Richman, J.E., Nicholson, S.B. and Gaines, C.S. (1990) 'A new visual-verbal saccadic test: the Developmental Eye Movement test (DEM)'. *J. Am. Optom. Assoc.*, **61**, 124–35.

Gibson, H.W. (1955) *Textbook of Orthoptics*. Hatton Press Ltd., London.

Giles, G.H. (1960) *The Principles and Practice of Refraction*. Hammond, Hammond and Co. Ltd., London.

Gilman, G. (1990) 'The behavioral model of vision', in *Conference Notes: First International Congress of Behavioral Optometry*, Monte Carlo, 2nd–5th November.

Grisham, D. and Simons, H. (1990) 'Perspectives on reading disabilities', in *Principles and Practice of Pediatric Optometry*. Lippincott, Philadelphia.

Helveston, E.M. (1987) 'Management of dyslexia and related learning disabilities'. *J. Learn. Disab.*, **20**, 415–21.

Hennessey, D., Iosue, R.A. and Rouse, M.W. (1984) 'Relation of symptoms to accommodative infacility of school-aged children'. *Am. J. Optom. Physiol. Opt.*, **61**, 177–83.

Holland, K.C. (1988) 'Reading with vision (Eleventh Turville Memorial Lecture)'. *Optometry Today*, 2 Jan.

Hulme, C. (1988) 'The implausibility of low-level visual deficits as a cause of children's reading difficulties'. *Cognitive Neuropsychology*, 5, 369–74.

Hynd, G.W. and Semrud-Clikeman, M. (1989) 'Dyslexia and brain morphology'. *Psychol. Bulletin*, 106, 447–82.

Irlen, H. and Lass, M.J. (1989) 'Improving reading problems due to symptoms of scotopic sensitivity syndrome using Irlen lenses and overlays'. *Education*, 109, 413–17.

Jenkins, T.C.A., Pickwell, L.D. and Yekta, A.A. (1989) 'Criteria for decompensation in binocular vision'. *Ophthal. Physiol. Opt.*, 9, 121–5.

Keogh, B.K. (1974) 'Optometric vision training programs for children with learning disability: review of issues and research'. *J. Learn. Disab.*, 7, 36–48.

Lovegrove, W., Frances, M. and Slaghuis, W. (1986) 'A theoretical and experimental case for a visual deficit in specific reading retardation'. *Cognitive Neuropsychology*, 3, 225–67.

Lyle, T.K. and Wybar, K.C. (1967) *Lyle and Jackson's Practical Orthoptics in the Treatment of Squint (and Other Anomalies of Binocular Vision)*. Lewis, London.

Mallett, R. (1988) 'Techniques of investigation of binocular vision anomalies', in *Optometry* (K. Edwards & R. Llewellyn, eds). Butterworth, London, 238–69.

Miles, T., Wheeler, T.J. and Haslum, M.N. (1994) 'More dyslexic boys after all'. Presented at: *3rd International Conference of the British Dyslexia Association*, UMIST, Manchester, April 5th–8th.

Miles, T.R. and Miles, E. (1991) *Dyslexia: a Hundred Years On*. Open University Press, Milton Keynes.

Millodot, M. (1986) *Dictionary of Optometry*. Butterworth, London.

Pavlidis, G.T.H. (1981) 'Sequencing eye movements and early objective diagnosis of dyslexia' in *Dyslexia Research and its Application to Education*. (G.T.H. Pavlidis & T.R. Miles, eds). John Wiley & Sons, Chichester, 98–16.

Pennington, B.F. and Smith, S.D. (1983) Genetic influences on learning disabilities and speech and language disorders. *Child Development*, 54, 369–87.

Pickwell, D. (1989) *Binocular Vision Anomalies: Investigation and Treatment*. Butterworth, London.

Pierce, J.R. (1977) 'Vision therapy and academic achievement: Part 1'. *Review of Optometry*, June 1977, 48–63.

Rosenfield, M., Ciuffreda, K.J., Ong, E., Super, C. (1995) 'Vergence adaptation and the order of clinical vergence range testing'. *Optom. Vis. Sci.* 72, 219–223.

Rutter, M. (1978) 'Prevalence and types of dyslexia', in *Dyslexia, an Appraisal of Current Knowledge*. (A.L. Benton & D. Pearl, eds) (5–28). Oxford University Press, New York.

Shaywitz, S.E., Escobar, M.D., Shaywitz, B.A., Fletcher, J.M. and Makuch, R. (1992) 'Evidence that dyslexia may represent the lower tail of a normal distribution of reading ability'. *N. Engl. J. Med.*, 326, 145–50.

Sheedy, J.E. and Saladin, J.J. (1983) 'Validity of diagnostic criteria and case analysis in binocular vision disorders', in *Vergence Eye Movements: Basic and Clinical Aspects*. (C.M. Schor & K.J. Ciuffreda, eds). Butterworth, Boston, 517–38.

Siderov, J. and DiGuglielmo, L. (1991) 'Binocular accommodative facility in prepresbyopic adults and its relationship to symptoms'. *Optom. Vis. Sci.*, 68, 49–53.

Stanovich, K.E. (1991) 'Discrepancy definitions of reading disability: Has intelligence led us astray'. *Reading Research Quarterly*, 26, No. 1, 7–29.

Stein, J. and Fowler, S. (1985) 'Effect of monocular occlusion on visuomotor perception and reading in dyslexic children'. *The Lancet*, 13 July, 69–73.

Stein, J.F. (1991) 'Visuospatial sense, hemispheric asymmetry and dyslexia', in *Vision and Visual Dysfunction: Vision and Visual Dyslexia*. (J.F. Stein. & J.R. Cronly-Dillon, eds). CRC Press, Boca Raton, USA.

Stidwill, D. (1990) *Orthoptic Assessment and Management*. Blackwell Scientific Publications, Oxford.

Sucher, D.F. (1991) 'Variability of monocular visual acuity during binocular viewing'. *Optom. Vis. Sci.*, **68**, No. 12, 966–71.

Wilkins, A., Milroy, R., Nimmo-Smith, I., Wright, A., Tyrell, R. and Holland, K. (1992) 'Preliminary observations concerning treatment of visual discomfort and associated perceptual distortion'. *Ophthal. Physiol. Opt.*, **12**, 257–63.

Wilkins, A.J. (1995) *Visual Stress*. Oxford University Press, in press.

Wilkins, A.J., Evans, B.J.W., Brown, J., Busby, A., Wingfield, A., Jeanes, R. and Bald, J. (1994) 'Double-masked placebo-controlled trial of precision spectral filters in children who use coloured overlays'. *Ophthal. Physiol. Opt.* **14**, 365–70.

Wilkins, A.J., Nimmo-Smith, I. and Jansons, J.E. (1992) 'Colorimeter for the intuitive manipulation of hue and saturation and its role in the study of perceptual distortion'. *Ophthal. Physiol. Opt.*, **12**, 381–5.

Wilkins, A.J., Nimmo-Smith, I., Tait, A., Mc Manus, C., Della Sala, S., Tilley, A., Arnold, K., Barrie, M., and Scott, S. (1984) 'A neurobiological basis for visual discomfort'. *Brain*, **107**, 989–1017.

Yekta, A.A., Pickwell, L.D. and Jenkins, T.C.A. (1989) 'Binocular vision, age and symptoms'. *Ophthal. Physiol. Opt.*, **9**, 115–20.

Yule, W. (1988) 'Dyslexia – not one condition but many'. *Brit. Med. J.*, **297**, 501–502.

Useful addresses

British Dyslexia Association, 98, London Road, Reading, Berkshire, RG1 5AU; Dyslexia Institute Head Office: 133, Gresham Road, Staines, TW18 2AJ.

CHAPTER 10

Examining Children for Colour Deficiency

Jennifer Birch

10.1   Introduction

In the normal eye, the retinal cones contain three classes of photopigment which have maximum sensitivity in the long-wave (red), medium-wave (green) and short-wave (blue) parts of the spectrum. Colour deficiency arises when one of these photopigments is missing (dichromatism), or when an abnormal photopigment is present which differs in sensitivity from the corresponding normal pigment (anomalous trichromatism). Photopigment abnormalities vary from slight to severe. There are three types of colour deficiency and differences in severity within each type; protan and deutan defects are known collectively as red–green colour deficiency.

(a)   Protan defects   The long-wave photopigment is either missing or abnormal, causing loss of sensitivity to red light.
(b)   Deutan defects   The medium-wave photopigment is either missing or abnormal, causing loss of sensitivity to green light.
(c)   Tritan defects   The short-wave photopigment is either missing or abnormal, causing loss of sensitivity to blue light.

The number of cone photopigments and their spectral sensitivity is genetically determined. Genes which specify the long-wave and medium-wave sensitive photopigments are located on the X chromosome and the inheritance of protan and deutan defects is X-linked. About 8% of males (one in 12) and 0.4% of females (1 in 200) are affected. The different types of colour deficiency do not occur with the same frequency and deuteranomalous trichromatism predominates in both males and females (see Table 10.1).

The gene specifying the short-wave photopigment is located on chromosome 7 and tritan colour deficiency is inherited as an autosomal dominant trait. An equal number of males and females are affected. The prevalence of congenital tritan defects has not been firmly established. The prevalence of tritanopia is probably not greater than 1 in 10 000 and tritanomalous trichromatism not greater than 1 in 500. Many clinical colour vision tests are designed to identify red–green colour deficiency only.

Table 10.1 **Frequency of different types of red-green deficiency in males and females.**

Type of deficiency	Frequency in males	Frequency in females
Protanopia	1%	0.01%
Protanomalous trichromatism	1%	0.03%
Deuteranopia	1%	0.01%
Deuteranomalous trichromatism	5%	0.35%
Total	8%	0.40%

10.2 Assessment of colour vision in children under four years of age

Photopigments are genetically determined, but the visual pathway is not mature until about three months of age. Infant colour vision can be examined objectively using electrodiagnostic techniques, optokinetic nystagmus, or by measuring the pupil response to suitably designed coloured targets. Preferential looking is the method of choice for the examination of babies and toddlers. Subjective examination involving either a verbal or motor response can be attempted from about three years of age.

Pease and Allen (1988) have designed a pseudoisochromatic test for pre-ferential looking. There are four plates all with 'vanishing' designs. Vanishing designs are constructed so that people with normal colour vision can distinguish a coloured figure but this cannot be seen by colour deficient individuals. Iso-chromatic colours for different types of colour deficiency are used in the design (Birch, 1993). Two plates are for demonstrating the visual task, and are used to show that the child is responding correctly. One plate is for detecting red–green colour deficiency and one plate for identifying tritan defects. The colour design is based on that of the Farnsworth F2 plate (Taylor, 1975). The contained figure is a square. Each plate is shown a number of times with the square positioned on either the right or left side. A number of repetitions are needed to confirm the test result.

Subjective examinations present a problem in logistics. Tests designed for adults contain a variety of visual tasks which may be too difficult for a child to complete without assistance. Pseudoisochromatic plates require verbal identi-fication of a contained figure and are the simplest tests to use. If a child has difficulty naming the figure the examiner either rehearses the possible alternative names, offers replicas from which the child can select the one to match the figure seen or encourages the child to draw over the figure using a clean paintbrush or cotton bud. These methods always increase the viewing time. Most pseudoisochromatic plates are intended to be viewed for three or four seconds only and the verbal response should be immediate. Prolonging the viewing time reduces the efficiency of the test as it assists colour deficient people to obtain the correct result.

Several special pseudoisochromatic tests for children have been produced with simple figures, such as familiar geometric shapes or pictures, which are easier for a child to name quickly. However, the majority of these tests have poor colour design and give an unacceptable number of false positive results. Other visual tasks such as colour matching games, selecting similar colours or finding the odd one out have also been tried. These need to be given by an experienced examiner and take quite a long time to complete. Small colour differences are too subtle for young children and tests, or games, made with large colour differences can only identify individuals with severe colour deficiency.

Games composed of dominoes, lotto counters or mosaic patterns painted with isochromatic colours have all been devised to examine three year-olds (Verriest, 1981). The Fletcher-Hamblin Simplified colour vision test consists of three ceramic tiles with mosaic patterns. The child has to point to colours which look different from the majority in the mosaic, or select the colour which looks most like a reference colour. Ceramic is used so that the tiles can be handled and wiped clean. Children enjoy this test, but the screening efficiency is variable (Marre *et al.*, 1989).

10.3   Routine colour vision screening

Colour deficiency occurs in families, and parents may know that a child is likely to be colour deficient if another family member is affected. In an X-linked inheritance the most common transmission is from maternal grandfather to grandson. Boys with a colour-deficient brother have a 50% chance of being similarly affected and boys with a colour deficient uncle have a 25% chance. Colour-deficient girls must have a colour deficient father as well as colour-deficient maternal relatives. Children with severe colour deficiency often make colour naming mistakes or choose incorrect colouring materials at an early age. However, children with slight colour deficiency are unlikely to make obvious mistakes and, if there is no close relative affected, the first indication of colour vision problems is failure of a screening test.

Many occupations require good colour vision and careers advisors need to be aware of colour deficiency. However, if screening is delayed until adolescence the child may already have been placed at an educational disadvantage. Hall (1992) advocates initial colour vision screening at 11 years of age, but this also seems much too late as colour coding is used extensively in primary schools.

Colour vision assessment can easily be undertaken in stages. Ideally the first examination should be made when the child begins school at four or five years of age and a second examination after seven years of age when the child is capable of responding to adult screening methods. This second examination confirms the initial screening result, and aims to estimate the type and severity of colour deficiency. A final more comprehensive examination, which includes tests of practical hue discrimination ability, can be given when career options need to be considered.

Colour is an important coding dimension and is frequently used as a teaching aid, especially in the first years of formal education. Young children are taught colour names, and colour codes are often included in reading programmes. Colour is used to identify shapes and building blocks in number games. Ten different colours are needed for arithmetic and for computations in decimal systems. Most children are able to use a variety of colour names correctly by five to six years of age and colours of varying hue, saturation and chroma can be matched with almost 100% accuracy by six year-olds. Facility with colours is therefore assumed in teaching materials intended for pupils in this age group.

The aim of initial colour vision screening is therefore to identify pupils who would benefit from methods of instruction which do not rely exclusively on colour recognition (Bacon, 1971). Children with severe colour deficiency are most at risk and it is important that they are identified. Identification of slight colour deficiency in young children requires expertise. However, some false negative screening results are acceptable at this stage, providing that another more accurate examination is planned when the children are older. False positive results, however, are unacceptable at any age. A report of colour deficiency should be included in personal academic records which are transferred from one school to another as the child progresses through the educational system. The child's parents need to be informed and occupational limitations discussed well before career options are being considered and a choice made. It is important that the facts are explained in a tactful and informative way. A child should not be made to feel 'defective', and should not be exposed to ridicule from peers. Poor handling of the situation can lead to psychological trauma, resentment, or denial.

Clinical colour vision tests are designed to perform different functions. Screening tests identify individuals with normal or abnormal colour vision. Grading tests estimate the severity of colour deficiency. Both screening and grading tests classify colour deficiency into protan, deutan or tritan but tests composed of pigment colours are not able to distinguish dichromats and anomalous trichromats. Vocational tests examine practical hue discrimination or colour recognition. There are four test design categories each involving a different visual task (Table 10.2). Pseudoisochromatic tests require identification of a coloured figure. These tests are simple to use and have the widest application for screening. Most seven year-olds are able to complete standard tests, such as

Table 10.2   The function of different types of colour vision test.

Function	Test type	Example	Visual task
(1) Screening (identification of colour deficiency)	Pseudoisochromatic designs	Ishihara plates	Identification of a figure
(2) Grading (identification of severe colour deficiency)	(a) Hue discrimination ability	Farnsworth D15 test	Arrangement of a colour order
	(b) Approximate colour matching	City University test	Choice of the most similar colour to a given example
(3) Diagnosis (identification of the exact type of colour deficiency)	Anomaloscopes	Nagel anomaloscope	Precise colour matching with spectral stimuli
(4) Practical ability (suitability for various occupations)	(a) Fine hue discrimination	Farnsworth– Munsell 100 hue test	Arrangement of a colour order and calculation of an error score
	(b) Lanterns	Holmes Wright lantern	Colour naming

the numeral designs of the Ishihara plates, but younger children may find this difficult. The Ishihara test for unlettered persons has the most easily understood format, and is the preferred test for children from four to seven years of age. Vocational tests and tests of practical hue discrimination ability, such as the Farnsworth-Munsell 100 hue test, are not suitable for young children and are only relevant when career options are being considered.

10.4   Screening four to seven year-old children

All colour vision tests require comprehension of the visual task and different tests become useful at different stages of development. Chronological age is less important than the attainment of the necessary cognitive skills.

The Ishihara test for unlettered persons is the most effective test for children under seven years of age (Birch & Platts, 1993). The test became available in the United Kingdom in 1990 but was originally produced in Japan in 1970 (Verriest, 1981). The test is intended for use with four to six year-olds. The same colour combinations are used as in the most accurate designs of the standard Ishihara test (Birch & McKeever, 1993). There are eight plates in all; four plates contain symbols, either a circle or a square, and four plates contain pathways. Two of the four symbol designs are for introduction and two plates are transformation designs containing either a circle or a square. One of the pathway designs is for introduction, two plates contain transformation designs and one plate is for protan/deutan classification. The pathways are less complex than those of the standard Ishihara plates except for the classification plate which is the same as plate 26 in the 38-plate edition. The symbol designs are more effective than the pathway designs. A clean paint brush or cotton bud is needed to draw over the pathway designs. The longer viewing time needed to draw over the figure helps children with normal colour vision to see both the correct and 'confusion' pathways in transformation designs, especially on plate 6.

Although Plate 6 correctly identifies colour deficiency, it is probably better not to include it in the examination. Similarly, there is no need to include the classification plate (Plate 8) unless colour deficiency is found. The test therefore consists of six plates only, three for demonstration and three for screening, and takes only a few minutes to complete. The test can be used with children under four years of age but the plates may have to be shown twice to confirm the first result if the child is hesitant or makes an error. Printed replicas of a circle and square are included with the test. These can be used as an aid to identification if needed but most children over four years of age can respond verbally even if circles are sometimes described as rings or 'O's.

Several other special pseudoisochromatic tests for children have been produced. The Matsubara test contains pictures and the Guy's colour vision for children test contains upper-case letters. Both these tests have poor colour design and children with normal colour vision often fail (Hill *et al.*, 1982). Poor results are also obtained with the Velhagen Pflugertrident test (Birch & Platts, 1993). The Pflugertrident test was published in Leipzig in 1980 and is the recommended test for kindergarten children in the former German Democratic Republic (Marre *et al.*, 1989). In this test the contained figure is a letter E and the child turns a hand-held replica to match the orientation of the figure seen.

All the plates have vanishing designs, and although the visual task appears to be simple, three responses are possible. These are: the correct result; an incorrect match (in which the E is positioned incorrectly); or nothing seen. Colour-deficient children are reluctant to report nothing seen and therefore guess, placing the replica correctly for some designs and incorrectly in others. Young children with normal colour vision also frequently mismatch the figure, and it is necessary to repeat the test, or refer the child to a specialist examiner, if mistakes are made (Mantyjarvi, 1992). Identification of adult deuteranomalous trichromats is unreliable with the Pflugertrident test (Mantyjarvi, 1991). A similar matching technique is used in a prototype 'anomaloscope' plate test made with light emitting diodes (Swanson & Everett, 1992). This test is also failed by a large number of children with normal colour vision suggesting that both the colour design and the examination method is unsatisfactory.

Children under seven years of age can be examined with adult pseudoisochromatic tests if a small number of carefully chosen plates are presented. Drawing over the figure, or selection of a matching replica, can be encouraged if verbal identification is difficult. A recommended selection of six of the most efficient designs from the Ishihara plates is shown in Table 10.3. These plates require the identification of only four numbers; 1, 2, 3, and 5. Two plates, the introduction and classification plates contain pairs of numerals but a card can be placed over half of the plate so that only one figure need be identified at a time. Two plates (Plates 6 and 7 of the standard test) are transformation designs and two are vanishing designs (Plates 10 and 14).

Children respond best to numbers up to their chronological age and plates containing higher numbers should be avoided. Replicas of the number six are often inverted by young children and plates containing sixes and nines should be avoided. About 50% of three to four year-olds choose to draw over the numbers and it is necessary to show the plates three times in about 25% of examinations to distinguish topographical mistakes from true errors. A small percentage of children in the five to seven age-group choose to draw over the design or to use replicas but usually only one showing of the plates is needed. Older children tend to complete the loops of the serif designs of the Ishihara test and may interpret the numbers three or five as eight. This should not be counted as an error on vanishing designs. A test consisting of six plates takes about five minutes to complete.

The Dvorine pseudoisochromatic plates are considered as comparable to the Ishihara plates for identifying red–green colour deficiency. However all the plates have vanishing designs, and failure to read any of the plates gives only negative information. This test is less useful for children since failure to read any numbers may be due to lack of comprehension as well as colour deficiency.

Table 10.3   Selection of six plates from the 38-plate Ishihara pseudoisochromatic test suitable for screening children between 4 and 7 years of age for red-green colour deficiency.

Plate	Numerals Contained	Design	Normal	Responses Red-Green Deficient
1	1 2	Introduction	1 2	1 2
6	2 5	Transformation	5	2
7	5 3	Transformation	3	5
10	2	Vanishing	2	–
14	5	Vanishing	5	–
24	3 5	Classification	3 5	Protans read 5
				Deutans read 3

Visibility of the confusion figure in transformation designs is a convincing positive demonstration of colour deficiency in young children. The standard Ishihara plates and the Dvorine plates contain designs with pathways which are intended for use with non-verbal subjects. These designs are more complex than those included in the Ishihara test for unlettered persons and are unsuitable for young children (Verriest, 1981).

It is important that pseudoisochromatic tests include at least one introductory design. The correct response to the introductory plate confirms that the child is able to complete the test. Failure to respond correctly means that the test cannot proceed. Occasionally, children with psychological problems simulate colour deficiency, either consciously or unconsciously (a visual conversion reaction). On these rare occasions, the examiner is alerted by inconsistent responses. For example, the child may be unable to interpret designs containing large colour differences intended to grade the degree of colour deficiency but be successful with plates containing small colour differences. Mixed protan, deutan and tritan results may be obtained and the introductory plate failed. Referral to the family physician is necessary in these cases.

All colour vision tests composed of pigment colours are designed to have the correct colour appearance when illuminated by standard source C, as defined by the Committee Internationale d'Eclairage. This is a bluish white light which corresponds with overcast North sky illumination in the northern hemisphere. Illumination with artificial daylight fluorescent light sources is satisfactory for colour vision tests, but tungsten light is too red and should not be used. The level of illuminance should exceed 200 lux (100 candelas per sq m).

Ishihara plates are only useful for screening and give no indication of the severity of colour deficiency. If an estimate of severity is required it is necessary to give a second test which has a grading function (Table 10.2). This can be either the American Optical Company (HRR) test, the Farnsworth D15 test or the City University test. The plates of the HRR test should be shown in reverse order, after the introductory plates, so that the test begins at an easy rather than a difficult level. In this age group it is only possible to grade the severity of red–green colour deficiency into two categories, slight or severe, rather than into three categories according to the test instructions. Moderate and severe tritan colour deficiency is also identified. Failure of either the D15 or the City University test identifies severe colour deficiency (Table 10.4). The recommended examination procedure may need to be modified for both these tests.

The concept of setting out a colour order is generally too difficult for children under 7 years of age and a step-by-step procedure is adopted with the D15 panel. The examiner asks the child to select the colour which looks most like the reference colour from the remaining colours, and subsequently the colour most like the last colour selected and placed in the box. The advantage of this test method is that the examiner can observe isochromatic colours being considered

Table 10.4   Severity of red-green colour deficiency shown by combined use of the Ishihara pseudoisochromatic plates and either the Farnsworth D15 test or the City University test.

Ishihara plates	Farnsworth D15 test	The City University test	Severity of red-green deficiency
Fail	Pass	Pass	Slight
Fail	Fail with partial errors	Fail with up to 4 errors	Moderate
Fail	Fail with complete errors	Fail with 5 or more errors	Severe

even if they are not eventually placed in position. Typical colour arrangements are obtained in protan, deutan and tritan deficiency.

The City University test was developed from the D15 test and is the preferred test for grading the severity of colour deficiency in young children. The test has the same colours as the D15 test but these are displayed on the pages of a book so that manipulation of the colours is not required. There are 10 plates. Each plate contains a central colour sample and four peripheral colours. The child selects the peripheral colour which looks most like the central test colour in each plate. Three of these colours represent typical isochromatic colour confusions in protan, deutan and tritan colour deficiency. The fourth colour is the next colour in the hue circle used in the D15 test and is the normal selection. Only plates 1–6 of the second edition of the City University test should be used in this age group. Plates 7–10 contain desaturated colours which are too difficult for young children to distinguish. The idea of choosing the most similar colour is quite a difficult concept for young children and the instructions may have to be repeated for each plate. Protan/deutan classification is not always reliable with this test and mixed protan/deutan responses frequently occur as an artifact of the test design.

Both the D15 test and the City University test fail about 5% of the male population compared to the known incidence of 8% with red–green colour deficiency.

10.5   Screening children of seven to eleven years of age

Colour-coding is used in many areas of the school curriculum after seven years of age. Colour changes may have to be distinguished in chemistry experiments and colours need to be matched in embroidery, woodwork, metalwork and in the graphic arts. Colour codes are used in electrical wiring and in electronics. If a child is severely colour deficiency it may be desirable to obtain permission for help to be given in practical examinations in subjects, such as chemistry, in which accurate hue discrimination is important. More time can be requested in geography examinations involving colour-coded maps.

After seven years of age it is usually possible to administer to the child standard pseudoisochromatic tests, such as the numeral designs of the Ishihara plates, in the manner of an adult examination with a short viewing time, and the examiner can be confident that accurate colour vision screening has been performed. Each pseudoisochromatic plate is shown for about 4 seconds and immediate verbal identification of the figure is required. Similarly, the visual task needed for the D15 test and the City University test is explained once only at the beginning of the examination and the test proceeds at the normal pace. Abbreviated editions of the Ishihara plates are available which contain a smaller number of plates than the standard test. Unfortunately these compilations do not contain the most efficient designs and it is better to select the best plates from the 38-plate test if a more rapid examination is needed (Birch & McKeever, 1993). The selection of plates is different from that recommended for younger children because there is no need to restrict the numerals included. The six most efficient screening designs of the 38-plate test are plates 2, 3, 5, 9, 12 and 16. This selection contains four transformation designs and two vanishing designs. The hidden-digit plates, in which people with colour deficiency can distinguish a figure which cannot be seen by people with normal colour vision, have poor screening efficiency and should be omitted. If colour deficiency is found, a classification plate should be given and a grading test performed.

Diagnosis of the exact type of red–green colour deficiency can only be made using spectral stimuli. The Nagel anomaloscope is the instrument of choice. The instrument consists of a Maxwellian-view spectroscope in which two halves of a 2° bipartite field are illuminated respectively by monochromatic yellow (589 nm), and a mixture of monochromatic red and green wavelengths (670 nm and 546 nm). Exact colour matches must be made by adjusting both the luminance of the yellow test field and the red–green matching ratio (Birch, 1993). Children enjoy making a colour match but many seven year-olds find it difficult to change both halves of the field simultaneously and the examiner has to assist by setting the red–green mixture ratio within the anticipated matching range using the results of other tests as a guide. The child then alters the yellow luminance control and reports if an exact match can be obtained. If the examination method is adapted in this way, there is no difficulty in distinguishing protan and deutan defects or in identifying dichromatism and anomalous trichromatism.

Few children under the age of 10 years have the necessary cognitive skills to complete the Farnsworth-Munsell 100 hue test. This test examines practical hue discrimination ability and is more appropriate for young people over 13 years of age when career options are being considered. A lantern test may also be appropriate at this stage if careers in transport or the armed services are being considered.

10.6   Occupational colour vision standards

Normal colour vision is required in occupations which make extensive use of connotative colour coding and in occupations where failure to use a colour code correctly might be a safety hazard (Table 10.5). Colour deficiency may be a disadvantage in a number of occupations. In these cases, the need for normal colour vision depends on the importance of the colour task, the frequency with which colour judgements have to be made and the availability of additional clues to aid colour recognition. Recruitment policies vary, and individual enquiries must be made to establish company policy. Some employers demand normal colour vision, whilst others accept recruits with slight colour deficiency. In some cases it is sufficient for a colour deficient person to be aware of likely problems, and to seek the advice of a colleague if difficulties arise.

Table 10.5   (a) Careers and occupations which may require normal colour vision.

The Armed Services:
  officers in the navy, air force, army and marine service,
  pilots, engineers and vehicle drivers.
Merchant Navy officers and seamen.
Customs and Excise officers.
Civil Aviation:
  airline pilots, engineers, airport technical and maintenance
  staff, air traffic controllers.
Railways:
  train drivers, engineers and maintenance staff.
Electrical and electronic engineers.
Hospital laboratory technicians and pharmacists.
Police and fire service officers.
Workers in paint, paper and textile manufacture, photography
  and fine art reproduction.
Workers in industrial colour quality assurance.

(b) Careers and occupations in which colour deficiency may be handicap.

Bacteriology	Interior design
Botany	Histopathology
Cartography	Horticulture
Chemistry	Geology and metallurgy

10.7   References and further reading

References

Bacon, L. (1971) 'Colour vision defect – an educational handicap'. *Med. Officer.*, **125**, 199–209.

Birch, J. and Platts, C.E. (1993) 'Colour vision screening in children; an evaluation of three pseudoisochromatic tests'. *Ophthal. Physiol. Opt.*, **13**, 344–9.

Birch, J. and McKeever, L.M. (1993) 'Survey of the accuracy of new pseudoisochromatic plates'. *Ophthal. Physiol. Opt.*, **13**, 35–40.

Hall, D.M.B. (1992) *Health For All Children*, 2nd edn. Oxford University Press, Oxford.

Hill, A.R., Heron, G., Lloyd, M. and Lowther, P. (1982) 'An evaluation of some colour vision tests for children'. *Docum. Ophthal. Proc. Ser.*, **33**, Junk, The Hague, pp 183–7.

Marre, M., Lange, C., Roitzsch, R., Buchmann, R. and Sender, R. (1989) 'Color vision screening in 4384 kindergarten children'. *Doc. Ophthalmol.*, [Suppl.] **52**, 113–16.

Mantyjarvi, M. (1991) 'Velhagen Pflugertrident pseudoisochromatic plates in screening red-green defects'. *Graefe's Arch. Clin. Exper. Ophthalmol.*, **229**, 145–56.

Mantyjarvi, M. (1992) 'Colour vision testing in pre-school aged children'. *Ophthalmologica*, **202**, 147–51.

Pease, P.L. and Allen, J. (1988) 'A new test for screening color vision'. *Amer. J. Optom. Physiol. Opt.*, **65**, No. 9, 728–9.

Swanson, W.H. and Everett, M. (1992) 'Colour vision screening of young children'. *J. Ped. Ophthalmol. Strab.*, **29**, 49–54.

Taylor, W.O.G. (1975) 'Constructing your own PIC test'. *Brit. J. Physiol. Opt.*, **30**, 22–4.

Verriest, G. (1981) 'Colour vision tests in children'. *Atti. Fond. G. Ronchi.*, **36**, 83–119.

Further reading

Birch, J. (1993) *Diagnosis of Defective Colour Vision*. Oxford University Press, Oxford.

CHAPTER 11

An Introduction to Visual Electrodiagnostic Testing

W. David Thomson

11.1   Introduction

The visual system of a neonate is strikingly immature and undergoes radical changes over the first few years of life. The complex cellular-level changes herald the emergence and development of visual function. These changes are far more than mere growth but constitute a significant remodelling and reorganization of neuronal synapses particularly in the visual areas of the brain. This is a time of great plasticity within the system and there is ample evidence that any form of visual deprivation during this critical period leads to functional amblyopia which cannot be reversed once the system becomes 'hard-wired' (see Chapter 4). For this reason it is vital that any potential obstacles to the normal development of vision are identified as early as possible.

Unfortunately it is notoriously difficult to obtain reliable information about the visual status of young children. Normal clinical techniques requiring subjective responses are of course useless, and the clinician is forced to rely on behavioural responses such as preferential looking (Teller, 1979), operant techniques (Mayer & Dobson, 1980, 1982) and various objective tests (Boothe *et al.*, 1985). The development of equipment and techniques capable of recording electrical responses relating to activity in various parts of the visual pathway, has provided a valuable new tool for studying the development of human vision and for the objective assessment of visual function.

This chapter will provide a basic introduction to the methodology of visual electrodiagnostics and an overview of its clinical applications with particular reference to infants. A detailed discussion of the origins of the various electrophysiological responses is beyond the scope of this book but further reading is given at the end of the chapter.

11.2   Electrophysiology

The absorption of light by the photoreceptors triggers off a complex train of electrical events as an array of nervous impulses is transmitted along the visual pathway from the retina to the visual cortex. Some of these events can be recorded by placing surface electrodes at various sites adjacent to the visual pathway.

The study of electrical changes in the eye dates back over 100 years to when Du Bois Reymond (1849) discovered that a small potential difference existed between the cornea and the posterior pole of the eye (Galloway, 1981). Later Holmgren (1865) noted that this resting potential changed when the retina was stimulated with light (Galloway, 1981). These early experiments were all conducted on experimental animals and it was not until the development of amplifiers that similar observations could be made on the human eye. The development of better electrodes, amplifiers and recording and analysis techniques has led to a dramatic improvement in the quality of the recordings and a far better understanding of the origins of the responses.

Three electrodiagnostic tests are now commonly used; namely the electro-oculogram (EOG), the electroretinogram (ERG) and visual evoked potentials (VEPs). The EOG and ERG are related to retinal function, whereas VEPs reflect the activity of the visual cortex.

Much of the methodology for recording these different responses is similar and for expedience will be dealt with together. Specific differences will be considered in the discussion of each response.

11.3   Recording techniques

11.3.1   Electrodes

Electrophysiological studies of the human visual system rely on the fact that potentials generated by visual cells are to some extent dissipated to adjacent tissues. At certain points along the visual pathway, these potentials can be picked up using skin electrodes. These are usually about 1 cm in diameter and made of silver, coated with a thin layer of silver chloride. The central portion is usually dome-shaped with a small hole at the top to allow the cavity to be filled with electrode jelly.

The electrode is attached to the skin using either an annulus of double-sided adhesive tape or glue, before being filled with the conductive jelly. It is vital that a low resistance connection is established between the electrode and the skin if contamination of the signal by 'noise' is to be avoided.

11.3.2   Amplifiers and recording devices

The potentials picked up by the electrodes are very small and must be amplified before they can be displayed or analysed. Most electrophysiological recording systems use differential amplifiers, the output from which is related to the difference between the two inputs. One input is attached to an electrode placed over an active site while the other is attached to a reference electrode placed over a relatively inactive site. Any potentials not related to the response being measured (i.e. noise) will tend to be picked up by both electrodes and will be subtracted from the signal by the differential amplification. Thus differential amplification provides a useful method for increasing the signal to noise ratio. The signal can be cleaned up further by passing it through electronic filters which selectively attenuate frequencies not contained in the response being investigated.

The resultant signal can be viewed on an oscilloscope or output to a pen recorder or other recording device. However, in recent years, computers have been used increasingly to record and analyse electrophysiological recordings. This is achieved by sampling the signal using an analog-to-digital (A/D) converter which transforms the continuously varying (analog) potential to a series of digital measurements at discrete time intervals. Once in this form, the data can be readily manipulated, displayed, analysed or stored by a computer.

11.3.3 Signal averaging

Even when extreme care is taken in setting up equipment, the electrophysiological responses are often too small to be detected against the background noise. The problem of extracting these small responses can be overcome by recording the response to a number of stimulus presentations and averaging signals which are time-locked to the stimulus. In other words, the response following each consecutive stimulus presentation (flash, pattern reversal etc.) is stored (usually in computer memory) and at the end of the recording the responses are averaged. Background noise will not be correlated with the stimulus presentation and will tend to cancel out leaving just that part of the signal which is related to the visual stimulation.

This technique has been applied in many studies of the ERG and is vital for extracting VEPs.

11.4   The electro-oculogram (EOG)

In the normal eye, there is a potential difference of approximately $+10\,mv$ between the cornea and the posterior pole. This is variously referred to as the corneo-retinal, standing or resting potential.

If electrodes are placed on either side of the globe (Fig. 11.1), the potential difference between them is found to change as the eye rotates towards or away from each electrode respectively (Fig. 11.2). Thus by recording between electrodes at the inner and outer canthi or above and below the eye, both horizontal and vertical components of eye movements can be measured. This technique is one of the few methods for recording eye movements which does

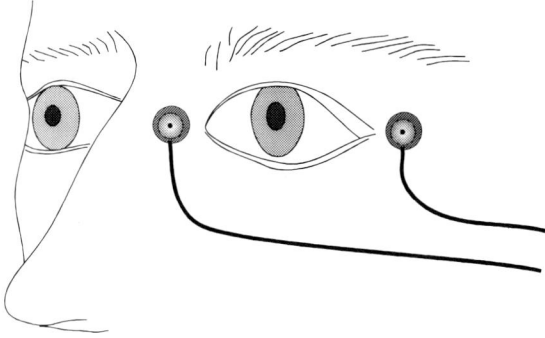

Fig. 11.1 To record an electro-oculogram (EOG), electrodes are placed on either side of the eye. As the eyes move, the potential difference between the two electrodes changes as the relatively positive corneas move towards or away from each electrode respectively.

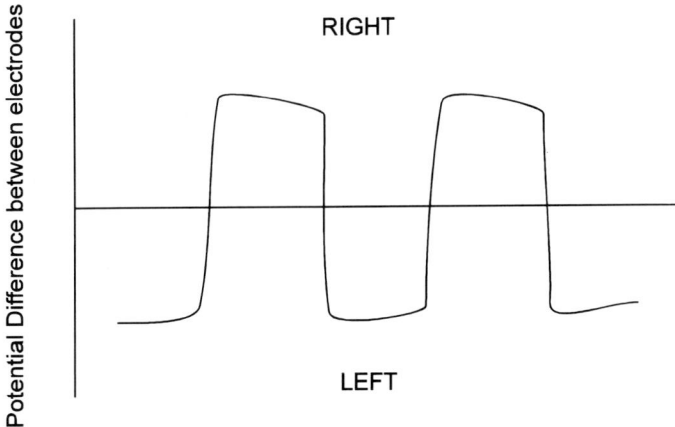

Fig. 11.2 Schematic representation of the potential difference between two electrodes placed at the inner and outer canthi as the subject makes a series of horizontal saccadic movements. With careful calibration eye movements of less than 1° can be recorded.

not involve an attachment to the globe or some invasion of the visual field. With careful calibration, eye movements of less than 1° can be reliably recorded using this method.

However, the corneo-retinal potential is not stable and varies with a number of factors, in particular the level of light or dark adaptation (Francois *et al.*, 1955; Ten Doesschate & Ten Doesschate, 1956). While this seriously limits the usefulness of the EOG as a method for obtaining data for quantitative eye movement analysis, it forms the basis of a valuable clinical test (Arden *et al.*, 1962).

Typically the patient is asked to make a series of eye movements between two fixation lights set approximately 30° apart. The lights are usually alternately illuminated for 1 second each, ten times each minute. The patient first carries out eye movements for 12 minutes in the dark and then for a further 10 minutes while exposed to a bright background light (Arden *et al.*, 1962).

As the amplitude of the eye movements remains constant throughout, any change in the potential recorded must reflect a change in the corneo-retinal potential. In normal eyes, the corneo-retinal potential is found to decrease during the dark adaptation phase and to increase rapidly during the first seven to ten minutes of light adaptation before falling again slightly (Fig. 11.3). This fall is followed by a further rise with the response thereafter taking the form of damped oscillation (Kris, 1958).

The maximum amplitude during the light phase is usually about twice the minimum amplitude recorded during the dark phase. This light/dark ratio, known as the Arden index, has been shown to change in a number of retinal diseases (Arden *et al.*, 1962).

The change in the corneo-retinal potential appears to arise mainly from the photoreceptor-retinal pigment epithelium complex. As such, the test is particularly sensitive to conditions which affect these structures, e.g. retinitis pigmentosa and retinal detachment. In some cases of retinitis pigmentosa, changes in the EOG may be detected in advance of changes in the dark adaptation function or the ERG (Arden & Fojas, 1962).

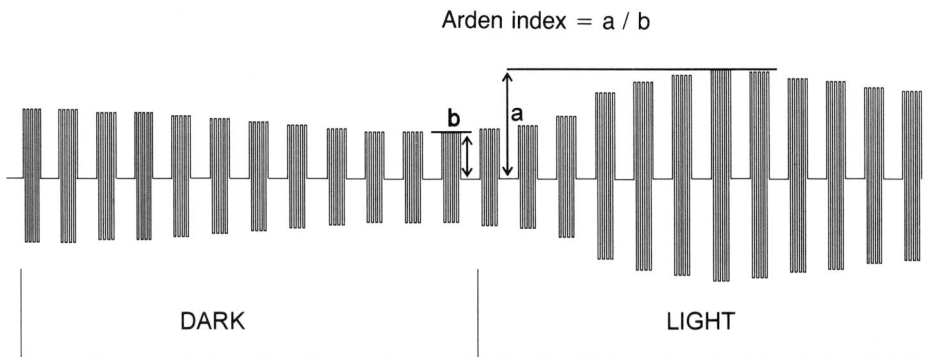

Arden index = a / b

DARK   LIGHT

Fig. 11.3 Schematic representation of a typical EOG obtained during dark, then light adaptation. The subject makes a series of eye movements between two points set approximately 30° apart while in the dark, and subsequently against a bright background. The change in the amplitude of the trace reflects variations in the corneo-retinal potential. The potential is found to decrease during the dark adaptation phase and then to rise rapidly during the first 7–10 minutes of light adaptation before decreasing again. The ratio of the maximum amplitude to the minimum amplitude (a:b) is known as the Arden index and has been shown to change in a number of retinal diseases.

The EOG is a useful method for obtaining a qualitative assessment of the eye movements of children. As a test of retinal function, it requires considerable cooperation on behalf of the patient and is therefore unsuitable for young children. It is also unsuitable for those with very poor vision as they will be unable to make accurate eye movements between the targets.

11.5   The electroretinogram (ERG)

An electroretinogram is a recording of the transient change in the standing potential of the eye in response to visual stimulation.

The ERG was first discovered by Holmgren in 1865 working on frogs (Armington, 1974). The human ERG was recorded as early as 1877 by Dewar, but substantial human ERG research did not become possible until the development of contact lens electrodes in the 1940s (Karpe, 1945; Henkes, 1951; Riggs, 1986).

An ERG is recorded by placing the active electrode on or close to the cornea, and the reference electrode on a relatively inactive site, usually the forehead. Several types of corneal electrodes have been developed over the years. Early designs were based on large scleral contact lenses with silver electrodes imbedded within the cup of the lens. Smaller contact lenses based on the Henkes (1951) and Burian-Allen (1954) designs are still used particularly in research. However, all contact lens electrodes interfere with vision to some extent, and are not easily tolerated, especially by young children.

Several less 'invasive' electrodes are now available. The gold leaf electrode (Arden *et al.*, 1979) consists of a strip of gold coated foil which is inserted into the lower conjunctival fornix and hooked over the lower lid so that it lies in contact with the anaesthetized cornea (Fig. 11.4). This type of electrode pro-

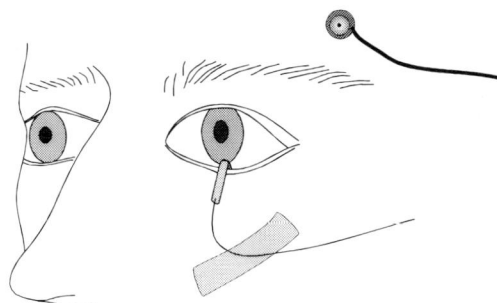

Fig. 11.4   The gold leaf electrode consists of a strip of gold coated foil which is inserted into the lower conjunctival fornix and hooked over the lower lid so that it lies in contact with the anaesthetized cornea. This type of electrode produces excellent results and is used extensively for clinical electroretinography.

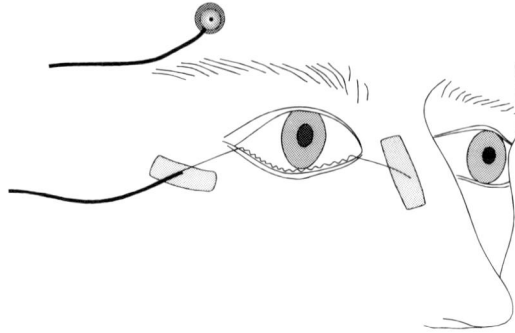

Fig. 11.5 The DTL fibre electrode is made up of filaments of silver-impregnated nylon. The fibre is placed along the lower lid margin so that it floats on the corneal tear film.

duces excellent results and is used extensively for clinical electroretinography.

The DTL fibre electrode (Dawson *et al.*, 1979) is made up of filaments of silver-impregnated nylon. The fibre is placed along the lower lid margin so that it floats on the corneal tear film (Fig. 11.5). The fibre is very well-tolerated (Dawson *et al.*, 1982) and in some cases can be used without a corneal anaesthetic. The amplitude of potentials recorded with the DTL electrode is smaller than those recorded using either contact lens electrodes (Dawson *et al.*, 1982) or gold foil electrodes (Wright *et al.*, 1985). However, in general, its wider patient acceptability outweighs the reduction in response amplitude (Thompson & Drasdo, 1987).

Despite the improvements in corneal electrode design, in many cases the problems of inserting any form of electrode into a child's eyes are insurmountable. In these cases, an ERG can be obtained by using a skin electrode placed on the lower lid (Giltrow-Tyler *et al.*, 1978). However, the amplitude of the ERG response recorded by this method is greatly reduced and signal averaging may be necessary.

The ERG is a complex response arising from potentials generated in a variety of retinal cells. The shape of the ERG depends on many factors, in particular the nature of the retinal stimulation and the state of retinal adaptation. Its clinical value arises from the fact that both the shape and amplitude of the response are affected in a number of retinal diseases.

11.5.1   The flash ERG

The bulk of research has been concerned with the ERG response to flashes of light (the flash ERG). Although the shape of the flash ERG depends on many factors, three main components, known as the a-, b- and c-waves, can usually be identified.

Granit (1933) proposed that the ERG is the sum of three components which he called PI, PII and PIII (Fig. 11.6). According to Granit's analysis, PI develops principally from the pigment epithelium and constitutes the c-wave. PII consists of two components, a positive peak which forms the b-wave and a slow positive DC shift. This potential is thought to arise mainly from the Müller (glial) cells. PIII is a negative potential, the leading edge of which forms the a-wave of the ERG. The a-wave originates in the photoreceptors and both rod and cone contributions can be demonstrated under appropriate conditions. The a-wave is also sometimes referred to as the late receptor potential.

The advent of more sensitive recording methods led to the discovery of a number of other components, in particular the early receptor potential (ERP) and oscillatory potentials (Fig. 11.7). The normal ERP occurs before the a-wave and can only be elicited by very bright flashes. It consists of a positive peak with a very short latency (<0.1 ms), followed by a negative trough followed by a smaller positive phase. The entire ERP is complete within 5 ms. The spectral sensitivity and time course of the ERP correlate with visual pigment activity, and ERP amplitude is linearly related to the number of photoisomerizations of photopigment (Pak & Cone, 1964).

Oscillatory potentials (OPs) are small wavelets superimposed on the rising phase of the b-wave. The OPs have an almost fixed latency over a wide range of intensities whereas the latency of the a- and b-waves decreases as the intensity is increased. This suggests that the OPs have a different origin to the a- and b-waves and although the matter is not yet resolved, there is some evidence that they arise from the retinal amacrine cells (Wachtmeister, 1972; Wachtmeister & Dowling, 1978).

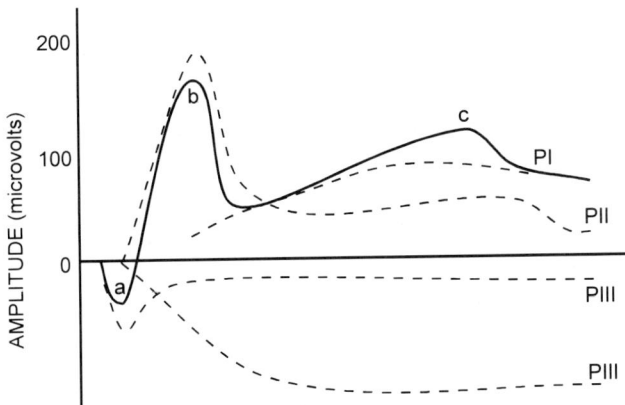

Fig. 11.6 A typical flash ERG consists of three main components known as the a, b, and c waves. Also shown are the components underlying the ERG according to Granit's analysis (PI, PII and PIII).

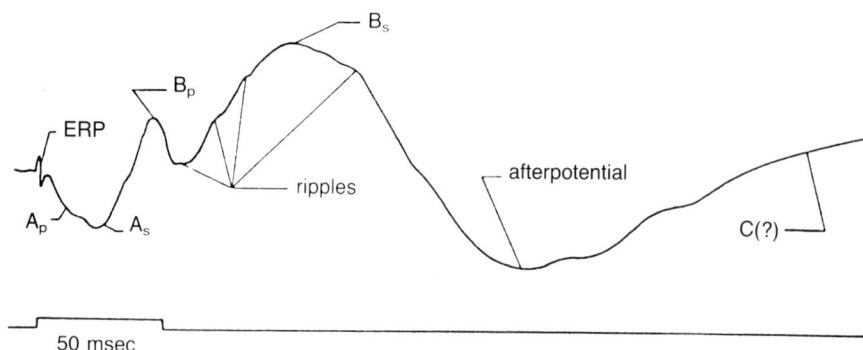

Fig. 11.7 An idealized ERG waveform showing the early receptor potential (ERP), the photopic and scotopic a-waves (A_p and A_s), the photopic and scotopic b-waves (B_p and B_s) and the c-wave. Oscillatory potentials (ripples) can occur throughout the entire response but are usually seen on the rising phase of the b-wave. *NB*: not all these components would be seen in any single recording condition. (From Armington, J.C. (1974) *The Electroretinogram.* Academic Press, New York.)

The flash ERG therefore, reflects the functional integrity of a variety of retinal cells. By varying various stimulus parameters, it is possible to selectively stimulate some retinal cells more than others (Armington, 1986). For example, by using a red flash flickering at 30 Hz, a cone-dominated ERG can be recorded. Conversely, by presenting dim blue flashes to a dark-adapted eye at a frequency of 2 Hz, a rod-dominated ERG can be obtained.

The flash ERG has been shown to be of diagnostic value in a variety of retinal conditions. As the ERG represents the sum of the potentials generated over a large area of the retina, its amplitude is related to the proportion of functioning retina within the stimulated area (Crews *et al.*, 1978). For example, if only half of the stimulated area is functioning, the ERG response would be halved. Since the amplitude of the ERG seems to be related to retinal area rather than cell density, large field ERG responses are not particularly sensitive to macular changes, since the macula only represents a small area of the retina.

The flash ERG has also been used to evaluate the status of the retina in patients with media opacities (corneal opacities, cataracts, vitreous haemorrhages, etc.). If a sufficiently intense flash is used, some light will penetrate the opacity and, if the retina is functional, an ERG will be recorded.

The flash ERG is affected at an early stage in a number of hereditary retinal degenerations, allowing early diagnosis and counselling. For example, the ERG is often affected at a very early stage in retinitis pigmentosa (recessive form), when fundus changes and changes in visual function may be minimal (Armington *et al.*, 1961). Other conditions which have been shown to affect the flash ERG include, retinal detachment (Rendahl, 1961), vitamin A deficiency (Gombas *et al.*, 1970), high myopia (Dhanda, 1966) and ocular trauma (Crews *et al.*, 1978).

11.5.2 The pattern electroretinogram (PERG)

Riggs (1966) was among the first to study the ERG to patterned stimuli. Some years later, a resurgence of interest in pattern stimulation was sparked by new evidence that PERGs may reflect activity at a more proximal level in the retina than the flash ERG (Maffei & Fiorentini, 1981). Maffei & Fiorentini demonstrated that the PERG gradually disappeared following section of the optic nerve, suggesting that the response was, at least in part, mediated by retinal ganglion cells (ganglion cell activity does not contribute significantly to the flash ERG). Since then, a wide variety of patterned stimuli have been used including gratings, bars and checks. Usually, the pattern is periodically reversed so that the black areas become white and vice versa, while the overall luminance remains constant.

The PERG is a relatively small response and signal averaging techniques are often required to elicit good results. The amplitude of the PERG has been shown to be sensitive to optical blur (Odom, 1982; Hess & Baker, 1984) and therefore it is vital that the subject wears a spectacle correction (if required) and obtains a clear and unobstructed view of the stimulus. For this reason, gold leaf or DTL fibre electrodes are usually preferred for recording PERGs.

The morphology of the PERG is dependent on a number of factors, particularly the configuration of the patterned stimulus. Several studies have found that the PERG is spatially-tuned, i.e. a mid-range of check sizes produces a larger response than either larger or smaller checks (Odom *et al.*, 1982; Korth, 1983). This evidence is considered to support the claim that the origin of the PERG is different to the flash ERG.

There has been much debate as to the exact origin of the PERG but there is now a preponderance of evidence that the PERG is affected in conditions such as glaucoma (Wanger & Persson, 1983; Marx *et al.*, 1986), optic neuritis (Plant *et al.*, 1986; Vaegan & Billson, 1987), optic atrophy (Maffei *et al.*, 1985; Harrison *et al.*, 1987), and amblyopia (Arden & Wooding, 1985), all of which have in common the loss of ganglion cells. In general, it can be said that an abnormal PERG in the presence of a comparatively normal flash ERG would normally indicate ganglion cell dysfunction.

11.6 Visual evoked potentials (VEPs)

The EOG and ERG provide valuable information about the integrity of the retina but are largely unaffected by post-retinal lesions. However, the integrity of the entire visual pathway can be investigated by recording Visual Evoked Potentials (VEPs).

VEPs are recorded by placing electrodes on areas of the scalp juxtaposed to visually-active areas of the brain – principally the occipital poles. The nature of the potentials recorded is dependent on the exact placement of electrodes and therefore some form of standardization is necessary. A variety of standards have been proposed, some based on measurements from various bone structures (e.g. the Queen's Square system), others based on proportional measurements (e.g. the 10/20 system) (see Regan, 1989).

The visually-evoked component of the recording is usually small compared with the background electroencephalogram (EEG). To extract the VEP, the responses to 30–100 stimulus presentations must be recorded and averaged. The background EEG will not be time-locked to the stimulus presentation and will tend to cancel out leaving just that part of the EEG which is systematically related to the visual stimulation, i.e. the VEP.

Many different visual stimuli have been used to generate VEPs although in a clinical environment three types of stimuli are commonly employed: a diffuse flash stimulus; a patterned stimulus which reverses in contrast at fixed intervals (pattern-reversal); and a patterned stimulus which is alternated with a uniform grey field of the same space-averaged luminance (pattern appearance). The three types of stimulation produce very different VEPs. The flash VEP is complex and shows considerable intra-subject variability. Small wavelets, possibly of subcortical origin, with a latency of around 25 ms sometimes precede the main response. A typical response is shown in Fig. 11.8. Various labelling schemes

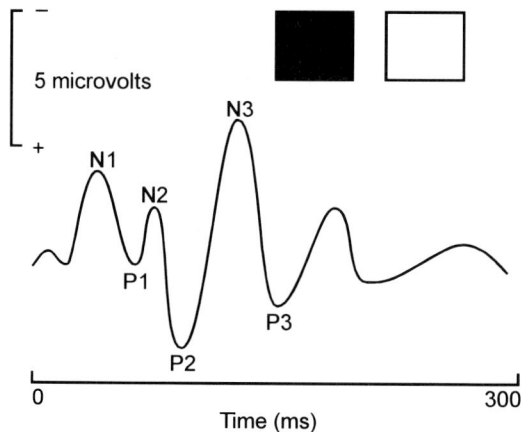

Fig. 11.8   A typical flash VEP. Note that negativity is shown as upwards. Components are usually labelled according to their polarity (positive = P, negative = N) and in order of occurrence.

have been proposed but the most common method describes the polarity (positive, P; negative, N) and order of the components, for example, P2 refers to the second positive peak. Interpretation of VEPs is further confused by the convention of clinical studies to record negative as upwards while other studies use the opposite convention.

The amplitude of the flash VEP is commonly quantified as N2–P2, and its latency is measured from the onset of the flash to P2. Although the amplitude of the flash VEP tends to be variable, its latency is relatively stable at around 100 ms. The flash VEP does not require accurate focusing or fixation and is therefore more suitable for assessing young or uncooperative children than the pattern VEPs where these factors are far more important.

The pattern-reversal VEP is generally much simpler than that obtained in response to a flash and tends to produce more repeatable responses. Again, the morphology of the response depends on electrode placement and the nature of the stimulus. A typical pattern-reversal VEP is shown in Fig. 11.9. The most notable feature of the response is a positive peak with a latency of around 100 ms often referred to as the P_{100} component.

The pattern-onset VEP is more complex than the pattern-reversal VEP and enjoys yet another nomenclature (Fig. 11.10), the onset components being referred to as CI, CII and CIII. These components are affected in different ways by subject and stimulus variables. For example, CII appears to be particularly sensitive to defocus of the retinal image whereas CI is more sensitive to contrast.

Both pattern-reversal and pattern-onset VEPs are dependent on the subject's ability to resolve the visual stimulus. Therefore, by gradually reducing the size of the checks until a VEP is no longer elicited, the technique can be used to

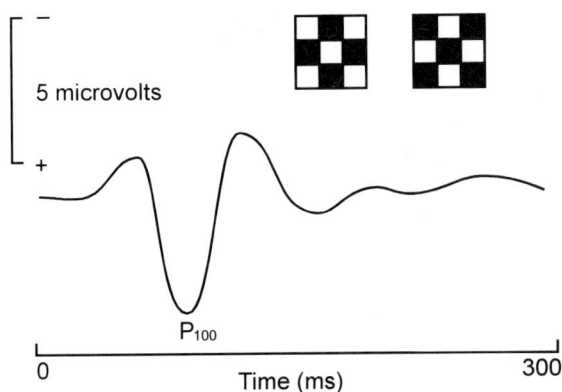

Fig. 11.9 A typical pattern reversal VEP. Note that negativity is shown as upwards. The response is much simpler than the flash VEP with the most notable feature being a positive peak with a latency of 100 ms (P_{100}).

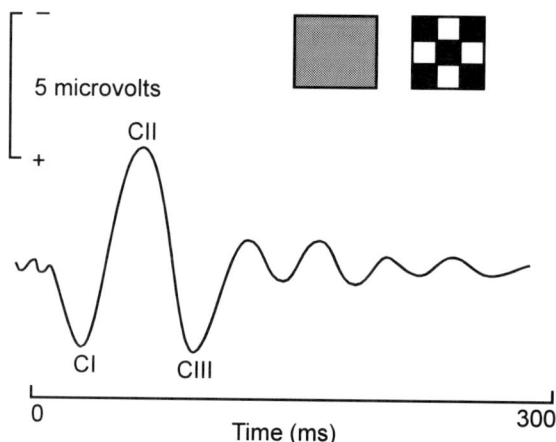

Fig. 11.10 A typical pattern appearance VEP. Note that negativity is shown as upwards. The exact shape of the response depends on many factors, but the three components (CI, CII and CIII) can usually be identified.

obtain an objective estimate of visual acuity (Sokol, 1978, 1980). Contrast sensitivity can also be estimated by extrapolating a straight line plot of VEP amplitude versus stimulus contrast (Atkinson *et al.*, 1979). Likewise, optical defocus has been shown to affect the latency and amplitude of pattern VEPs (but not flash VEPs) (Sokol & Moskowitz, 1981). Indeed, by placing lenses of different powers in front of the eye and determining the lens which produces a pattern VEP with the minimum latency and maximum amplitude, a crude objective refraction can be carried out (Millodot & Riggs, 1970; Duffy & Rengstorff, 1971). Regan (1973) has shown that by rotating a stenopaic slit in front of the cornea while recording a pattern VEP, the axes of astigmatism can be determined. Millodot & Newton (1981) measured the amplitude of accommodation by recording pattern-reversal VEPs while placing negative lenses in front of the eyes.

VEPs provide a gross measure of the integrity of the entire visual pathway including the retina, the optic nerves, the optic chiasma, the optic tracts and the optic radiations. Used in combination with other electrodiagnostic tests, VEPs can provide valuable information about the location of a lesion. For example, an abnormal VEP in the absence of any change in the ERG or EOG would generally indicate a post-retinal lesion.

However it is important to note that the ERG gives approximately equal weighting to the entire retina, while VEPs tend to reflect the importance given to the fovea by the visual cortex. Therefore small macular lesions which have little effect on the ERG, may have a devastating effect on VEPs. The site of post-retinal lesions can be investigated further by comparing the VEPs from both visual cortices and investigating the responses obtained by stimulating each eye in turn or by presenting stimuli in different parts of the visual field.

Although the VEP may be affected in a number of retinal diseases, VEPs are of particular value in the investigation of conditions affecting the post-retinal visual pathway. For example, Halliday *et al.* (1972) showed that the latency of the VEP is often increased in patients suffering from optic neuritis. Furthermore, the response may be abnormal for several years following an acute attack, long after the clinical signs and symptoms have subsided. VEPs are affected in a largely predictable manner by lesions at other levels of the visual pathway and by combining half-field or quadrant stimulation with careful electrode placement, objective information about visual field status can be obtained.

The principal challenge when testing infants is to maintain their cooperation for long enough to obtain a result. A technique which has been used with some success is to present the visual stimulus (grating, etc.) over a more interesting picture such as a cartoon (Regan, 1977). Although, the background picture will itself produce a VEP, and therefore add some noise to the signal, the noise will not be time-locked to the stimulus and will tend to cancel out with averaging. Even so, young infants cannot be relied on to maintain steady fixation or accommodation and for this reason flash VEPs are often preferred.

Another problem encountered when assessing young children is the time taken to obtain results. Conventional VEP techniques require the averaging of many responses to obtain a single VEP. To obtain an estimate of, for example, visual acuity, VEPs must be recorded using a range of stimuli and the process can become very lengthy. A technique known as stimulus sweeping (or zooming) can greatly reduce the time taken to investigate the effect of specific stimulus parameters on the VEP (Regan, 1986, 1989). For example, to assess visual acuity, the subject would be presented with a counterphasing grating or check pattern modulated at a high temporal frequency while the spatial frequency (size of the bars/checks) is slowly ramped up or down. VEPs can be extracted from the resulting responses using narrow-band synchronous filter techniques (Regan, 1989).

VEPs have been used extensively to study the development of various aspects of vision, including visual acuity (Norcia & Tyler, 1985), contrast sensitivity (Atkinson *et al.*, 1979; Norcia *et al.*, 1986, 1989), binocularity (Braddick *et al.*, 1980) and stereopsis (Petrig *et al.*, 1981). In general, data obtained by VEP methods is comparable to results obtained using behavioural techniques (such as preferential looking), though in some cases there is substantial disagreement between the time scale of development predicted by the two methods (Sokol, 1978; Sokol & Moskowitz, 1987; Dobson & Teller, 1978). The reasons for this are not clear although the following are among the suggested explanations:

(a) Behavioural techniques confound motor, cognitive and visuo-sensory development whereas the VEP assesses sensory development alone.
(b) VEP studies use temporally-modulated stimuli (flashed, pattern reversal, pattern onset, etc.) whereas stationary patterns are usually used in behavioural tests.
(c) VEP estimates of visual thresholds (acuity, contrast sensitivity) are obtained indirectly by extrapolating data obtained using suprathreshold stimuli.

It remains to be seen which of the various methods provides the best indication of the visual status in infants.

11.7   Summary

The ability to measure electrophysiological responses associated with visual processes has provided a powerful tool for studying the development of human vision. The same techniques are being used increasingly in clinical practice for providing objective information about the visual status of infants.

At present, the practice of electrodiagnostics tends to be limited to a few hospitals, specialist centres and research laboratories. However, as recording and analysis techniques develop and understanding of the responses improve, the use of electrodiagnostics is likely to become more widespread particularly in the field of pediatric optometry.

11.8   References and further reading

References

Arden, G.B., Barrada, A. and Kelsey, J.H. (1962) 'New clinical test of retinal function based upon the standing potential of the eye'. *Brit. J. Ophthal.*, **46**, 449–82.
Arden, G.B., Carter, R.M., Hogg, C.R., Siegel, I.M. and Margolis, S. (1979) 'A gold foil electrode extending the horizons for clinical electroretinography'. *Invest. Ophthal. Vis. Sci.*, **18**, 421–6.
Arden, G.B. and Fojas, M.R. (1962) 'Electrophysiological abnormalities in pigmentary degenerations of the retina'. *Arch. Ophthal.*, **68**, 369–89.
Arden, G.B. and Wooding, S.L. (1985) 'Pattern ERG in amblyopia'. *Invest. Ophthalmol. Vis. Sci.*, **26**, 88–96.
Armington, J.C. (1974) *The Electroretinogram*. Academic Press, New York.
Armington, J.C. (1986) Electroretinography, in *Electrodiagnosis in Clinical Neurology*, 2nd edn. (M.J. Aminoff, ed.). Churchill Livingstone, New York, 403–40.
Armington, J.C., Gouras, P., Tepas, D. and Gunkel, R. (1961) 'Detection of the electroretinogram in retinitis pigmentosa'. *Exper. Eye Res.*, **1**, 74–80.
Atkinson, J., Braddick, O. and French, J. (1979) 'Contrast sensitivity of the human neonate by the visual evoked potential'. *Invest. Ophthalmol. Vis. Sci.*, **18**, 210–13.

Boothe, R.G., Dobson, V. and Teller, D.Y. (1985) 'Postnatal development of vision in human and non-human primates'. *Annu. Rev. Neurosci.*, **8**, 495–545.

Braddick, O.J., Atkinson, J., Juliez, B., Kropfl, W., Bodis-Wollner, I. and Raab, E. (1980) 'Cortical binocularity in infants'. *Nature*, **288**, 363–5.

Burian, H.M. and Allen, L.A. (1954) 'A speculum contact lens for electroretinography'. *Electroenceph. Clin. Neurophysiol.*, **6**, 509–11.

Crews, S.J., Thompson, C.R.S. and Harding, G.F.A. (1978) 'The ERG and VEP in patients with severe eye injury', in *Documments Ophthalmologica Proceedings Series*, **15**, Junk, The Hague, 203–209.

Dawson, W.W., Trick, G.L. and Litzgow, C.A. (1979) 'Improved electrode for electro-retinography'. *Invest. Ophthal. Vis. Sci.*, **18**, 988–91.

Dawson, W.W., Trick, G.L. and Maida, T.M. (1982) 'Evaluation of the DTL corneal electrode', in *Docum. Ophthal. Proc. Ser.*' (G. Niemeyer & Huber, eds), **31**, 81–8. Junk, The Hague.

Dhanda, R.P. (1966) 'Electroretinogram and dark adaptation study in myopic retinal degeneration'. *Pro. All-India Ophthal. Soc.*, **23**, 77–82.

Dobson, V. and Teller, D.Y. (1978) 'Visual acuity in human infants: A review and comparison of behavioural and electrophysiological studies'. *Vis. Res.*, **18**, 1469–83.

Duffy, F.H. and Rengstorff, R.H. (1971) 'Ametropia measurements from the visual evoked response'. *Am. J. Optom.*, **48**, 717.

Francois, J., Verriest, G. and De Rouck, A. (1955) 'Modification of the amplitude of the human electro-oculogram by light and dark adaptation'. *Brit. J. Ophthal.*, **39**, 398–408.

Galloway, N. (1981) *Ophthalmic Electrodiagnosis*. Lloyd-Luke Medical Books Ltd, London.

Giltrow-Tyler, J.F., Crews, S.J. and Drasdo, N. (1978) 'Electroretinography with non-corneal and corneal electrodes'. *Invest. Ophthalmol. Vis. Sci.*, **17**, 1124–7.

Gombas, G., Hornblass, A. and Vendeland, J. (1970) 'Ocular manifestations of vitamin A deficiency'. *Annal of Ophthalmol.*, **2**, 680–4.

Granit, R. (1933) 'The components of the retinal action potential in mammals and their relation to the discharge in the optic nerve'. *J. Physiol.*, **77**, 207–39.

Halliday, A.M., McDonald, W.I. and Mushin, J. (1972) 'Delayed visual evoked responses in optic neuritis'. *Lancet*, **1**, 982–5.

Harrison, J.M., O'Connor, P.S., Young, R.S.L., Kincaid, M. and Bentley, R. (1987) 'The pattern ERG in man following surgical resection of the optic nerve'. *Invest. Ophthalmol. Vis. Sci.*, **28**, 492–9.

Henkes, H. (1951) 'Use of electroretinography in measuring the effects of vasodilation'. *Angiography*, **2**, 125.

Hess, R.F. and Baker, C.L. (1984) 'Human pattern-evoked electroretinogram'. *J. Neurophysiol.*, **51**, 939–51.

Karpe, G. (1945) 'The basis of clinical electroretinography'. *Acta Ophthalmol.*, Suppl. **24**, 1–118.

Korth, M. (1983) 'Pattern evoked and luminance evoked response in the human electro-retinogram'. *J. Physiol.*, **237**, 451–69.

Kris, C. (1958) 'Corneo-fundal potential changes during light and dark adaptation'. *Nature*, **182**, 1027–8.

Maffei, L. and Fiorentini, A. (1981) 'Electroretinographic responses to alternating gratings before and after section of the optic nerve'. *Science*, **211**, 953–5.

Maffei, L., Fiorentini, A., Bisti, S. and Hollander, H. (1985) 'Pattern ERG in the monkey after section of the optic nerve'. *Exp. Brain Res.*, **59**, 423–5.

Marx, M.S., Bodis-Wollner, I., Podos, S.M., Teitelbaum, C.S. (1986) 'The pattern ERG and

VEP in glaucomatous optic nerve disease in monkey and human', in *Evoked Potential*. (R.Q. Cracco & I. Bodis-Wollner, eds). A.R. Liss, New York, 117–26.

Mayer, D.L. and Dobson, V. (1980) 'Assessment of vision in young children: a new operant approach yields estimates of acuity'. *Invest. Ophthalmol. Vis. Sci.*, **19**, 566–70.

Mayer, D.L. and Dobson, V. (1982) 'Visual acuity development in infants and young children as assessed by operant preferential looking'. *Vis. Res.*, **22**, 1141–51.

Millodot, M. and Newton, I. (1981) 'VEP measurement of the amplitude of accommodation'. *Brit. J. Ophthalmol.*, **65**, 294–8.

Millodot, M. and Riggs, L.A. (1970) 'Refraction determined electrophysiologically'. *Arch. Ophthalmol.*, **84**, 272–8.

Norcia, A.M. and Tyler, C.W. (1985) 'Spatial frequency sweep VEP: Visual acuity during the first year of life'. *Vis. Res.*, **25**, 1399–408.

Norcia, A.M., Tyler, C.W. and Allen, D. (1986) 'Electrophysiological assessment of contrast sensitivity in human infants'. *Am. J. Optom. Physiol. Opt.*, **63**, 12–15.

Norcia, A.M., Tyler, C.W. and Hamer, R.D. (1988) 'High visual contrast sensitivity in the young human infant'. *Invest. Ophthalmol. Vis. Sci.*, **29**, 44–9.

Odom, V.J., Maida, T.M. and Dawson, W.W. (1982) 'Pattern-evoked retinal responses (PERR) in humans: effects of spatial frequency, luminance and defocus'. *Curr. Eye. Res.*, **2**, 99–108.

Pak, W.L. and Cone, R.A. (1964) 'Isolation and identification of the initial peak of the early receptor potential'. *Nature*, **204**, 836–8.

Petrig, B., Juliez B., Kropfl, W., Baumgartner, G. and Anliker, M. (1981) 'Development of stereopsis and cortical binocularity in human infants: electrophysiological evidence'. *Science*, **213**, 1402–5.

Plant, G.T., Hess, R.F. and Thomas, S.J. (1986) 'The pattern evoked electroretinogram in optic neuritis'. *Brain*, **109**, 469–90.

Regan, D. (1973) 'Rapid objective refraction using evoked brain potentials'. *Invest. Ophthalmol.*, **12**, 669–79.

Regan, D. (1977) 'Speedy assessment of visual acuity in amblyopia by the evoked potential method'. *Ophthalmologica*, **175**, 159–64.

Regan, D. (1989) 'Rapid and precise recording techniques based on sine/cosine Fourier series analyzer', in *Human brain electrophysiology: evoked potentials and evoked magnetic fields in science and medicine*. Elsevier Science Publishing Co., New York, 112–23.

Rendahl, I. (1961) 'The clinical electroretinogram in detachment of the retina'. *Acta Ophthalmologica.*, **64**, 1–83.

Riggs, L.A. (1986) 'Electroretinography'. *Vis. Res.*, **26**, 1443–60.

Riggs, L.A., Johnson, E.P. and Schick, A.M.L. (1966) 'Electrical responses of the human eye to changes in wavelength'. *J. Opt. Soc. Am.*, **56**, 1621–7.

Sokol, S. (1978) 'Measurement of infant visual acuity from pattern reversal evoked potentials'. *Vis. Res.*, **18**, 33–41.

Sokol, S. (1980) 'Pattern visual evoked potentials: their use in pediatric ophthalmology', in *Electrophysiology and Psychophysics: their use in Ophthalmic Diagnosis*. (S. Sokol, ed.). Little Brown, Boston, 251–68.

Sokol, S. and Moskowitz, A. (1981) 'Effect of retinal blur on the peak latency of the pattern evoked potential'. *Vis. Res.*, **21**, 1279–86.

Sokol, S. and Moskowitz, A. (1987) 'Comparison of pattern VEPs and preferential looking behaviour in three-month-old infants'. *Invest. Ophthalmol. Vis. Sci.*, **126**, 359–65.

Teller, D.Y. (1979) 'The forced-choice preferential looking procedure: a psychophysical technique for use with human infants'. *Infant Behav. Dev.*, **2**, 135–53.

Ten Doesschate, G. and Ten Doesschate, J. (1956) 'The influence of the state of adaptation on the resting potential of the human eye'. *Ophthalmologica*, **132**, 308–20.

Thompson, D.A. and Drasdo, N. (1987) 'An improved method for using the DTL fibre in electroretinography'. *Ophthal. Physiol. Opt.*, **7**, 315–19.

Vaegan and Billson, F.A. (1987) 'The differential effect of optic nerve disease on pattern and focal electroretinograms'. *Doc. Ophthalmol.*, **65**, 45–56.

Wachtmeister, L. (1972) 'On the oscillatory potentials of the human electroretinogram in light and dark adaptation'. *Acta Ophthal.*, **116**.

Wachtmeister, L. and Dowling, J. (1978) 'The oscillatory potentials of the mudpuppy retina'. *Invest. Ophthalmol. Vis. Sci.*, **17**, 1176–86.

Wanger, P. and Persson, H.E. (1983) 'Pattern reversal electroretinograms in unilateral glaucoma'. *Invest. Ophthalmol. Vis. Sci.*, **24**, 749–53.

Wright, C.E., Williams, D.E., Drasdo, N. and Harding, G.F.A. (1985) 'The influence of age on the electroretinogram and visual evoked potential'. *Docum. Ophthalmol.*, **59**, 365–84, Junk, Holland.

Further reading

Carr, R.E. and Siegel, I.M. (1982) *Visual electrodiagnostic testing*. Williams and Wilkins, Baltimore & London.

Galloway, N. (1981) *Ophthalmic Electrodiagnosis*. Lloyd-Luke Medical Books Ltd, London.

Halliday, A.M. (ed.) (1982) *Evoked Potentials in Clinical Testing*. Churchill Livingstone, Edinburgh.

Harding, G.F.A. (1988) 'Neurophysiology of vision and its clinical application', in *Optometry*. (K. Edwards. & R. Llewellyn, eds). Butterworth, London.

Regan, D. (1989) *Human brain electrophysiology: evoked potentials and evoked magnetic fields in science and medicine*. Elsevier Science Publishing Co., New York.

SECTION 3
ABNORMAL NEUROLOGICAL, OCULAR AND ORBITAL CONDITIONS

CHAPTER 12
Diseases of the Eye and Orbit
Baljean Dhillon & Brian Fleck

12.1   Introduction

Increasingly optometrists are seen by the public as the primary source of advice on eye problems. Children with a wide range of eye diseases may be first seen by an optometrist, who must be able to detect signs of significant disease and refer appropriately.

12.2   Trauma

Ocular injury is particularly common in childhood. The variety is wide, from blunt trauma with stones (thrown or catapulted) to penetrating injury with sharp objects.

Children who have accidents may be reluctant to report them to the parents or health worker because they are afraid of punishment, therefore the history should be taken (as always) with patience and sympathy.

Periorbital bruising

The lids and orbit are good protectors of the eyeball. A 'black eye' is the result of bleeding in and around the eyelids (Plate 1) and is a common cause of ptosis (i.e. lowering of the upper eyelid).

The upper lid should always be lifted to check that the eyeball is healthy and the eye movements should be checked to ensure they are full. No treatment is needed and the blood usually is absorbed over one or two weeks, with full recovery of the function and appearance of the lids.

Lid lacerations

If superficial and clean these can be treated using surgical adhesive tape. However full-thickness, dirty wounds require cleansing, careful examination and repair under general anaesthetic. Involvement of the lacrimal canaliculi may lead to scarring and later to watering eye problems, which may require further surgery.

Subconjunctival haemorrhage

Minor trauma or severe coughing can cause rupture of small blood vessels and produce a subconjunctival haemorrhage, which resolves without local treatment.

Corneal abrasions

These may easily be diagnosed with fluorescein dye. Antibiotic ointment, a mydriatic to dilate the pupil and reduce painful ciliary muscle spasm, and a pad to aid rapid healing.

Chemical injuries

Disinfectants, detergents, paints, glues and perfumes if splashed into the eye, should be immediately irrigated with sterile isotonic saline or clean tap water.

Most chemicals found in the home are harmless, though strong bleach and alkaline solutions (Plate 2) can burn the lid margin, conjunctival, and corneal surface which can later lead to scarring. Children so affected need urgent ophthalmological evaluation and treatment.

Subtarsal foreign body

This diagnosis may be suggested by a history of exposure to dust or sand, on a beach visit for example. The eye is red and very painful, and following instillation of fluorescein dye an 'ice rink' pattern of epithelial scratches is seen in the superior cornea. Eversion of the upper lid is a simple procedure, and removal of the foreign body brings instant relief.

Corneal foreign body

Any foreign body can embed itself into the corneal epithelium. If superficial, the foreign body can be lifted off after instilling local anaesthetic drops and using a cotton tipped bud, or a needle (Plate 3). Deeper metallic particles may erode into the stroma and leave a 'rust ring', and the surrounding corneal tissue forms a scar. The rust remnant is best removed by an ophthalmologist, who can view the cornea through a microscope, or slit lamp, and safely remove deeply embedded material. In the very young, or uncooperative child, a short general anaesthetic allows safe removal. The resulting corneal abrasion heals quickly with topical antibiotic ointment, a mydriatic, and a pad, if tolerated.

Hyphaema

A red fluid level in the anterior chamber suggests blood and is called a hyphaema (Plate 4). Haemorrhage into the anterior chamber following blunt trauma often completely absorbs within a few days, but even a small bleed may be followed some hours or days later by a haemorrhage of much greater severity. All cases should therefore be referred urgently to an ophthalmologist. An unreactive, semi-dilated pupil due to iris bruising is often present.

Bleeding into the vitreous cavity and retina can occur with severe blunt trauma to the eye, or rapid decelerating head injuries. In the absence of a convincing history, 'non-accidental' or 'battered-baby' syndrome should be suspected (see Chapter 14) (Harcourt, 1971). The retina may become torn leading to retinal detachment which requires surgery. Milder concussion injuries causing white patches of retinal oedema usually resolve with no sequelae.

Orbital 'blow out' fracture

A direct blow on the eye can cause a sudden rise in orbital pressure and fracture either the thin bone forming the orbital floor, or the medial wall, with incarceration of fat or extraocular muscle (Plate 5). This can be the result of a tennis ball or a fist impact onto the orbit. The child will have lid bruising, diplopia (if both eyes are open), a 'sunken' eye (enophthalmos), and lower lid sensation impairment if the infraorbital nerve is damaged. Periorbital bruising is invariable.

In mild cases no surgical intervention is required and the appearance and movements of the eye are good once bruising has resolved. However, early surgery is needed in more severe cases (Dutton, 1991).

Perforating injuries

Sharp projectiles of metal or glass, or sharp-pointed instruments such as knives, scissors or sharp pointed toys can perforate the cornea or sclera. Sometimes the only evidence of a small perforation at the corneoscleral limbus is a protruding knob of iris tissue, and a distorted pupil. An eyepad should be applied gently, and the child sent directly to a hospital eye department. A general anaesthetic is needed to fully establish the extent of the injuries and to repair the eye.

12.3   The red eye

A constellation of eye diseases can present as a red eye. The key in discriminating the serious from the trivial and self limiting, is attention to other signs.

Orbital cellulitis

An acute inflammation in the superficial tissues anterior to the orbital septum is called a preseptal cellulitis. True orbital cellulitis (Plate 6) occurs deep to the septum and can be life-threatening, spreading backward to produce a cavernous sinus thrombosis. To distinguish between a pre- and postseptal infection, the reddened and swollen eyelids must be prised open to allow examination of the eyeball and assessment of vision. If the eye can see reasonably well, is free to move in all directions of gaze, the conjunctiva pristine white and the pupil reactive to light, the infection is preseptal. However if examination shows that the eye has poor vision, limited movement, tensely swollen conjunctiva, is painfully protruding or proptosed, and has a poorly reactive pupil, the infection is postseptal (Weiss, 1983).

Neonatal conjunctivitis ('ophthalmia neonatorum')

Conjunctivitis occurring soon after birth may be particularly severe (Pierce, 1982). The lids are oedematous and swollen but lid retractors allow the eyeball to be examined. The cornea should be examined for signs of ulceration, for it is this which can lead to blindness. All babies suspected of suffering from such an infection need urgent referral to an ophthalmology and/or pediatric team, as certain pathogens, gonococcus in particular, can melt away the cornea and perforate the eye within 24 hours.

Bacterial conjunctivitis

A sticky discharge is always present in bacterial conjunctivitis. The infection settles quickly with topical antibiotic drops instilled every two hours for the first two days, then every four hours for five days, prescribed by the family doctor. Infection spread by fingers should be minimized, and simple hygiene observed to limit spread generally.

Viral conjunctivitis

This presents with bilateral redness and watering, and accompanies an upper respiratory infection; no treatment is indicated. In some cases there is intense photophobia related to small areas of inflammation deep in the corneal epithelium. These cases should be referred to an ophthalmologist.

Allergic conjunctivitis

Conjunctivitis associated with hayfever is characterized by itching, watering and eye rubbing. Avoiding grass pollens if possible, and using sodium cromoglycate

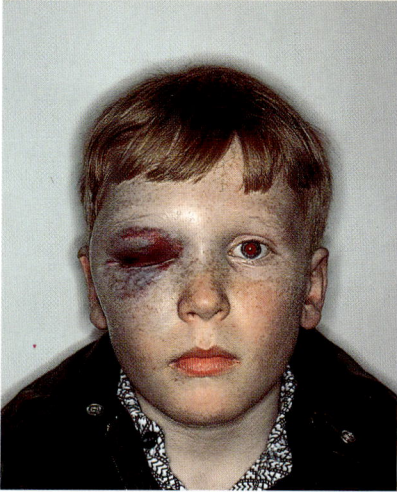

Plate 1 Periorbital bruising.

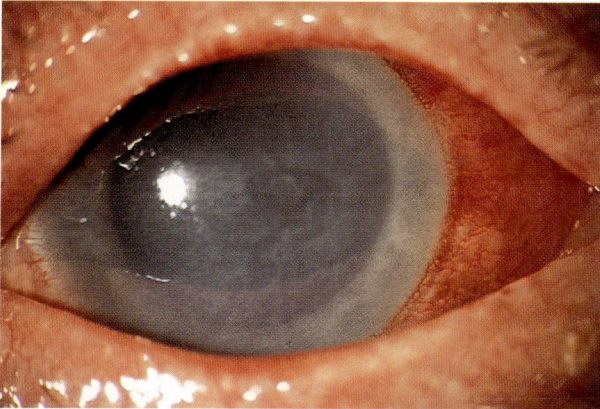

Plate 2 Corneal scar due to alkaline burn.

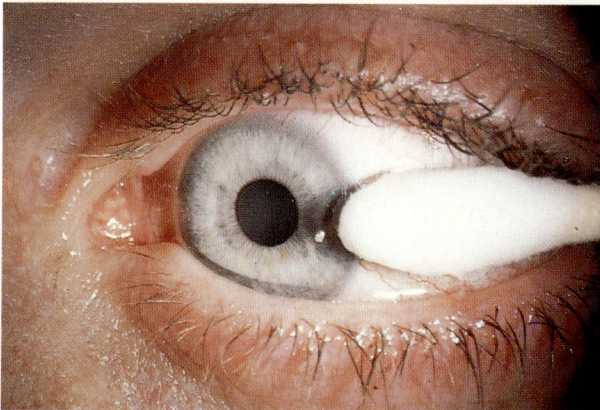

Plate 3 Removing a corneal foreign body using a cotton wool bud, following instillation of a topical anaesthetic.

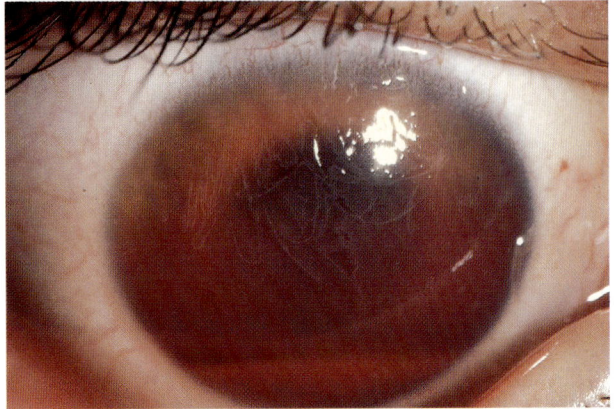

Plate 4 Hyphaema. Blood is present in the anterior chamber.

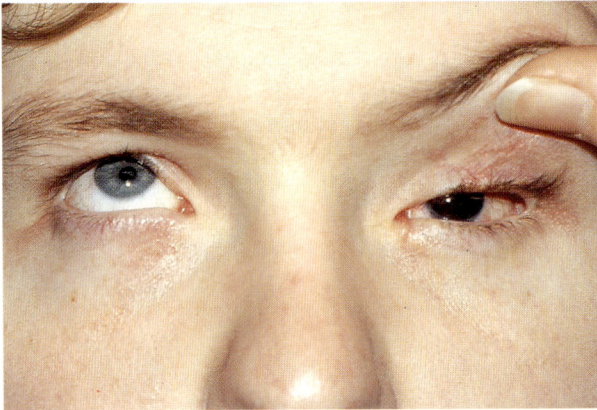

Plate 5 Orbital 'blow out' fracture. The left eye is sunken, and fails to elevate on upgaze.

Plate 6 Orbital cellulitis, secondary to sinusitis.

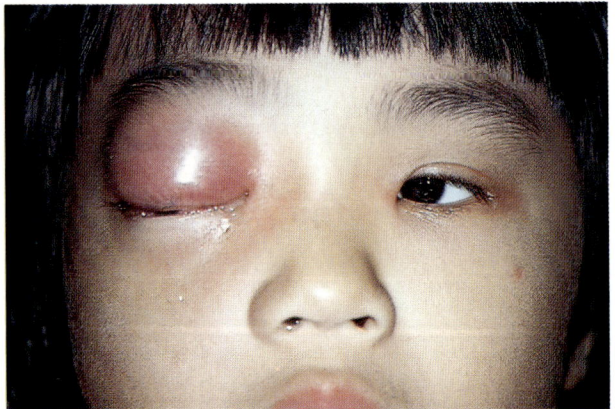

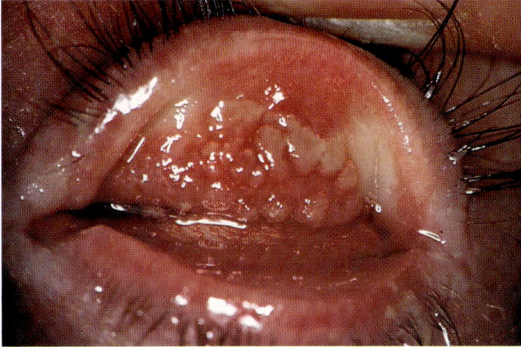

Plate 7 (above) Giant papillae in vernal keratoconjunctivitis.

Plate 8 (right) Dendritic corneal ulcer, stained with fluorescein and rose bengal.

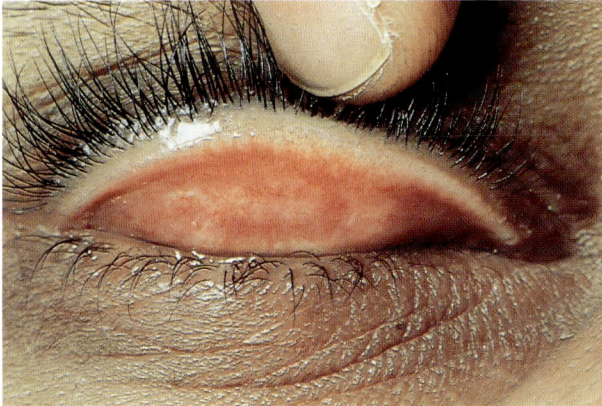

Plate 9 Subtarsal scarring due to trachoma.

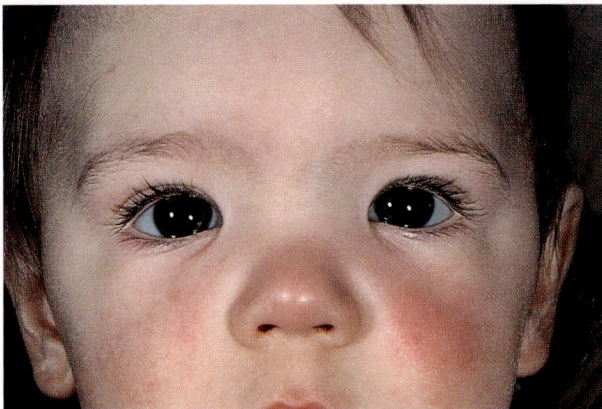

Plate 10 Epicanthus.

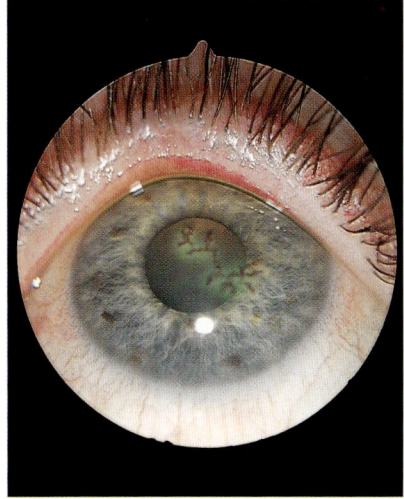

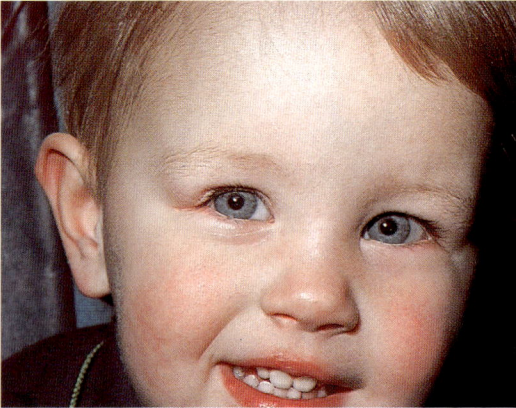

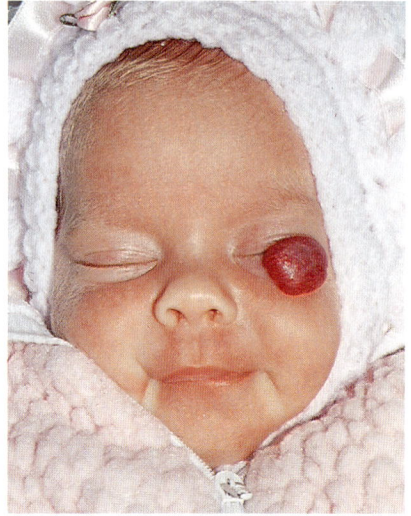

Plate 11   (above) Angular dermoid.

Plate 12   (right) Capillary haemangioma.

Plate 13   Blepharitis.

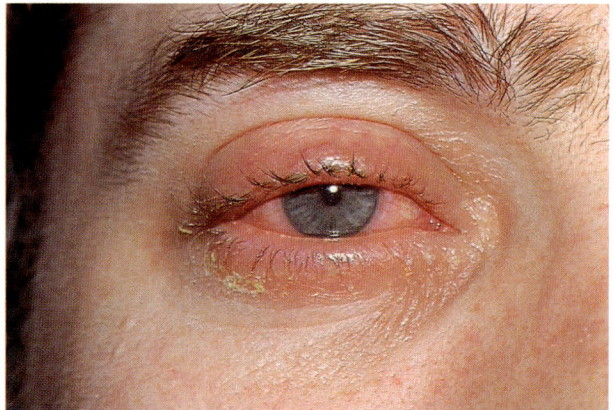

Plate 14   Tarsal cyst.

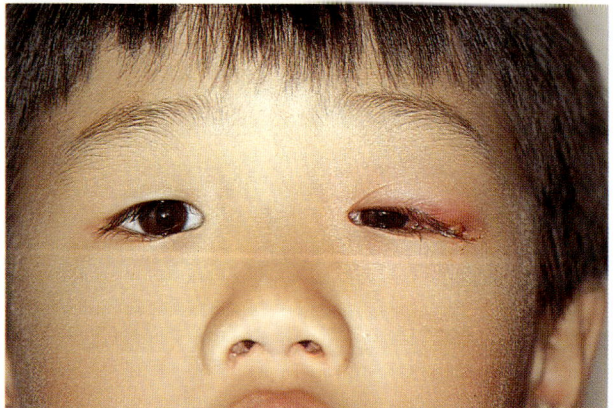

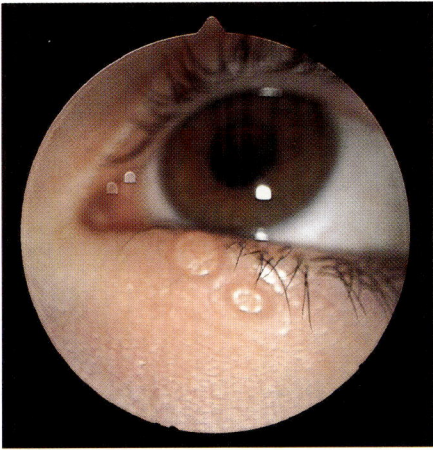

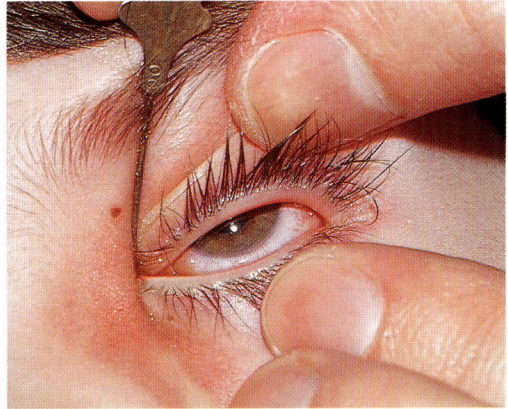

Plate 15   (left) Molluseum contagiosum.

Plate 16   (above) Nasolacrimal duct probing. A metal probe has been inserted through the lower canaliculus, and pushed down through the nasolacrimal duct.

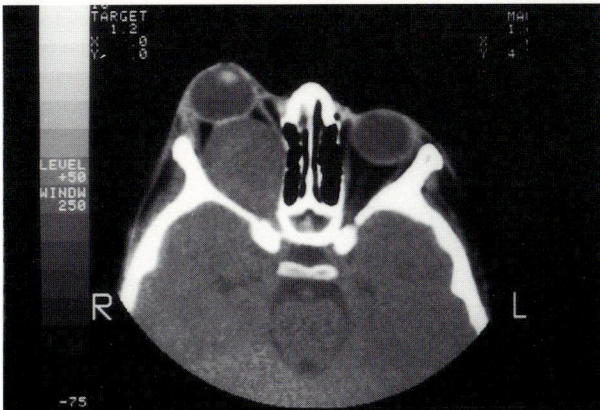

Plate 17   Enlarged cornea in congenital glaucoma.

Plate 18   CT scan of optic nerve glioma.

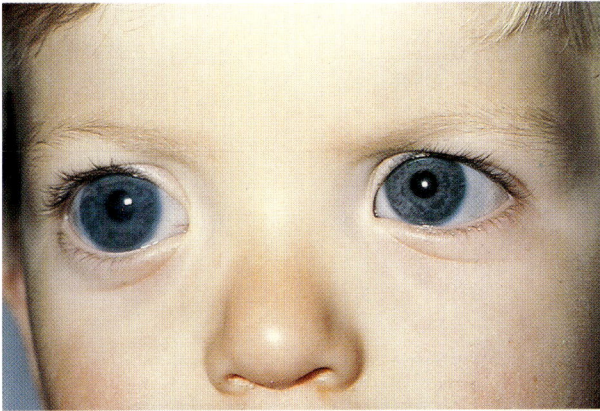

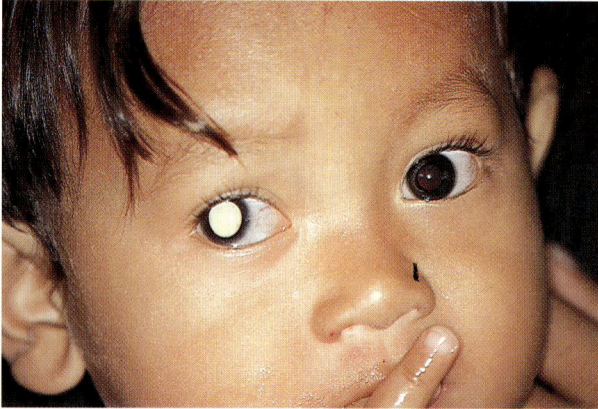

Plate 19 Retinoblastoma causing a white pupil reflex.

Plate 20 Retinal traction band caused by retinopathy of prematurity.

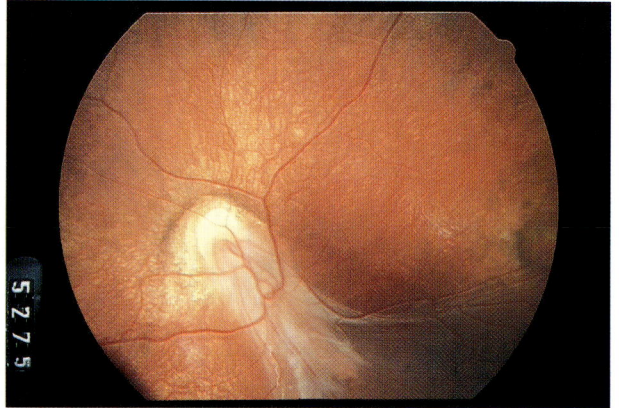

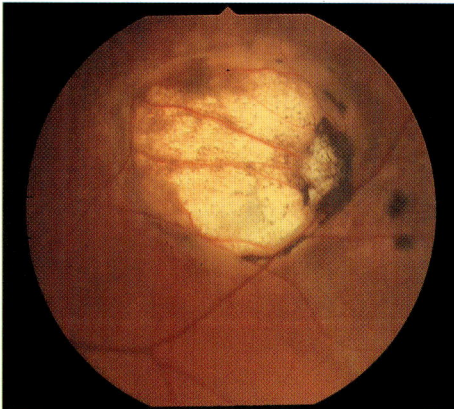

Plate 21 Retinal scar as a result of toxocara infestation.

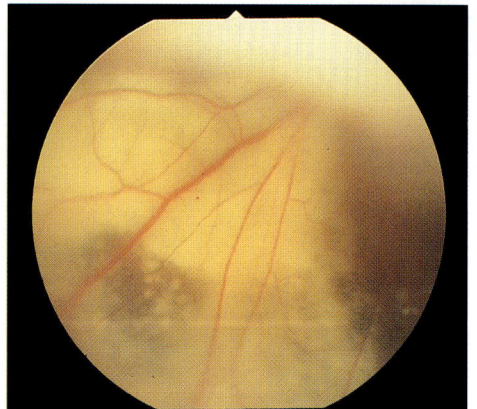

Plate 22 Subretinal lipid and exudates in Coats' disease.

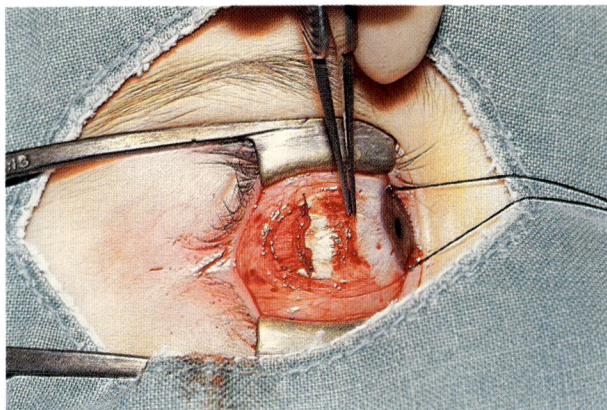

Plate 23 Surgical recession of the lateral rectus muscle. The forceps are holding the original muscle insertion. The muscle has been detached from the eye and sutured on again more posteriorly.

Plate 24 Brown's syndrome affecting the left eye, which depresses on adduction.

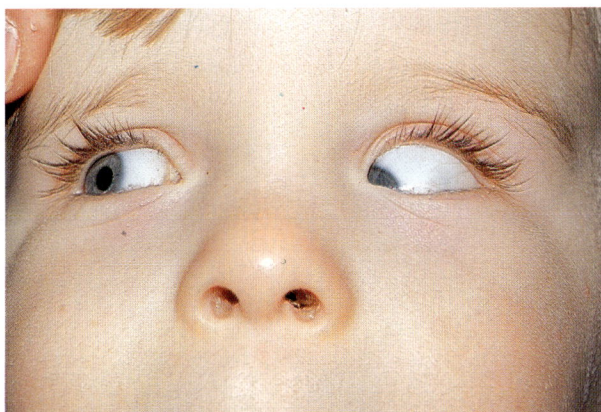

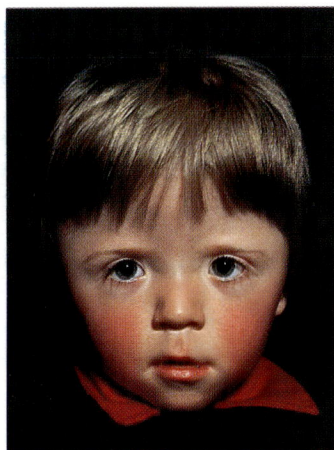

Plate 25 Craniofacial dysostosis, with widely spaced eyes.

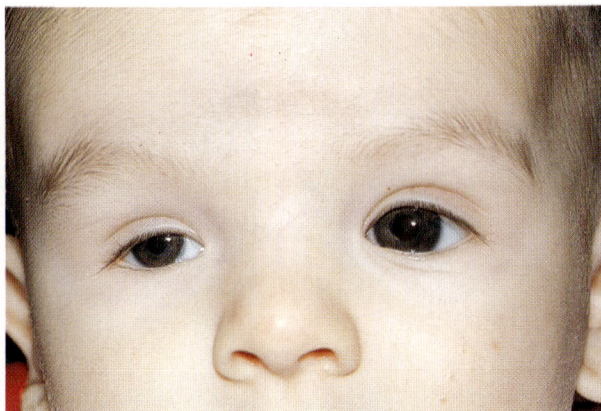

Plate 26 Right microphthalmos.

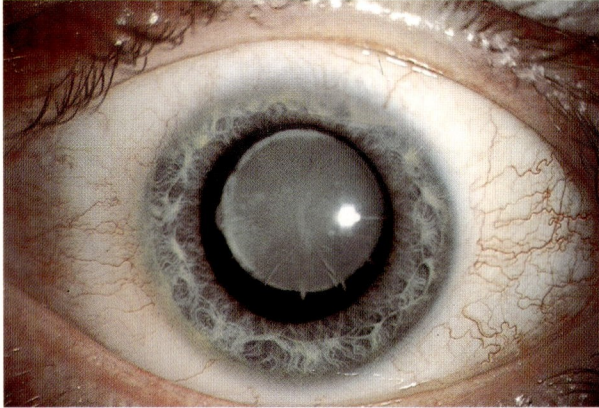

Plate 27 Congenital cataract. Only the central part of the lens is opaque in this case.

Plate 28 Keratoconus.

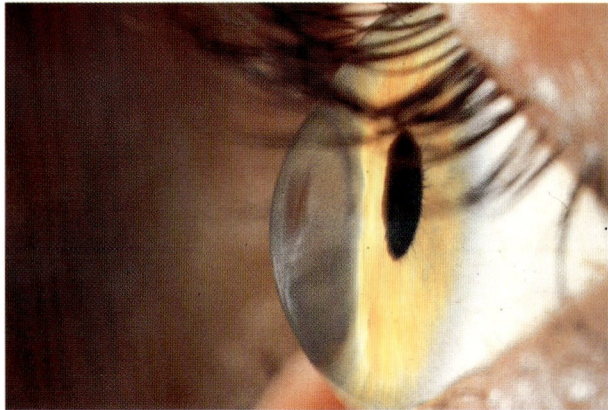

Plate 29 Inferior iris coloboma.

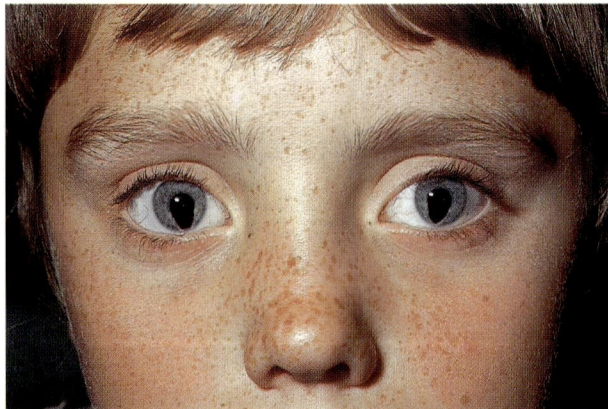

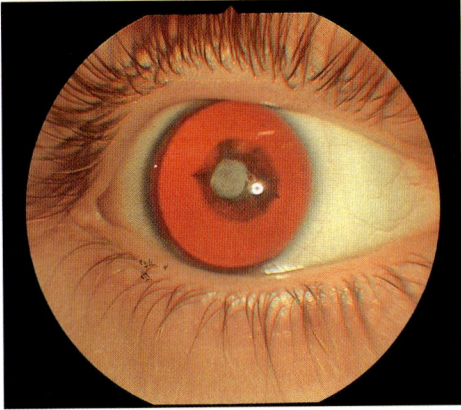

Plate 30 Aniridia, with anterior polar cataract.

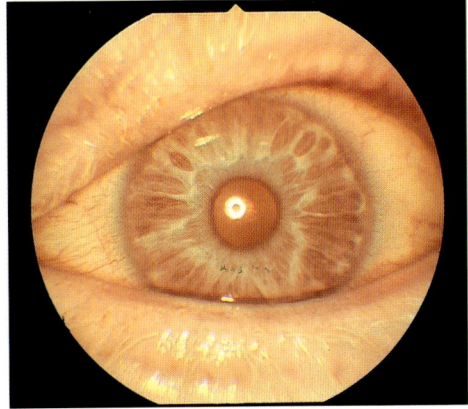

Plate 31 Albinism. The iris appears pink on transillumination.

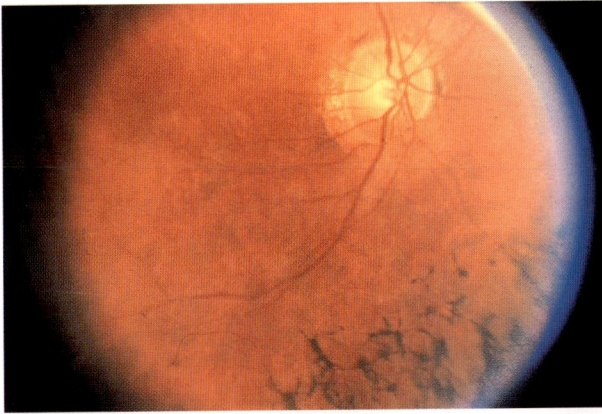

Plate 32 (left) Retinitis pigmentosa. Bone spicule retinal pigmentation.

Plate 33 (below left) Cone dystrophy with 'bull's eye' pigment disturbance at the macula.

Plate 34 (below) Toxoplasma retinal scarring with adjacent reactivation.

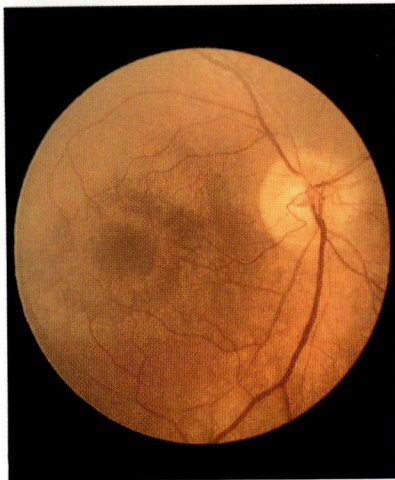

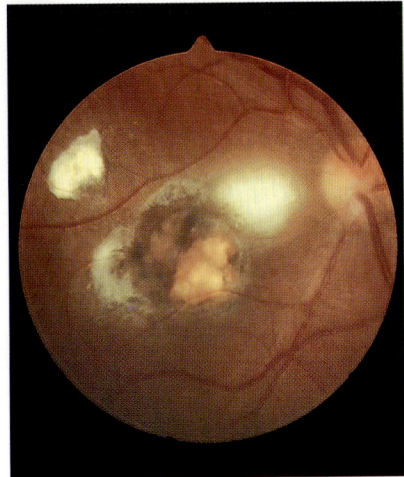

Plate 35 Optic nerve hypoplasia.

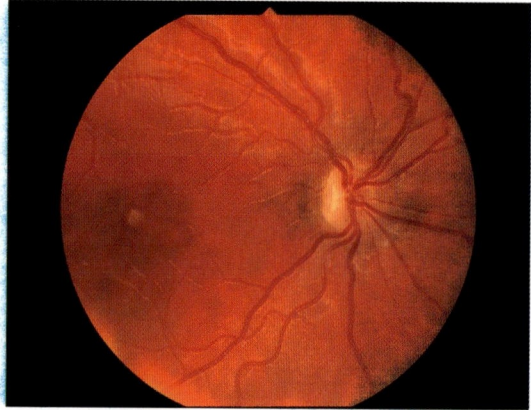

Plate 36 Optic disc pit.

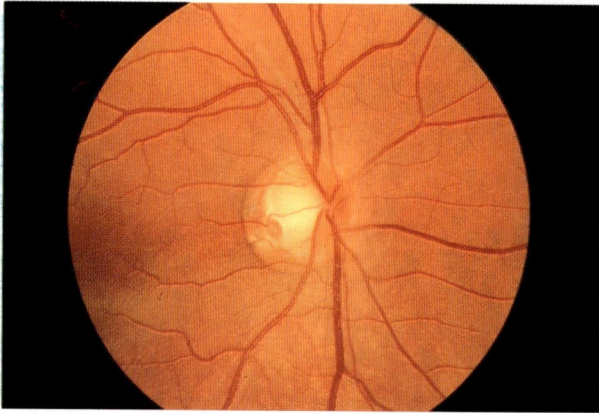

Plate 37 Optic disc drusen.

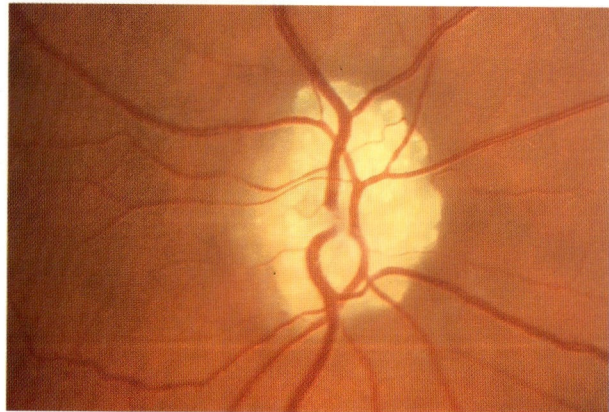

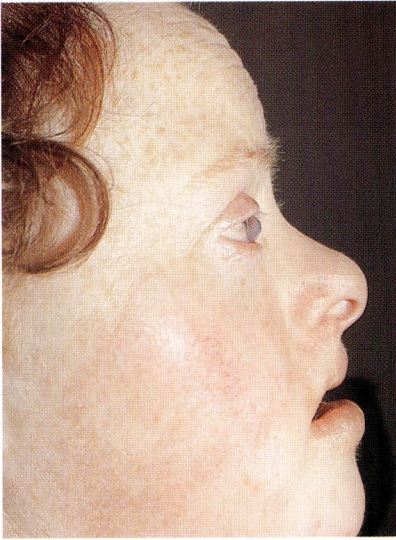

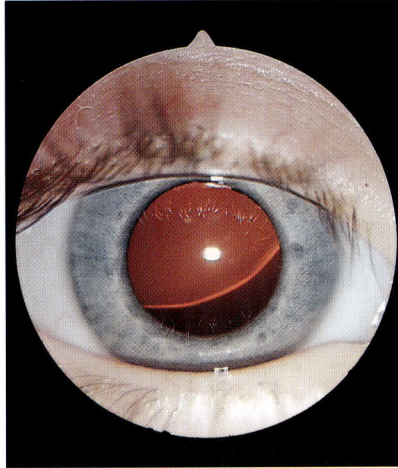

Plate 38 (above left) Down's syndrome with keratoconus.

Plate 39 (above) Dislocated lens in Marfan's syndrome.

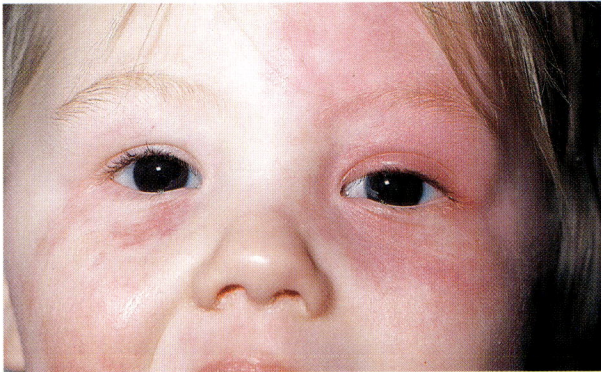

Plate 40 (left) 'Port wine stain' in Sturge-Weber syndrome.

Plate 41 Stevens-Johnson syndrome.

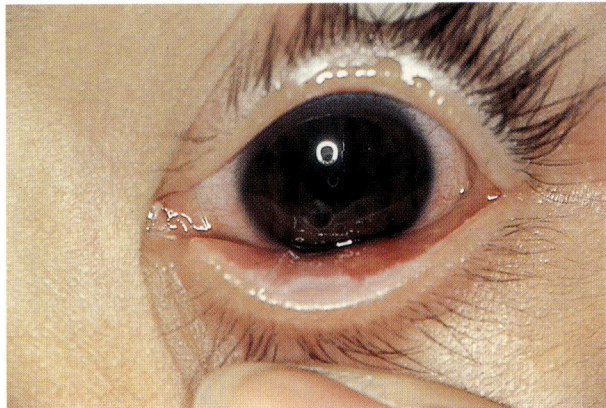

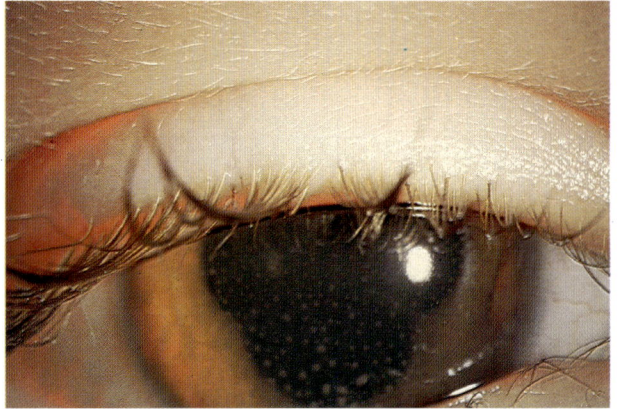

Plate 42 Iritis in a patient with juvenile chronic arthritis.

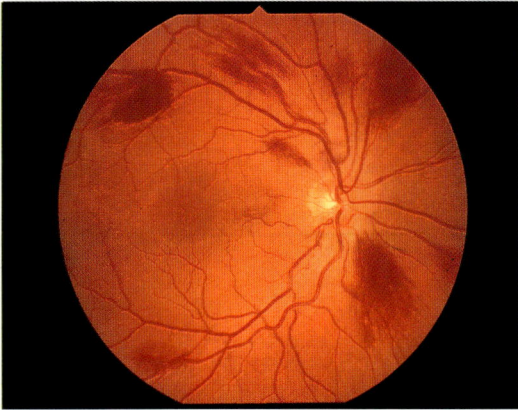

Plate 43 Leukaemia.

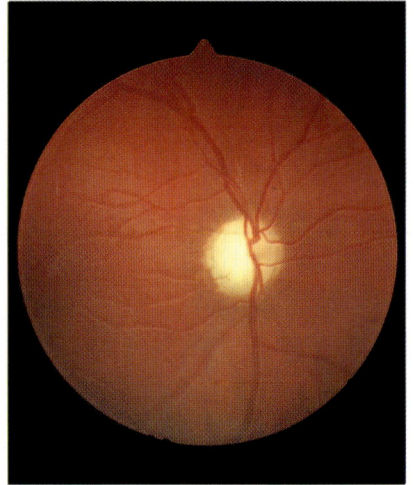

Plate 44 Optic atrophy.

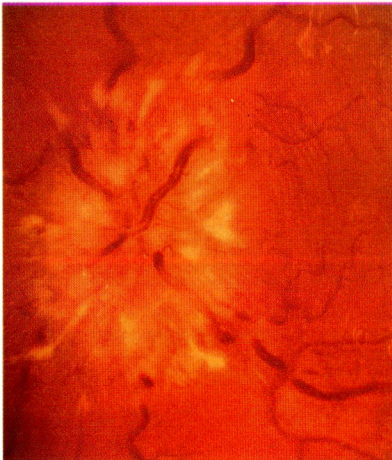

Plate 45 Papilloedema.

eyedrops helps prevent symptoms. Combined antihistamine/decongestant eye-drops give temporary relief from symptoms and are available without prescription.

Vernal keratoconjunctivitis

This inflammation of cornea and conjunctiva can be a severe disease and can produce debilitating corneal problems (Buckley, 1981). Children suffering from this should be managed by an ophthalmologist. Pain, photophobia and watering are intense and the large corneal ulcers can scar and permanently impair vision. Giant papillae are one sign of vernal conjunctivitis (Plate 7) and treatment includes the use of sodium cromoglycate drops (which prevent histamine release), and reducing the intense inflammatory reaction with steroid eyedrops.

Corneal ulcer

This is a very common problem in developing countries (Omerod, 1986), where predisposing factors include malnutrition (Vitamin A deficiency), debilitating infections (measles), neglected trauma (corneal foreign body, abrasion), and pre-existing eye disease (vernal keratoconjunctivitis).

In developed countries the herpes simplex virus is the most common cause of corneal infection. This produces a characteristic 'branching' or dendritic ulcer (Plate 8) which is easily identified with the help of fluorescein. The child may also have a cold sore on the lip or small blistering lesions on the eyelid skin.

If a viral etiology is suspected urgent referral is advisable – treatment should include a topical antiviral. It is important to note that inappropriate steroid treatment encourages viral replication, causing overwhelming corneal destruction and blindness.

Trachoma

This infection, caused by *Chlamydia trachomatis* is endemic in many parts of the developing world, and is a cause of blindness in later life (Taylor, 1993). The organism is spread by flies, fingers and contaminated linen, and produces a recurrent conjunctivitis mainly affecting the area hidden beneath the upper lid. Subsequent scarring (Plate 9) pulls the eyelash-bearing upper lid margin inwards which abrades the corneal surface with subsequent ulceration. Prevention of acute infections involves face washing with clean water – still a luxury in many parts of the world. Acute infections may be treated using tetracycline ointment.

Glaucoma

Very rarely glaucoma secondary to retinoblastoma or retinopathy of prematurity can produce a painful red eye. However the adult form of primary-angle closure glaucoma does not occur in childhood, and dilating the pupils of a child will not produce this problem.

12.4   Eyelids

The eyelids and eyelashes are often overlooked during the eye examination but, if diseased, they are a potent source of irritation, and eye-rubbing, and if untreated can cause conjunctival and corneal problems. Allergy and infection should be diagnosed early and treated quickly to prevent these complications.

Skin allergies

Local irritants such as atropine, cosmetics, nickel and plant pollens can produce an allergic moist swelling of the eyelids in susceptible individuals. The offending substance should be identified and removed. If the local reaction is severe, topical steroids and antihistamine drugs can be used under the careful supervision of an ophthalmologist. Inappropriate and unsupervised steroid treatment can lead to blindness through steroid-related cataract and glaucoma, or encouragement of viral replication in a child with unsuspected herpetic eye disease (see also under corneal ulcer).

Epicanthus

This semilunar fold of skin (Plate 10) is usually bilateral and gives the appearance of a wide nasal bridge which hides the nasal sclera and can produce an appearance of convergent strabismus. The mother can be reassured that as the child grows, and the nasal bridge extends forwards, the folds will be drawn out and disappear. No treatment is required.

A more severe form of epicanthus occurs in association with congenital ptosis and severe narrowing of the palpebral fissure (belpharophimosis). Surgical correction is often required.

Epiblepharon

A prominent fold of skin on the lower lid inverts the lower eyelid so that the lashes rub on the cornea. This causes irritation, but the condition resolves spontaneously over a period of months with growth of the eyelids.

Ptosis

Ptosis in children is most often caused by congenital weakness of the levator muscle (Collin, 1989).

A unilateral ptosis covering the pupil leads to deprivation amblyopia. However, if the lid is lifted and the visual axis cleared at an early stage full visual recovery is possible. Bilateral ptosis will encourage tilting the head back, allowing the child to see, and is less likely to lead to amblyopia.

Marcus Gunn jaw-winking is a fascinating condition where unilateral ptosis is present, but when the jaw is moved away from the side of the affected lid the ptosis disappears or the upper lid may be retracted! The cause is abnormal connections between the 3rd and 5th cranial nerves.

A child with such ptosis should be referred to an ophthalmologist. If the pupil is covered the type of surgery depends on the function of the levator palpebrae superioris, assessed by observing upper lid excursion. Mild ptosis can be corrected by tightening of the levator but if the levator function is poor, the frontalis muscle of the forehead may be used to elevate the eyelid.

Angular dermoid

This benign developmental tumour appears as a mobile subcutaneous lump in the upper outer part of the eyelid (Plate 11). Surgical excision may be performed for cosmetic reasons.

Capillary haemangioma

The 'strawberry naevus' lesion (Plate 12) can grow rapidly in the newborn but spontaneously involutes and diminishes in size later in childhood. If the pupil is covered, swift intervention can avert amblyopia, and the treatment options include injection of corticosteroid, dye-laser treatment, or surgical excision (Kushner, 1982a).

12.5   Eyelid margin problems

The eyelids contain meibomian glands which in health produce secretions vital for the formation of a healthy tear film. The lid margins, tears and corneal surface act as one in protecting, cleansing and lubricating the exposed part of the eye. Disruption or infection of one of these structures impairs the function of the other two, for instance infection of the eyelids alters the quality of the tears, which in turn causes drying of the corneal surface. Infection from the lids can provoke a hypersensitivity reaction in the peripheral cornea and 'marginal' keratitis.

Blepharitis

This is an inflammation of the eyelid margins, with the associated signs of itching and reddening of the delicate, thin skin of the lid (Plate 13). Secondary bacterial infection can be recognized by golden-yellow crusting and discharge, which should be treated with lid cleansing with a moist, cotton-tipped bud and topical antibiotics. Herpes simplex blepharitis produces weeping vesicles and is treated with antiviral cream.

Stye

This local infection of a superficial lash follicle requires topical antibiotic drops, and warm compresses, and will 'come to a head' to rupture onto the skin surface. Surgery is not needed.

Tarsal cyst

Also called Chalazion or Meibomian cyst, the infected meibomian gland may produce an acute red swelling of the lid or a chronic fibrous mass (Plate 14). Multiple or recurrent chalazia may be the result of chronic staphylococcal blepharitis. Such cysts often resolve or discharge spontaneously. Topical antibiotics are only needed if conjunctivitis develops.

If the cyst does not resolve spontaneously, or is large enough to interfere with vision, incision into the lesion from the conjunctival surface and currettage of the contents under general anaesthesia may be performed.

Molluscum contagiosum

If present on the lid margin, this virus-shedding, umbilicated lesion causes a recurrent follicular conjunctivitis which does not improve with topical medicines (Plate 15). Treatment options include currettage or excision to remove the site of viral production.

12.6 Watering eye

Nasolacrimal duct blockage

Approximately 1–2% of infants have delayed patency of their nasolacrimal ducts. This is usually unilateral and resolves by 9–12 months.

Pooling of tears with overflow, in the absence of a patent nasolacrimal system, predisposes to recurrent bacterial conjunctivitis, which should be treated with lid cleansing. Antibiotic treatment is rarely needed. If the symptoms of watering and recurrent conjunctivitis persist after 9–12 months of age, syringing and probing of the nasolacrimal system is indicated under general anaesthesia (Plate 16) (Kushner, 1982b).

Congenital glaucoma

An infant with watering eyes, photophobia, plus enlargement and cloudiness of the corneas, is likely to have congenital glaucoma (Plate 17). The intraocular pressure is very high. The eye may remain 'white' till the late stages of the disease, when congestion of the conjunctival blood vessels occurs. The alternative name 'buphthalmos', meaning 'bull's eye', refers to the appearance of the enlarged corneas. Urgent referral to an ophthalmologist is indicated. The condition results from insufficient drainage of aqueous, typically due to a fine membrane occluding the surface of the trabecular meshwork. Goniotomy (Barkan, 1942) and trabeculotomy (Quigley, 1982) procedures surgically create an internal fistula between the anterior chamber and Schlemm's canal. Trabeculectomy surgery as performed in adults tends to have little success in children as the operation site quickly heals over and drainage of fluid out of the eye ceases.

12.7 Proptosis

Masses behind the eye can displace the eyeball forwards and this sign is called proptosis. A diagnosis of true proptosis must be distinguished from causes of an appearance of a protruding or prominent eye. These include true eye enlargement in myopia or ptosis of the fellow upper lid. It is important to ask about pain and speed of progression, and to check the visual acuity, the direction of protrusion, the degree of inflammation and any impairment of ocular motility. All children with proptosis should be evaluated by an ophthalmologist. Treatment may involve surgical biopsy to establish the diagnosis, followed by further surgical, drug or radiation treatment.

Orbital cellulitis

This is the commonest cause of acute onset proptosis in children (see Section 12.3), and responds well to antibiotic treatment.

Orbital pseudotumour

A non-specific granuloma which has the features of painful proptosis, lid and conjunctival swelling, limitation of ocular motility and diplopia. Ultrasound and CT scans aid diagnosis, which is confirmed by biopsy.

Rhabdomyosarcoma

This is the commonest orbital malignancy in children (Ghafoor, 1985) and presents in a 6–7 year old with rapidly progressing proptosis displacing the eye down and outward. As the lids can no longer protect the eye, exposure produces conjunctival swelling and corneal ulceration. Treatment consists of biopsy, radiotherapy and chemotherapy.

Orbital dermoid cysts

These cystic lesions are usually located in the upper outer aspect of the orbit and contain sebaceous material, hair and fat. The external 'lump' may represent only the 'tip of the iceberg' which can extend deep into the orbit.

Optic nerve glioma

This presents in the first few years of life with a slowly progressive proptosis and gradual visual deterioration due to optic atrophy (Plate 18).

12.8   Leukocoria (white pupil)

This sign should NEVER be overlooked as the eye may harbour a life-threatening tumour, amongst other possibilities, and a child displaying the sign needs urgent referral to an ophthalmologist.

Retinoblastoma

This malignant tumour of the retina occurs sporadically or as a dominantly inherited disease (Plate 19). It usually arises in the first three years of life and is often fairly advanced when first detected on routine examination or when a squint is present. Other late presenting features may be hyphaema, and the red and painful eye of glaucoma. In the early stages, the tumour looks like a white elevation of the retina. The tumour may spread beneath the retina or burst into the vitreous. Spread into the orbit or into the brain along the optic nerve is life-threatening. The fellow eye should always be repeatedly examined, as should the eyes of other members of the family for active tumour in the siblings, and regressed tumour in the parents. In advanced cases when there is no prospect for salvaging vision, enucleation with excision of as much optic nerve as possible is the only treatment. Smaller tumours or recurrences may be treated by external beam irradiation, radioactive scleral plaques, or cryotherapy (Shields, 1981). Chemotherapeutic agents are available to treat metastatic disease. Genetic counselling is important in this devastating condition.

Retinopathy of prematurity

The term 'retinopathy of prematurity' (ROP) refers to all retinal changes seen in premature babies, from mild peripheral vascular changes to advanced retinal scarring and shrinkage (Plate 20). The older term 'retrolental fibroplasia', which referred to advanced cases with white scar tissue immediately behind the lens, is no longer used. Mild ROP can lead to high myopia, amblyopia and squint. Progression to severe scarring disease is not common, but when it occurs it is blinding, and prevention of this by screening examinations and treatment with cryo- or laser-therapy is now performed in most neonatal intensive care units (Cryo-ROP Study Group, 1990).

Toxocara infestation

Eggs of this parasitic worm are found in puppy faeces and toddlers may occasionally ingest these eggs (Ellis, 1986). Intense inflammation occurs in the retina if a worm reaches the eye, and permanent retinal scarring results (Plate 21). While generalized infection may require drug treatment in hospital, there is no effective treatment for ocular involvement.

Persistent hyperplastic primary vitreous (PHPV)

This condition is normally unilateral, the affected eye is small, and white fibrous tissue is seen behind the lens (Pollard, 1985).

Coats' disease

This vascular anomaly can destroy vision by producing a creamy coloured exudative retinal detachment through leakage from abnormal retinal blood vessels (Plate 22). Freezing the lesion with a cryoprobe can be effective (Ridley, 1982).

12.9   Strabismus surgery

Strabismus operations may be performed in order to help a child regain binocular vision, or to improve cosmetic appearance. In every case the limitations of strabismus surgery must be fully explained to the parents. There is a common belief that an operation will 'cure' a squint. The need for continued spectacle wear, and further occlusion treatment for amblyopia must be explained. When a 'functional' result with binocular vision is not anticipated, the presence of a small residual deviation and the possibility of late consecutive divergence must be discussed.

Timing of strabismus operations

Optimal results for infantile esotropia (Chapter 19) are obtained if surgery is performed by the age of 18 months. Surgery for acquired esotropia is usually performed at the age of 3–4 years, once any refractive error or amblyopia have been treated. Intermittent exotropia, if symptoms are severe enough to justify surgery at all, is best treated at about the age of five years as earlier surgery risks secondary convergence with amblyopia. Earlier surgery is needed if the deviation is becoming constant, with loss of binocularity.

Operations

Most strabismus operations in children are performed as day cases, using a short-acting general anaesthetic. Absorbable sutures are used, and the eye is not padded after surgery. The eye is red and watery for one to two weeks after the operation.

Surgical technique

The conjunctiva is opened at the corneoscleral limbus and dissected back to the muscle insertion.

Muscle-weakening operations

Recession (Plate 23). The muscle is detached from the eye and sutured to the sclera more posteriorly.

Muscle-strengthening operations

In a resection, the muscle is detached from the eye, a short portion is cut off, and the muscle is sutured back onto the eye at its normal site of insertion. This tightens the muscle.

Horizontal strabismus

A convergent strabismus may be treated by recession of the medial rectus muscle plus resection of the lateral rectus muscle of one eye, or by recession of the medial rectus muscle of each eye. When the angle of a convergent strabismus is greater for near than for distance, recession of the medial rectus muscle of each eye is the preferred operation. A divergent strabismus may be treated by recession of the lateral rectus muscle plus resection of the medial rectus muscle of one eye, or by recession of the lateral rectus muscle of each eye. When the angle of a divergent strabismus is greater for distance than for near, recession of the muscle of each eye is the preferred operation.

Posterior fixation suture ('Faden') operation

In convergent strabismus with a high AC/A ratio non-surgical treatments such as bifocal spectacles or miotic eyedrops may prove impractical for some children. An alternative treatment is a 'Faden' operation (von Noorden, 1978). The medial rectus muscle is sutured to the sclera just posterior to the equator of the eye. This has little effect in the primary position of gaze, but limits adduction. The effect is therefore to reduce selectively excessive convergence for near vision.

Vertical strabismus

Relative overaction of the inferior oblique muscles is often seen in children with convergent strabismus, especially in infantile esotropia. The eye deviates upwards when adducted. The condition is normally bilateral. The inferior oblique muscles may be weakened by a recession operation. Less commonly either eye may drift upwards when it is not fixing – dissociated vertical deviation (DVD). The vertical deviation is present in abduction and adduction and the recovery movement is relatively slow. Recession of both superior rectus muscles may be performed to correct this condition.

Botulinum toxin

Muscles may be temporarily weakened by injecting botulinum toxin directly into the muscle, under local anaesthetic in adults and general anaesthetic in children. This is particularly useful in lateral rectus paralysis, prior to a definitive operation (Riordan-Eva, 1992). Botulinum toxin is injected into the medial rectus muscle to weaken it, allowing assessment of residual lateral rectus function. One cause of congenital lateral rectus palsy is Mobius syndrome, in which the sixth and seventh cranial nerves are absent. Weakness of the facial muscles accompanies a large angle convergent squint.

Adjustable suture

In cooperative teenagers more accurate alignment may be obtained using 'adjustable suture' strabismus surgery. The suture attached to the eye muscle is tied with a bow knot during the operation and left exposed on the surface of the eye. The next day the bow may be undone after instilling local anaesthetic eyedrops, and the suture loosened or tightened as necessary in order to obtain optimal eye alignment (Rosenbaum, 1977).

Duane's syndrome

Classically, this consists of marked limitation of abduction, with widening of the palpebral fissure; and slightly defective adduction, with narrowing of the palpebral fissure and globe retraction. Abnormal innervation of the medial and lateral recti muscles is the cause of the abnormality in most cases. Surgery is required if there is a large deviation in the primary position, or a troublesome abnormal head posture (Pressman, 1986).

Brown's superior oblique tendon sheath syndrome

This is caused by 'sticking' of the superior oblique tendon within its sheath at the trochlea. The problem is mechanical rather than neurological or muscular. There is absence of elevation in adduction, and the eye may become depressed in adduction (Plate 24).

The syndrome may result in an abnormal head posture with diplopia in certain directions of gaze, and surgery is needed in some cases (von Noorden, 1982).

12.10   Nystagmus

The term nystagmus refers to rhythmic involuntary movements of the eyes. Nystagmus may be pendular, with oscillations of the eyes of equal speed in each direction. Alternatively, nystagmus may be jerking, with a fast movement in one direction followed by a slower recovery movement in the opposite direction. Nystagmus may be primary, with no underlying cause, in which case treatment is aimed at maximizing visual potential. Alternatively, nystagmus may be secondary to underlying disease. It is vital that every new case of nystagmus is fully assessed by an ophthalmologist, and often in addition by a pediatric neurologist, in order that underlying disease may be detected and treated (Castells, 1992).

Latent nystagmus

Latent nystagmus refers to a form of nystagmus which occurs when one eye is covered and does not occur, or is minimal, during binocular vision. Latent nystagmus is often seen in infantile esotropia, and is of the jerking type. The 'jerk' phase of the nystagmus is away from the occluded eye.

Nystagmus due to visual deprivation

The fixation reflexes develop within the first three to four months of life. Profound visual deprivation during this period leads to a rather characteristic 'searching' nystagmus. The eyes wander around as if they are attempting to fix. The movements are relatively slow, and normally some underlying cause such as congenital cataracts, Leber's congenital amaurosis, retinopathy of prematurity, or cortical blindness is evident on further examination.

Primary congenital nystagmus

Nystagmus as an isolated condition has certain characteristic features. Recognition of these features can be helpful in reaching a diagnosis and avoiding unnecessary neurological investigation. Primary 'congenital' nystagmus becomes apparent within the first three months of life. The key characteristic is that the nystagmus only occurs in a horizontal direction, in all directions of gaze. Sometimes the nystagmus has a much lower amplitude when the child looks to one side – the 'null point' and this may lead to a compensating head posture.

In primary congenital nystagmus, the visual acuity is usually within the range of 6/12–6/36. Hypermetropic astigmatism is often present and should be fully corrected. Near vision is often disproportionally good. Mainstream education can be recommended, although some patients do not achieve the visual acuity required for a driving licence. Contact lens optical correction improves vision in some cases (Dell'Osso, 1988), and biofeedback training has been reported to produce improvement in some cases (Abadi, 1980). Albinism produces this type of nystagmus.

Nystagmus secondary to neurological disease

Nystagmus acquired in infancy and early childhood may be secondary to a range of ocular and neurological diseases. Various patterns of nystagmus may occur, but a common feature is that the nystagmus has a vertical component. Diseases affecting the visual pathways, and particularly the optic chiasma, may result in nystagmus. While individually rare, these diseases are very significant as they include optic nerve glioma, craniopharyngioma and other tumours. Young children with recently-acquired nystagmus and visual loss must therefore be investigated urgently.

12.11   Congenital abnormalities and syndromes

A child with a developmental abnormality in the eyeball, eyelid or orbit should
be examined for other systemic malformations. Unfortunately, many congenital
eye defects are not treatable.

Craniofacial dysostoses

Abnormal skull development may lead to abnormal orbit shape and position
(Plate 25). This may lead to strabismus.

Microphthalmos

This is a small eye, often resulting from intra-uterine infections such as rubella,
cytomegalovirus and toxoplasmosis, and is usually associated with other ocular
abnormalities (Plate 26).

Congenital cataract

This can be a result of heredity (often autosomal dominant), or prenatal infections such as rubella (Plate 27). Metabolic disorders such as galactosaemia can
cause cataract. Investigation of congenital cataract should include a careful
family history, and examination of blood and urine for electrolyte and amino
acid abnormalities (Kohn, 1976). However, in 50% of patients, the cause is
unknown.

Complete bilateral cataracts require early surgical extraction and visual rehabi-
litation to prevent amblyopia from stimulus deprivation (Taylor, 1981). Ideally,
surgery should be performed before the age of three months. Optical correction
is by soft contact lenses during infancy, followed by spectacles or contact lenses
during childhood (Hoyt, 1986). Surgery is associated with the later complications
of secondary glaucoma and retinal detachment. Unilateral aphakia following
cataract surgery carries a poorer outlook for visual acuity as contact lens wear,
and occlusion of the fellow eye, is difficult for a child to tolerate and the results
of treatment are disappointing. Partial cataracts can be left as the visual acuity
may be good. Cooperation and understanding between parents, optometrist,
orthoptist, pediatrician and ophthalmologist is essential for optimal management
of congenital cataract.

Congenital glaucoma

This is frequently genetically acquired and can be associated with other iris and
corneal malformations (see Section 12.6).

Corneal dystrophies

Congenital corneal dystrophies are rare, and present with cloudy corneas at birth. Congenital hereditary endothelial dystrophy (CHED) (Kirkness, 1987) and posterior polymorphous dystrophy (PPD) (McCartney, 1988) account for most cases. Other causes of cloudy corneas in infancy include congenital glaucoma, congenital rubella syndrome and some metabolic diseases. The corneal epithelial and stromal dystrophies rarely develop before adulthood. Thygeson's epithelial dystrophy causes irritation, watering and photophobia and is occasionally seen in teenagers.

Keratoconus

Keratoconus may first develop in teenagers (Plate 28). Typically, increasing myopic astigmatism is found on repeated refractions. Retinoscopy, keratoscopy and keratometry images are irregular. There may be a history of allergy, and eye-rubbing may contribute to development of the condition. The central cornea protrudes slightly ('cone' shaped) and the central corneal stroma becomes thin. Fine lines of scarring may develop in the deep stroma. Acute episodes of pain, redness and watering may occur in advanced cases due to corneal oedema following localized splitting of Descemet's membrane (acute hydrops).

Treatment in most cases is optical. Spectacles may provide adequate vision in mild cases and are the preferred treatment. Increasingly, irregular astigmatism may eventually lead to reduced acuity with spectacle correction, and gas permeable contact lenses will then improve acuity. Scleral contact lenses or 'piggy back' hard-on-soft contact lens combinations may be useful in some cases. Corneal transplant surgery is only considered when all reasonable attempts at contact lens fitting have failed (Smiddy, 1988).

Coloboma

This is due to the failure of fusion of the choroidal fissure during the seventh week of development. Usually the iris is involved, but the defect may extend into the ciliary body, retina, choroid, and optic nerve (Plate 29).

Persistent pupillary membrane

An embryological remnant, this consists of strands of tissue suspended in front of the lens, and usually causes little visual impairment.

Aniridia

This is a genetic disease with absence of the iris, nystagmus, reduced visual acuity, and sometimes glaucoma or peripheral corneal scarring (Plate 30) (Nelson, 1984). Photochromic spectacles aid patient comfort.

Albinism

A genetic disease resulting in reduced production of the pigment melanin. In oculocutaneous albinism there is little or no skin pigmentation or eye pigmentation. The eyes look pink due to the absence of iris, retinal pigment epithelium and choroidal pigmentation (Plate 31). The patient is photophobic, and is more comfortable while wearing tinted or photochromic spectacles. There is associated nystagmus, reduced visual acuity, poorly formed foveae, and abnormal nerve crossing at the optic chiasma. Ocular albinism refers to a milder form of albinism in which hair, skin and iris pigmentation are relatively normal, but fundal pigmentation is reduced. Again, there is nystagmus, reduced visual acuity, poorly formed foveae, and abnormal nerve crossing at the optic chiasma (Kinnear, 1985).

Myelinated nerve fibres

These have no effect on vision and require no treatment. Retinal nerve fibres are normally unmyelinated until they enter the optic nerve, but myelination of retinal nerve fibres adjacent to the optic disc occurs in some individuals as a normal variant.

Retinitis pigmentosa

This can be inherited as an autosomal dominant, recessive or X-linked disease. The dominant form has the best prognosis, and the recessive disease the worst, with early visual loss. The underlying defect is a bilateral and irreversible degeneration of the rod, and at a later stage cone, photoreceptors. Typically an adolescent complains of poor vision in dim illumination, and the diagnosis is confirmed by retinal examination. In the early stages clumps of pigment are seen in the peripheral retina and these progress centrally (Plate 32). The visual fields contract progressively until only 'tunnel vision' remains. Eventually even this is lost. There is no cure at present.

Leber's congenital amaurosis

This may be considered as a congenital form of retinitis pigmentosa, in which the baby is blind, nystagmus develops secondary to poor acuity and the electroretinogram shows absent retinal electrical activity. Pigment changes similar to those seen in retinitis pigmentosa develop later.

Macular dystrophies

These affect central vision, and present with nystagmus, photophobia and poor colour vision. The diagnosis is confirmed by the clinical appearance of pigmentary disturbance at the macula, and electrophysiological testing (Plate 33).

Toxoplasma chorioretinitis

In most cases the original infection was prenatal or occurred in early childhood, leaving scars in the retina. Dormant cysts persist within the lesions and very occasionally reactivate during adult life, producing creamy-white fluffy opacity of the retina and vitreous adjacent to the scar (Plate 34) (Noble, 1982). Treatment of a reactivated lesion, using combinations of antibiotics, is only required if the lesion is near the optic disc or macula and is significantly reducing vision. Inactive scars are seen frequently and no active treatment is needed for these. However the patient should be told that there is inactive toxoplasmosis scarring of the retina and that they should seek urgent medical advice in the (very unlikely) event of future acute visual loss.

Optic nerve hypoplasia

An under developed optic nerve (Plate 35) is seen in association with midline brain defects e.g. septo-optic dysplasia which is associated with small stature. The 'double ring' sign refers to a rim of bare sclera which is sometimes seen surrounding the very small optic nerve head.

Optic disc pit

A structural abnormality of the optic disc in which a small area of deep cupping of the disc is seen, usually on the temporal side (Plate 36). Central serous chorioretinopathy may develop in these eyes.

Optic disc drusen

These are small particles of protein material which look like sugar granules embedded in the optic nerve head (Plate 37). Arcuate field defects can develop in these eyes.

Scleral crescent

This term refers to the area of bare sclera which can sometimes be seen adjacent to the optic nerve head. It is of no functional significance.

12.12   Systemic disease and the eye

Diabetes mellitus (DM)

DM is a chronic disorder of carbohydrate metabolism, and is the most common endocrine disorder of childhood. Most diabetic children have Type 1, insulin-dependent diabetes mellitus (IDDM). The peak ages of onset for IDDM are between about six years and puberty, with frequency increasing with age from about one case in 1500 at five years of age, to about one case in 350 at 16 years of age. Whilst there are a number of ocular manifestations of diabetes, optometrists are particularly concerned with monitoring diabetics for retinal signs, the prevalence of which rises with increasing duration of the disease. Diabetic retinopathy in childhood is uncommon. Rarely neovascularization is observed in adolescents, where diabetes is poorly controlled. If a child is under the care of an optometrist, referral for ophthalmological opinion should be made whenever maculopathy, preproliferative retinopathy or proliferative retinopathy is detected.

Rubella

Ocular involvement is common in congenital rubella syndrome, particularly if the mother contracted rubella in the first four weeks of pregnancy.

The common ocular features are: microphthalmia; cataract, usually bilateral nuclear cataract which become denser as the child grows older; congenital glaucoma; corneal opacity; uveitis – the pupil tends to be small and cannot be widely dilated; pigmentary retinopathy – typically referred to as 'salt-and-pepper' retinopathy which is usually non-progressive and is compatible with good visual acuity (Givens, 1993).

Down's syndrome

Also known as trisomy 21, this is associated with staphylococcal blepharitis, broad epicanthal folds, keratoconus and cataract (Plate 38).

Marfan's syndrome

A dominantly inherited condition associated with lens dislocation and cataract, high myopia and retinal detachment (Plate 39). The skeletal features of arachnodactyly (long, thin spindly fingers and toes) and hyperextensible joints are typical.

Neurofibromatosis

An autosomal dominant genetic disorder which gives rise to multisystem benign tumours of neuroectodermal tissue (Ragge, 1993). Café-au-lait pigmented skin patches and small neurofibroma skin lumps are present in most cases, and 'Lisch nodules' appear on the irises during childhood. Occasionally benign optic nerve glioma tumours develop, with reduced acuity.

Sturge-Weber syndrome

This normally presents with 'port-wine stain' skin lesion in infancy (Plate 40). If the upper eyelid is involved, glaucoma may develop in the eye during childhood.

Stevens-Johnson syndrome

A drug-induced allergy, usually due to sulphonamide derivatives, causing conjunctival ulceration and scarring which may lead to dry eye and corneal scarring (Plate 41).

Juvenile chronic arthritis (JCA)

Children with certain forms of arthritis may develop iritis (Kanski, 1984) (Plate 42). While iritis normally presents with a red, photophobic eye in the adult, a child with JCA-related iritis may have a white and painless eye. Blurred vision is the only symptom and may not be detected in young children. Regular screening examinations using a slit lamp are therefore needed in these children. Band keratopathy, glaucoma and cataract develop if treatment is delayed.

Leukaemia

This can result in retinal haemorrhages and creamy white retinal infiltrates (Plate 43).

Non-accidental injury

Also known as battered baby syndrome. Retinal haemorrhages are a key feature of shaking injuries (see Chapter 14).

12.13   Neurological disease and the eye

Visual acuity

Progressive deterioration of visual acuity can be the earliest sign of a range of neurological diseases including brain tumours and degenerative diseases of the brain. Young children adapt quickly to reduced vision and their behaviour may remain apparently normal even when quite severe visual loss is present. Conversely, it can sometimes be difficult to determine whether apparent reduction of visual acuity in a child is genuine or is due to poor attention during testing. Electrical tests of retinal function (electroretinogram) and optic nerve function (visually-evoked potential) can be helpful in this situation (Kriss, 1992).

Visual field

As with visual acuity young children adapt remarkably to reduced visual field, and a defect may not become apparent until visual loss is quite severe. Constricted visual fields may result from optic nerve damage in hydrocephalus. Right or left homonymous defects may be found in some children with cerebral palsy.

Cortical blindness

This refers to reduced acuity due to disease of the optic radiations or occipital cortex of the brain. The condition should be suspected in a child with reduced acuity if there is a history of cerebral palsy, seizures, or general developmental delay.

Delayed visual development

This can occur in an otherwise normal baby. The baby appears to be blind during the first few months of life but later develops normal vision (Fielder, 1985). Electroretinogram, visually-evoked potential and EEG testing excludes major organic disease and the diagnosis is made by simply waiting for a few months and reassessing visual behaviour regularly.

Optic atrophy

A typical presentation is a child who fails the school eye test with a below-par visual acuity. Optic atrophy may be an inherited disorder, or as a result of neonatal anoxia, trauma, inflammation, compression by a tumour, or following papilloedema associated with hydrocephalus (Plate 44).

Papilloedema

Papilloedema refers to oedema of the optic disc. The rim of the disc is blurred, the disc is pink, and small splinter shaped haemorrhages may be present at the edge of the disc (Plate 45). The term 'choked disc' can be used to describe the appearance of the optic nerve head. Visual acuity and pupil reactions are normal until a late stage in the condition. Visual fields are initially normal apart from enlarged blind spots, but later become constricted if the condition is not adequately treated. Papilloedema is most often caused by raised intracranial pressure (Ghose, 1983), and other neurological defects may be present such as headaches, nausea and weakness of abduction of one or both eyes due to sixth cranial nerve weakness.

If optic nerve head abnormality is detected, urgent referral to an ophthalmologist or pediatric neurologist is advised. The optic discs often appear pink and raised in hypermetropes, and refraction is a key part of the assessment of a child with possible papilloedema.

12.14   References and further reading

References

Abadi, R.V., Carden, D. and Simpson, J. (1980) 'A new treatment for congenital nystagmus'. *Brit. J. Ophthalmol.*, **64**, 2–6.

Barkan, O. (1942) 'Operation of congenital glaucoma'. *Am. J. Ophthalmol.*, **25**, 552–6.

Buckley, R.J. (1981) 'Vernal keratopathy and its management'. *Trans. Ophthalmol. Soc. UK.*, **101**, 234–8.

Castells, I., Harris, C.M., Shawkat, F. and Taylor, D. (1992) 'Nystagmus in infancy'. *Brit. J. Ophthalmol.*, **76**, 434–7.

Collin, J.R.O. (1989) 'Ptosis', in *A Manual of Systematic Eyelid Surgery*, 2nd edn. Churchill Livingstone, 41–72.

Cryotherapy for retinopathy of prematurity cooperative group. (1990) Multicentre trial of cryotherapy for retinopathy of prematurity. Three-month outcome'. *Arch. Ophthalmol.* **108**, 195–204.

Dell'Osso, L.F., Traccis, S., Abel, L.A., Erzurum, S.I. and Donin, J.F. (1988) 'Contact lenses and congenital nystagmus'. *Clin. Vis. Sci.*, **3**, 229–32.

Dutton, J.J., Manson, P.N., Iliff, N. and Putterman, A.M. (1991) 'Management of blow-out fracture of the orbital floor'. *Surv. Ophthalmol.*, **35**, 279–98.

Ellis, G.S., Pakalnis, V.A. and Worley, G. (1986) 'Toxocara canis infestation. Clinical and epidemiological associations with seropositivity in Kindergarten children'. *Ophthalmol.*, **93**, 1032–8.

Fielder, A.R., Russell-Eggitt, I.R., Dodd, K.L. and Meller, D.H. (1985) 'Delayed visual maturation'. *Trans. Ophthalmol. Soc. UK*, **104**, 653–61.

Ghafoor, S.Y. and Dudgeon, J. (1985) 'Orbital rhabdomyosarcoma: improved survival with combined pulsed chemotherapy and irradiation'. *Brit. J. Ophthalmol.*, **69**, 557–61.

Ghose, S. (1983) 'Optic nerve changes in hydrocephalus'. *Trans. Ophthalmol. Soc. UK*, **103**, 217–20.

Givens, K.T., Lee, D.A., Jones, T. and Ilstrup, D.M. (1993) 'Congenital rubella syndrome: ophthalmic manifestations and associated systemic disorders'. *Brit. J. Ophthalmol.*, **77**, 358–63.

Harcourt, R.B. and Hopkins, D. (1971) 'Ophthalmic manifestations of the battered baby syndrome'. *Brit. Med. J.*, **3**, 398–403.

Hoyt, C.S. (1986) 'The optical correction of pediatric aphakia'. *Arch. Ophthalmol.*, **104**, 6541–2.

Kanski, J.J. and Shun-shin, G.A. (1984) 'Systemic uveitis syndromes in childhood – an analysis of 340 cases'. *Ophthalmology*, **91**, 1247–51.

Kinnear, P.E., Jay, B. and Witkop, C.J. Jr. (1985) 'Albinism'. *Surv. Ophthalmol.*, **30**, 75–101.

Kirkness, C.M., McCartney, A.C.E., Rice, N., Garner, A. and Steele, A. McG. (1987) 'Congenital hereditary corneal oedema of Maumenee: its clinical features, management and pathology'. *Brit. J. Ophthalmol.*, **71**, 130–45.

Kohn, B.A. (1976) 'A differential diagnosis of cataracts in infants and childhood'. *Am. J. Dis. Child*, **130**, 184–91.

Kriss, A. and Russell-Eggitt, I. (1992) 'Electrophysiology assessment of visual pathway function in infants'. *Eye*, **6**, 145–53.

Kushner, B.J. (1982a) 'Intralesional corticosteroids injection for infantile adnexal hemangioma'. *Am. J. Ophthalmol.*, **93**, 496–506.

Kushner, B.J. (1982b) 'Congenital nasolacrimal system obstruction'. *Arch. Ophthalmol.*, **100**, 597–600.

McCartney, A.C.E. and Kirkness, C.M. (1988) 'Comparison between posterior polymorphous dystrophy and congenital hereditary endothelial dystrophy of the cornea'. *Eye*, **2**, 63–71.

Nelson, L.B., Spaeth, G.L. and Nowinski, T.S. (1984) 'Aniridia, a review'. *Surv. Ophthalmol.*, **28**, 621–42.

Nobel, K. and Carr, R. (1982) 'Disorders of the fundus: toxoplasma retinochoroiditis'. *Ophthalmology*, **89**, 1289–91.

Omerod, L.D., Murphee, A.L., Gomez, D.S., Schanzlin, D.J. and Smith, R.E. (1986) 'Microbial keratitis in children'. *Ophthalmology*, **93**, 449–55.

Pierce, J.M., Ward, M.E. and Seal, D.V. (1982) 'Ophthalmia Neonatorum in the 1980s: incidence, aetiology and treatment'. *Brit. J. Ophthalmol.*, **66**, 728–31.

Pollard, Z. (1985) 'Treatment of persistent hyperplastic primary vitreous'. *J. Pediatr. Ophthalmol.*, **22**, 180–3.

Pressman, S.H. and Scott, W. (1986) 'Surgical treatment of Duane's syndrome'. *Ophthalmology*, **93**, 29–38.

Quigley, H.A. (1982) 'Childhood glaucoma: the results with trabeculotomy and the study of irreversible cupping'. *Ophthalmology*, **89**, 219–25.

Ragge, N. (1993) 'Clinical and genetic patterns of neurofibromatosis 1 and 2'. *Brit. J. Ophthalmol.*, **77**, 662–72.

Ridley, M.E., Shields, J.A., Brown, G.C. and Tasman, W. (1982) 'Coat's disease evaluation and management'. *Ophthalmology*, **89**, 1381–7.

Riordan-Eva P. and Lee, J.P. (1992) 'Management of VIth nerve palsy – avoiding unnecessary surgery'. *Eye*, **6**, 386–90.

Rosenbaum, A.L., Metz, H.S., Carlson, M. and Jampolsky, A.J. (1977) 'Adjustable rectus muscle recession surgery. A follow-up study'. *Arch. Ophthalmol.*, **95**, 817–20.

Shields, J.A. and Augsburger, J.J. (1981) 'Current approaches to the diagnosis and management of retinoblastoma'. *Survey. Ophthalmol.*, **25**, 347–71.

Smiddy, W.E., Hamburg, T.R., Kracher, G.P. and Stark, W.J. (1988) 'Keratoconus: contact lens or keratoplasty?'. *Ophthalmology*, **95**, 487–93.

Taylor, D. (1981) 'Choice of surgical technique in management of congenital cataracts'. *Trans. Ophthalmol. Soc. UK*, **101**, 114–18.

Taylor, H.R. (1993) 'Trachoma – the future for a disease of the past'. *Brit. J. Ophthalmol.*, **77**, 66.

Weiss, A., Friendly, D., Eglin, K., Chang, M. and Cold, B. (1983) 'Bacterial periorbital and orbital cellulitis in childhood'. *Ophthalmology*, **90**, 195–203.

Von Noorden, G.K. (1978) 'Indications of the posterior fixation operation in strabismus'. *Ophthalmology*, **85**, 512–20.

Von Noorden, G.K. and Oliver, P. (1982) 'Superior tenectomy in Brown's syndrome'. *Ophthalmology*, **89**, 303.

Further reading

Taylor, D. (1990) *Pediatric Ophthalmology*. Blackwell Scientific Publications Inc., Boston.

von Noorden, G.K. (1990) *Binocular Vision and Ocular Motility*, 4th edn. CV Mosby Co., St. Louis.

CHAPTER 13

Pediatric Neurodevelopmental Disorders

Elizabeth Green

13.1 Cerebral palsy

This is a non-progressive neurological disorder resulting from damage occurring to the immature brain *in utero*, during or after birth. Some hereditary forms have been demonstrated. Although the disorder is non-progressive, its clinical presentation tends to change as the child matures. The damage is rarely limited purely to the motor areas of the brain, so that associated handicaps are common, such as visual difficulties, mental handicap, and epilepsy.

The type of cerebral palsy is often described by the anatomical distribution of the motor impairment and the type of neurological signs predominating. Total body involvement is described as a quadriplegia, unilateral involvement as a hemiplegia and lower-limb involvement as a diplegia. In addition, the cerebral palsy may be described as spastic, athetoid, choreo-athetoid or ataxic, depending on the main neurological signs present. The movement disorder may involve the muscles of the eyes, especially if spasticity is present. If the neurological deficit is severe, the likelihood of damage to the visual pathways and visual cortex is high. The visual impairment is compounded by the lack of visual experience resulting from the poor positioning and mobility achieved by the child.

Studies of visual problems in children with cerebral palsy show a high incidence of visual anomalies. Probably because of differences in the nature of the groups studied, there is a wide variance in prevalence data (Duckman, 1987). Percentages of strabismus range from as low as 15% (Lossef, 1962) to as high as 60% (Guibor, 1953; Jones & Dayton, 1968). The frequent occurrence of strabismus in cerebral palsy has focused attention on this particular visual finding, but studies show a similarly high prevalence of other problems. Significant refractive error occurs much more frequently in the cerebral-palsied population than in equivalent age-groups of children without cerebral palsy. Reports range from a prevalence of 40% (Duckman, 1979; Wiesinger, 1964) to 76% (Altman *et al.*, 1966). Duckman (1979) found oculomotor dysfunction in 92% of a group of cerebral-palsied children, and accommodative insufficiency in 100% (Duckman, 1984). It is clear that the prevalence of visual anomalies in the population of children with cerebral palsy is significantly higher than those found in a normal population (Roberts, 1972, 1978).

13.2 Spina bifida and hydrocephalus

Spina bifida and hydrocephalus are developmental defects caused by failure of fusion of the neural tube occurring early in embryonic life. The neural tube may be affected anywhere along its length, although the thoracolumbar region is the most common. Hydrocephalus occurs in around 80% of children with spina bifida. The hydrocephalus is often caused by either a mixture of obstruction at the aqueduct and malabsorption or overproduction of cerebrospinal fluid, or one of these factors alone.

It is particularly important to document the extent of strabismus and visual acuity in any child with hydrocephalus as one of the signs of increased intracranial pressure is a change in visual signs or acuity. A prolonged rise in intracranial pressure may lead to optic atrophy. Nystagmus may be present, and an increase of nystagmus can also indicate a rise of intracranial pressure especially if the child has an Arnold-Chiari malformation. This is a defect of the spinal canal at the junction of the spinal cord and the brain. If the pressure inside the head increases, the brain stem and/or cerebellum may attempt to herniate through into the defect.

13.3 Coordination problems

Coordination problems are seen fairly commonly in childhood, especially in boys. Although they may occur alone, difficulties of coordination are often accompanied by other developmental problems such as delayed speech and language development, poor concentration, an inability to sit still and, sometimes, reading and writing difficulties. An alternative name for this group of difficulties is organizational problems. This describes the central difficulty of organization of the input and output of the various systems of the brain, as well as a difficulty in building some of the systems, for example that of language. The range of intelligence seen in children with organizational problems is the same as in other children, although some children may appear mentally slow as they may find it difficult to express themselves verbally or to act on instructions. Additional signs found in affected children such as a poor sense of laterality may be found also in the visual system, together with difficulty in maintaining coordination as in convergence of the eyes.

The etiology of the condition is variable. In many children it seems to be an inherited characteristic which has not yet been identified as a clear genetically derived condition whilst in other children it may result from perinatal damage or cerebral insults of other kinds. It is always important to make a precise initial examination as there are a very small number of children who prove to have the early stages of a progressive neurological disease. Repeat examination can demonstrate the deterioration. In other children there may be evidence of a mild connective tissue disorder leading to laxity of joints.

The clinical signs in a child with organizational problems may not be as clear as the above description suggests. It may be difficult to know exactly what is wrong with the child, although often a certain degree of suspicion may lead to an assessment of the relevant areas and so define the problem.

13.4 Autism

This is a disorder characterized by severe difficulties in social interaction, in verbal and non-verbal communication and concept formation, and with a variable non-verbal intelligence. It may be accompanied by some mild motor difficulties, especially later in childhood, and by epilepsy, especially in adolescence. Autism usually has a poor prognosis for complete adult independence. Prevalence studies have found two to four autistic children in every 10 000, with more if severely retarded children with autistic features are included (Rutter, 1985).

There are several different theories of causation, but recent research has shown considerable evidence of brain dysfunction. Two types of causal agents have been identified – those associated with brain damage and genetic factors (Folstein & Rutter, 1977). The clinical syndrome may be associated with single-gene or chromosomal abnormalities such as the fragile X chromosome, phenylketonuria, tuberolus sclerosis and neurofibromatosis; whilst in other cases there is a history of infections such as congenital rubella.

Assessment of children with autism is difficult as the lack of communication and indifference to other people limits the possibilities of cooperative activity. Some autistic people do have particular skills in one or two areas such as music, letters or numbers, whilst at the end of the autistic continuum approaching normality children with Asberger's syndrome (Wing, 1981a) show a lack of awareness of other's feelings and have deviant styles of both verbal and non-verbal communication. At the other end of the developmental continuum, about half the children with severe mental retardation have symptoms of autism (Wing, 1981b).

13.5 Attention deficit disorder or hyperactivity

As the name suggests, the prime disorder appears to be in the attentional system. An affected child therefore has a short attention span, is highly distractible with disruptive behaviour as a result. In the USA treatment with stimulant drugs is popular, whilst in the UK management is more often by behavioural modification. There does not appear to be a clear etiology, but in some children it may result from perinatal damage or other cerebral insults. Some affected children may show particular sensitivity to artificial colourings or other additives, but controlled trials of management of hyperactivity by restriction of such additives have proved difficult as there are so many other factors which cannot be tightly controlled.

13.6 Developmental delay

Mild or severe delay may result from many different etiologies. There are various genetic causes with chromosomal abnormalities. Different phenotypes give rise to different but often characteristic clinical pictures. There are often abnormalities in several organs of the body, and abnormalities of a particular organ, for example the eye, will be associated with certain abnormal phenotypes. Full details of such conditions as well as recognizable syndromes without a clear genetic etiology may be found in Smith (1988).

The description of physical differences around the eyes may lead to a definitive diagnosis of the child's condition. Important features to note are the shape of the eyebrows and orbital ridges, prominent eyes, ptosis, lacrimal defects, strabismus, nystagmus, myopia, blue sclera, microphthalmos, colobomata or unusual patterning or colourations of the iris, glaucoma, defects or opacities of the cornea, cataracts, lens dislocations and retinal pigmentation.

One cause of an inherited mental handicap has been shown to result from a 'fragile-site' on the X chromosome, the syndrome being called the fragile X syndrome. A considerable proportion of boys attending schools for the mildly educationally delayed have been shown to have this fragile site (Thake *et al.*, 1987). Other causes for developmental delay include metabolic disorders, maternal infections during pregnancy leading to infection of the fetus, for example rubella or cytomegalovirus. There is still a proportion of cases where a definite reason for the developmental delay cannot be found. Visual signs will vary according to the etiology of the condition, and may be particularly common in some conditions such as strabismus in chromosomal abnormalities.

13.7 Speech and language delay and disorder

Speech and language delay is one of the most common problems of childhood. It is more common in boys, usually resolves completely and can be distinguished from language disorder by the fact that progress occurs following the usual developmental sequence. In language disorder an atypical sequence may be found, with abnormalities of either expression or comprehension, or both. Mild neurological signs are sometimes found in a child with a language disorder, with an increased likelihood of coordination problems in the eyes (see also Chapter 9).

13.8 References

Altman, H.E., Hiatt, R.L. and Deweese, M.W. (1966) 'Ocular findings in cerebral palsy'. *South Med. J.*, **59**, 1015–18.

Duckman, R.H. (1984) 'Accommodation in cerebral palsy: function and remediation'. *J. Am. Optom. Assoc.*, **55**, No. 4, 281–3.

Duckman, R.H. (1987) 'Vision therapy for the child with cerebral palsy'. *J. Am. Optom. Assoc.*, **58**, No. 1, 28–35.

Folstein, S. and Rutter, M. (1988) 'Autism: familial aggregation and genetic implications'. *J. Autism Dev. Disord.*, **18**, 3–30.

Guibor, G.P. (1953) 'Some eye defects seen in cerebral palsy'. *Amer. J. Phys. Med.*, **32**, No. 6, 342–7.

Jones, M.H. and Dayton, G.O. (1968) 'Assessment of visual disorders in cerebral palsy'. *Arch. Ital. Pediatr.*, **25**, No. 3, 251–64.

Lossef, S. (1962) 'Ocular findings in cerebral palsy'. *Amer. J. Ophthalmol.*, **54**, No. 6, 1114–18.

Lyons, K. & Jones, W.B. (eds) (1988) *Smith's Recognizable Patterns of Human Malformation*, 4th edn. W.B. Saunders & Co., London.

Roberts, J. (1972) 'Eye examination findings among children'. *Vital and Health Statistics. US Dept. of HEW*, **11**, No. 115.

Roberts, J. (1978) 'Refraction status and motility defects of persons 4–74 years. *Vital and Health Statistics, US Dept. of HEW*, **11**, No. 206.

Rutter, M. (1985) 'Infantile autism and other pervasive developmental disorders', in *Child and Adolescent Psychiatry: Modern Approaches*. (M. Rutter & L. Hersov, eds). Blackwell, Oxford.

Thake, A., Todd, J., Webb, T. and Bundey, S. (1987) 'Children with the fragile X chromosome at schools for the mildly mentally impaired'. *Devel. Med. Child Neurol.*, **29**, 711–19.

Weisinger, H. (1964) 'Ocular findings in mentally retarded children'. *J. Pediatr. Ophthalmol.*, **1**, No. 3, 37–41.

Wing, L. (1981a) 'Asberger's syndrome: a clinical account'. *Pschol. Med.*, **11**, 115–29.

Wing, L. (1981b) 'Language, social and cognitive impairments in autism and severe mental retardation'. *J. Autism Dev. Disord.*, **11**, 31–44.

CHAPTER 14

Ocular Signs of Child Abuse

Simon Barnard

14.1 Introduction

The abuse of children is not an uniquely modern phenomenon but rather an ugly trait that has affected mankind from the earliest of times. Throughout the 1950s and 1960s there was a growing awareness that young children presenting with fractures and intracranial bleeding were the victims of abuse by a parent or guardian. However, it was not until 1962 that the topic of child abuse gained medical attention when Kempe *et al.* suggested the term 'battered child syndrome' and proposed that such abuse was a frequent, but unsuspected, cause of serious injury or death in children.

It has been estimated that 40% of cases of physically abused children exhibit ocular complications (Fontana *et al.*, 1963; Roberton *et al.*, 1982). Friendly (1971) found that 6% of the reported abuse cases were detected by eye-care practitioners.

14.2 Definition of child abuse

The term 'child abuse' covers many facets that consitute maltreatment of a child. A parent may harm a child by a deliberate act or by a failure to provide adequate care. It encompasses both physically and emotionally damaging influences that result from acts of commission (abuse) or omission (neglect) by a responsible parent or guardian (Davoren, 1982). The definition is wide enough to include the problem known as 'child sexual abuse'. Child abuse may be categorized into four sub-groups: emotional abuse and neglect, sexual abuse, physical neglect, and physical abuse.

Emotional abuse and neglect

Emotional abuse is an intangible and immeasurable entity that differs from child to child and is partly dependent on the personality and sensitivity of each child. However, if the emotional development and child's behaviour is severely affected

273

by the parent's neglect, rejection or attitude to the child then this may be defined as 'emotional abuse' (Gothard *et al.*, 1985; Meadow, 1989).

Sexual abuse

Child sexual abuse involves dependent, developmentally immature children and adolescents in sexual activities they do not truly comprehend, to which they are unable to give informed consent, and which violate the social taboos of family roles or are against the law (Valman, 1987).

Physical neglect

Every child has certain basic requirements and it is the duty of every parent not to deliberately withhold adequate food, love, shelter and protection. Indications of parental neglect of a child include inferior general health (Gothard *et al.*, 1985), lack of adequate medical, dental and optometric care, signs of malnutrition, low level of activity and begging or stealing of food.

Physical abuse

This category includes injury which occurs due to the failure to provide a safe environment, or injury inflicted deliberately. Physical abuse can present as a broad spectrum of injury which may result as an escalation of discipline or from a more sinister premeditated violence. Abuse of drugs during pregnancy can also be considered to be a form of abuse (Giese, 1984).

14.3   Epidemiology

In England in the year ending 31 March 1992 there were 38 500 children and young persons under the age of 18 years on child protection registers, a rate of 3.5 per thousand population under the age of 18 years (Department of Health, 1994). Giese (1994), cites a paper by Daro & McCurdy (1992) which suggests an estimated 2.7 million alleged cases of child abuse reported in a fifty-state survey in the USA.

Smith (1988) reviewed the risk factors associated with abuse within families and concluded that whilst unemployment, poverty and low socioeconomic status play important parts in abusive families, abuse dose occur in families where parents are well educated and financially and socially stable. Smith cites other factors contributing to a family being at risk, including marital discord, social isolation, alcoholism and drug abuse.

Maltreatment of children is prevalent amongst males and females and can occur with children of any age (see Table 14.1).

Table 14.1 Children and young persons on child protection registers in England for the year ending 31 March 1993 (Department of Health, 1994).

		Number
Sex	Male	18 800
	Female	19 700
Age groups (years)	Under 1	2 500
	1–4	1 200
	5–9	12 200
	10–15	10 400
	16 and over	1 500

14.3.1 General signs of child abuse and neglect

There are many possible indications that a child is a victim of physical abuse but the difficulty for health-care practitioners and social workers is to differentiate such signs from those of truly accidental injury. For example, every child becomes bruised and grazed on the elbows, shins and knees by everyday activities and the presence of lacerations, scratches and bruises is not necessarily indicative of abuse. However, the optometrist should be aware that suspicious bruises tend to be found around the cheeks, jaw, eyes, ears or any soft tissue such as upper arms, buttocks or thighs. Multiple bruises at different stages of healing may be suspicious (Meadow, 1989a; Gothard *et al.*, 1985).

Bone fractures (Worlock *et al.*, 1986), burns (Keen *et al.*, 1975) and bites may also be caused by abuse.

Table 14.2 summarizes both the general physical and behavioural signs of child abuse and neglect, some of which may be apparent to the optometrist.

Munchausen syndrome by proxy is a bizarre disorder in which the care-giver, most commonly the mother, has a need to be around a medical environment or be the subject of medical attention and obtains this end by inducing medical disorders in her child (Meadow, 1989). For example, this may be done by poisoning the child. The mother may be suffering from Munchausen syndrome herself in which she inflicts illnesses upon herself to obtain the same end.

14.3.2 Ocular manifestations of child abuse

It was Kiffney (1964), who first reported ocular injuries (retinal detachment, bilateral subretinal haemorrhages and bilateral partial cataracts) in a case of battered baby syndrome. Since then a host of ocular manifestations of abuse have been reported and some of these are noted in Table 14.3.

Table 14.2 Summary of the general physical, emotional and behavioural signs of abuse and neglect (after Smith, 1988).

General physical signs of abuse and neglect	Emotional and behavioural signs of abuse and neglect
Bruises around cheeks, jaw, eyes, ears or mastoid area	'Frozen watchfulness'
Soft-tissue bruises on upper arms, thighs, buttocks or genitals	Fear of strangers
	Indiscriminate attachment to strangers
Hair loss with or without subgaleal haematoma	Failure to thrive/grow
Torn frenum of upper lip	Generalized anxiety
Torn floor of mouth	Low intellectual performance
Burns on any posterior part of the body	Sad affect
particularly buttocks, perineum, hands or feet	Low self-esteem
Full thickness burns	Impaired ability to enjoy life
Multiple lesions or fractures in different stages of	Social withdrawal
healing	Learned helplessness
Poor hygiene	Suicidal ideation or attempts
Inferior general health	Drug and alcohol abuse
Signs of malnutrition	Misconduct in school
Child not properly immunized	Academic failure/poor school attendance
Venereal disease in a pre-adolescent child	Aggressive behaviour
	Sleeping problems
	Running away
	Low level activity
	Weight fluctuation
	Fatigue

14.4   The optometrist's role

It is not the optometrist's function to diagnose abuse. However, when a child presents with suspicious signs the optometrist should be aware of the possibility of abuse being the cause. The index of suspicion may be raised if there are case-history inconsistencies (see Table 14.4). The optometrist should never confront parents or accuse them of abuse.

In the USA the optometrist is required by law to report suspicious clinical findings to the proper child protective agency (Giese, 1994). This is not the case in the UK where, when an optometrist detects disease or injury to the eye, he or she is legally bound to refer the patient to a registered medical practitioner (Opticians Act, 1958). If a patient (or the parent or guardian of a child) refuses to allow the practitioner to refer, the optometrist must make a note of the reasons for the refusal. However, it should be noted that the General Optical Council will support any optometrist who acts correctly in the best interests of a patient (Wilshin, 1994).

Table 14.3 Ocular manifestations of abuse.

External eye	Solt-tissue swelling, periorbital bruising[1] and multiple small skin burns (Harcourt, 1973).
Eyelids	Ptosis (Quinn & Gammon, 1983).
Eyelashes and eyebrows	Eyelash infestation with *Phthirius pubis* (crab louse) linked to child abuse (Scott & Esterley, 1983).
Conjunctiva	Haemorrhages associated with periorbital bruising following direct trauma, secondary to fractures of the anterior cranial fossa or from compression of the chest cavity (Smith, 1988; Cameron & Rae, 1975).
Cornea and anterior chamber	Corneal perforation (Smith *et al.*, 1973), scarring, edema and opacification (Quinn & Gammon, 1983; Harley, 1980). Corneal vascularization mimicking interstitial keratitis (Harcourt, 1973). Hyphaema (Reece & Grodin, 1985). Secondary glaucoma (Tseng, 1976).
Iris and pupil	Anterior and posterior synechiae (Friendly, 1971). Miosis (Quinn & Gammon, 1983). Iridoplegia (Gaynon *et al.*, 1988). Cycloplegia in the absence of drops (Quinn & Gammon, 1983). Anisocoria (Harcourt, 1973).
Lens	Cataract (Kiffney, 1964; Fessard *et al.*, 1976; Friendly, 1971).
Vitreous	Haemorrhage into the vitreous (Elner *et al.*, 1990).

Retina	Haemorrhages associated with
	    (a) direct head trauma associated with subdural haematoma
	    (b) 'the shaken baby syndrome' (Gilkes & Mann, 1967)[2]
	    (c) Purtscher's retinopathy (Tomasi & Rosman, 1975)[3].
	Retinoschisis (Greenwald *et al.* 1986).
	Retinal and macular folds (Gaynon *et al.* 1988).
	Chorioretinal lesions (Fessard *et al.*, 1967; Harcourt, 1973).
	Retinal detachment (Weidenthal, 1976).

Optic disc	Papilloedema. Optic atrophy (Harcourt, 1973).
Visual pathway	Damage to visual pathway including visual cortex (Harcourt, 1973).
Oculomotor defects	Esotropia (Fontana, 1989). Nystagmus.

[1] Any child presenting with two 'black eyes' should cause the practitioner's index of suspicion to be raised especially if there is evidence of bruising elsewhere.
[2] Repeated shaking of a baby can cause 'whiplash'-type injuries giving rise to retinal and cerebral haemorrhages. There may be an absence of external signs of direct head trauma.
[3] This is caused by sudden compression of the thorax or abdomen giving rise to an increased intraocular and intracranial vascular pressure.

Table 14.4 Case history inconsistencies with respect to signs or symptoms.

No history offered
History vague or inconsistent with injuries
History changes during course of examination
History varies between parent and child, or between parents
Multiple hospital admissions for accidental injuries
Increase of severity of injuries
Delay in seeking medical attention

Withhold not good from those to whom it is due, when it is in the power of
thy hand to do it.

Proverbs 3, 27

14.5   References

Cameron, J.M. and Rae, L.J. (1975) *Atlas of the Battered Child Syndrome*. Churchill Livingstone, London.

Daro, D. and McCurdy, K. (1992) *Current trends in child abuse reporting and fatalities: the results of the 1991 annual 50-state survey*. Chicago, Il.: National Center on Child Abuse Prevention Research. Working Paper number 808, April.

Davoren, E. (1982) 'The profession of social work and the protection of children', in *Child Abuse*. (Newberger, ed.). Little Brown & Co. Boston.

Department of Health (1994) 'Children and Young People on Child Protection Registers', Year Ending 31 March 1993.

Elner, S.G., Elner, V.M., Arnall, M. and Albert, D.M. (1990) Ocular and associated systemic findings in suspected child abuse. *Arch. Ophthalmol.*, **108**, 1094–101.

Fessard, C., Maroteaux, P. and Lamy, M. (1967) 'Le Syndrome de Silverman; fractures multiples du nourisson'. *Arch. Franch. Ped.*, **24**, 651–6.

Fontana, V.J. (1989) 'Child abuse: the physician's responsibility'. *NYSJ Med.*, **89**, (Part III) 152–5.

Fontana, V.J., Donovan, M.D. and Wong R.J. (1963) 'The maltreatment syndrome in children'. *N. Engl. J. Med.*, **269**, 1389.

Friendly, D.S. (1971) 'Ocular manifestations of physical child abuse'. *Trans. Am. Acad. Ophthalmol. Otolaryngol.*, **75**, 318–32.

Gaynon, M.W., Koh, K., Marmor, M.F. and Frankel, L.R. (1988) 'Retinal folds in the shaken baby syndrome'. *Am. J. Ophthalmol.*, **106**, 423–5.

Giese, M.J. (1994) 'Ocular findings in abused children and infants born to drug abusing mothers'. *Optom. Vis. Sci.*, **71**, No. 3, 184–91.

Gilkes, M.J. and Mann, T.P. (1967) 'Fundi of battered babies'. *Lancet*, **2**, 468–9.

Gothard, T.W., Runyan, D.K. and Hadler, J.L. (1985) The diagnosis and evaluation of child maltreatment. *J. Emerg. Med.*, **3**, 181–94.

Greenwald, M.J., Weiss, A., Oesterle, C.S. and Friendly, D.S. (1986) 'Traumatic retinoschisis in battered babies'. *Ophthalmology*, **93**, 618–24.

Harcourt, B. (1973) The role of the ophthalmologist in the diagnosis and management of child abuse. *Ophthalmic. Surg.*, **4**, 37.

Harley, R.D. (1980) 'Ocular manifestations of child abuse'. *J. Paed. Ophthalmol. Strabismus*, **17**, 5–13.

Kempe, C.H., Silverman, F.N., Steele, B.F., Droegmueller, W. and Silver, H.K. (1962) 'The battered baby syndrome'. *JAMA*, **181**, 17–24.

Kiffney, G.T. (1964) 'The eye of the "battered child"'. *Arch. Ophthalmol.*, **72**, 231–3.

Meadow, R. (1989a) 'Epidemiology of child abuse'. *Brit. Med. J.*, **298**, 727–30.

Meadow, R. (1989b) 'Munchausen Syndrome by Proxy'. *Brit. Med. J.*, **299**, 248–50.

Opticians Act (1958) 'Rules relating to Disease or Injury of the Eye' (SI, 1960/1936).

Quinn, K.I. and Gammon, J.A. (1983) 'Children's eyes as indicators of physical abuse'. *Am. Orth. J.*, **33**, 99–104.

Reece, R.M. and Grodin, M.A. (1985) 'Recognition of non-accidental injury'. *Ped. Clinics N. Am.*, **32**, No. 1, 41–60.

Roberton, D.M., Barbor, P. and Hull, D. (1982) 'Unusual injury? Recent injury in normal children and children with suspected non-accidental injury'. *Brit. Med. J.*, **285**, 1399–401.

Scott, S. (1988) 'Child abuse and neglect: a diagnostic guide for the optometrist'. *J. Am. Optom. Assoc.*, **59**, No. 10, 760–6.

Smith, S.M., Hanson, R. and Noble, S. (1973) 'Parents of battered babies: a controlled study'. *Brit. Med. J.*, **4**, 388–91.

Tomasi, L.G. and Rosman, N.P. (1975) 'Purtscher retinopathy in the battered child syndrome'. *Am. J. Dis. Child*, **129**, 1335–7.

Valman, H.B. (1987) 'Child abuse'. *Brit. Med. J.*, **294**, 633–5.

Weidenthal, D.T. and Levin, D.B. (1976) 'Retinal detachment in a battered infant'. *Am. J. Ophthalmol.*, **81**, 725–7.

Wilshin, R. (1994) Personal communication (Registrar, General Optical Council).

SECTION 4
MANAGEMENT AND TREATMENT OF THE CHILD PATIENT

CHAPTER 15

Working with Parents: Concepts and Techniques

Stanley Klein

Working with parents is a critical aspect of pediatric optometric care. However, the training of pediatric optometrists, like the training of colleagues in other pediatric health-care disciplines, rarely includes specific content about the doctor/parent relationship or the role of the family in health care (Kerns & Turk, 1985). Rather, it seems to be assumed that working with parents in a clinical setting will develop 'naturally' in each clinician, and that neither concepts nor techniques related to interacting with parents need to be learned (Wolraich & Reiter, 1979). Typically, the one area of clinical literature in which parents are likely to be mentioned at all is in reference to children with disabilities such as learning disabilities or low vision.

This chapter presents specific concepts about the doctor/parent relationship and the communication of information, often called patient education information, to parents. My goal is for the skilled clinician to be able to integrate these concepts and techniques into his or her day-to-day work with parents in ways which fit with the individual personal style of the clinician, the demands and constraints of the health care setting in which the optometrist practises, and the needs of the parents.

15.1 Biases about parents

Many health care professionals view parents negatively – as nervous, guilty, anxious, depressed, and/or over-protective. Such negative stereotyping often begins to develop when inexperienced clinicians observe parents in health-care settings. These clinicians seem to unaware of the fact that the sample of behaviour they observe is not representative of any parent's everyday parenting; rather, it is an observation of parents under significant stress brought about by concerns for a child's eye-health and the potentially frightening implications of any vision assessment. After observing many parents under the stress of seeking eye-care for a child with a 'problem', many optometrists, as they gain more experience with children as patients, conclude that all parents are anxious, inept, inadequate, troubled adults all the time.

In addition to observing parents under the stress of clinical care, most optometrists undergo these clinical learning experiences at a developmental stage in their own personal lives, as young adults, during which they are in the process of establishing themselves as independent individuals – a time when it is common for individual young adults to blame their own perceived inadequacies on their own parents' lack of parenting abilities. Thus, the stage-specific complaints of young adults in reference to their own parents serve to confirm young optometrist's observations of their child patients' parents.

Finally, popular psychology as reported by the public media as well as a considerable body of professional literature continues to blame parents, especially mothers, for the problems of children and, retrospectively for the problems of adults, thereby validating the personal and clinical experiences of the developing optometrist. For example, in a review of 125 articles in reference to psychological disorders of children, mothers were held responsible for 72 different kinds of psychological disorder (Caplan, 1986). Despite increasing research and clinical evidence of the role of constitutional characteristics in the development of physical and mental illnesses, parents continue to be stigmatized in professional literature (Seligman & Seligman, 1980).

The unfortunate result of the observations and experiences described is that many young optometrists unwittingly bring negative stereotypes or prejudices about parents to their pediatric clinical encounters which interfere with their perceptions of parents and their ability to communicate constructively with them (Klein, 1982). That all this often takes place before professionals have become parents themselves probably also plays a part.

15.2   Parents as experts and partners

A far more appropriate perspective (albeit one which professionals often find uncomfortable to assimilate) in reference to the parents of young patients is to appreciate that: first, parents are experts about their child; and second, parents can be partners in the diagnostic and treatment processes. This view is clearly articulated in the recent federal legislation in the United States which seeks to establish early intervention and family support programmes for families which include an infant or toddler with a disability and/or serious medical condition (see Public Law 99–457, Education of the Handicapped Act Amendments, US Congress and related regulations prepared by the US Office of Education, 1986: see also Seligman & Darling, 1989; Zambone, 1990).

The concept of parents as experts is especially troubling for many clinicians. However, when parental abilities to assess a child, such as estimating developmental levels in specific areas for their own child, have been studied, parents do as well or better than professional 'experts' (Vincent, 1988; Schopler & Reichler, 1972).

The partnership concept is particularly relevant in pediatric optometric care because most clinical problems require long-term (or chronic) management and care, usually delivered or supervised by parents. In the literature on models of the doctor/patient relationship, the mutual participation model (Szasz & Hollender, 1975) is considered most appropriate for chronic conditions because the doctor and the patient (and/or parents) work together toward a mutual goal. This model is effective when there are common goals, common understanding of the problem, and a common plan for treatment (Alpert & Wittenberg, 1986). However, this model usually is not appropriate in acute illness situations in which the doctor tells the patient what to do and/or administers the treatment directly to a relatively passive participant – the patient (Mumford, 1985).

Studies of patient compliance support the partnership model even though the term compliance suggests an authoritarian approach by the provider (Billings & Stoeckle, 1989). In a pediatric setting, Korsch and Negrete (1972) demonstrated that the key factors in parental (particularly maternal) cooperation with physicians and in successful health outcome for the child included: the mother's perceptions that the doctor praised her as a mother; an active exchange between doctor and mother; and the physician's expression of concern for the mother's feelings.

From a practical point of view, the process of meeting the eye-care needs of a child will be enhanced when an optometrist believes that the interaction with the child's parents will be one of active reciprocal learning i.e. parents and optometrist learning from each other how to best help the child. However, in learning, the self-esteem of the learner is critical; therefore, to facilitate learning (and teaching) by parents, the optometrist needs to clearly demonstrate respect for the expertise of parents and explicitly acknowledge their role as active partners.

15.3 Principles for parental/optometrist interaction

15.3.1 Setting

Here it is assumed that it is usually important for the optometrist to meet with the parent(s) separately from the young patient (see below in reference to older children). The setting in which a discussion of the child's history or the clinical findings occurs conveys a mutual participation model of communication when it encourages a give and take among adults of equal status. Specifically this means: each participant should be seated in an equally comfortable chair; each seated adult's eyes should be on the same level; each should be seated at a conversational distance from the others; and each should be able to take notes comfortably (Klein, 1979). Accordingly, a separate office, or seating area, with a desk and chairs is more appropriate than using an examining chair and associated equipment nearby along with other chairs. In addition, parents are entitled to uninterrupted privacy according to a prearranged schedule that respects the value of their time as well as the doctor's and allows sufficient time for discussion with an opportunity to continue, if necessary, at another time (Billings & Stoeckle, 1989).

15.3.2 Involving the father

Whenever possible, encourage the child's father to participate. All too often, despite recent cultural awareness of sexism, the mother is expected to attend meetings in reference to a child's health as if she were at home with nothing else to do, while her traditional husband's work is too important to be interrupted by such trivial matters! In that same stereotyped scenario, the mother is expected to report to the father so that he can provide his stamp of approval and pay the bill. In contrast, involving the father, which may require a special invitation in order to counteract stereotypical behaviour, communicates that he too has an important parenting role.

Involving fathers is especially important when the patient is a boy and/or when parents are expected to carry out or supervise compliance or participate in a treatment programme at home. Even when divorced fathers do not share in child custody, they can play a role in supporting compliance.

> Traditionally, fathers have not been actively involved in the educational and health care needs of their children. By involving fathers from the start (including fathers who may not be living with their children), clinicians demonstrate to children as well as their parents that fathers are important. It is not unusual for a boy to get the idea, based on his observation of his mother and most of his teachers (usually women), that school is girl's work. At the same time, fathers, when confronted with a child who is awkward and/or somewhat disappointing, are more likely than mothers to withdraw their efforts to be with their son. This unfortunate cycle of disappointment, frustration and withdrawal can be altered by involving fathers from the beginning and letting fathers know just how important they are. Fathers are usually very responsive to this approach, often reporting that it is the first time they have not felt left out by health professionals.
>
> (Klein, 1982, pp 114–15)

Once children are 10 to 12 years' old, meeting with parents separately is not likely to be constructive because it creates the impression that parents and the optometrist are on the same 'side' at a time when the child is likely to need the optometrist as a supportive ally or advocate 'against' the parents. Since such separate meetings also create the impression that the clinician is communicating something different to parents than to the child. Meeting with the parents and the child together, while at the same time providing an opportunity for confidential doctor/patient communication for the child, will be more constructive as long as the optometrist, by words and by action, focuses attention on the child and the child's health-care needs; and also remembers to be attentive to parental feelings.

15.3.3   The parent/optometrist partnership

Since parents ordinarily serve only as informants in relation to health-care providers, the importance of their active participation as observers and experts needs to be stated early in the process. If parents have already provided a case history to another provider, it is helpful for the optometrist to begin by apologizing for the repetitiousness and to explain the purpose of taking a case history from an eye care perspective. In addition, to counteract the common parental experience that a doctor's office is a courtroom in which parents are on trial, the optometrist can make clear that parents are not being judged on the basis of whatever they did or did not do and that it is unrealistic to expect parents to remember developmental details for each child. Rather, one purpose of the discussion is for parents to share their observations as well as their questions and concerns.

Another technique to address parental worries about being judged is for the optometrist to explicitly *empathize* with the parents by acknowledging that parenting is always difficult and that parenting a child with a problem (vision impairment, learning disability, etc.) can result in parents feeling upset, frustrated, angry, and/or discouraged – other feelings are also possible. Via specific empathic comments, an optometrist conveys understanding of the parental dilemma and addresses the common complaint of many parents that health-care providers do not really appreciate the day-to-day challenges of caring for children with health problems. For a discussion of empathy and under-standing, see Bernstein and Bernstein (1985), Korsch and Negrete (1972), Klein (1979) (1982) and Selig (1983).

By acknowledging the negative feelings parents experience, the clinician also helps the parents become more active because in the doctor's office many parents believe they are expected to be mature, objective, and stoic.

> ... parents are likely to actively suppress their feelings of frustration and worry. This process takes a great deal of psychic energy which is then unavailable for active participation in the diagnostic process. The clinician begins the process of freeing up this energy and thereby facilitating com-munication and understanding by providing parents with an opportunity to talk about their feelings and by responding with empathy and attention rather than with implied or explicit criticism, or impatience to get on with the procedures.

The clinician's goal is not to cure parents of their frustrations. Rather, as parents have an opportunity to express their feelings to the doctor and to each other, new energy for the task at hand becomes available, energy previously expended on keeping these feelings hidden. In a sense, the parents' emotional block to talking and learning is being treated. During such discussions, parents need to be assured that they are the most valuable people in their child's life and that they can be invaluable in all efforts on behalf of their child . . .

(Klein, 1982, p 116)

A useful technique for actively involving parents is to enquire about parental observations, in everyday interactions, of the child's visual acuity, colour discrimination, and other areas that the clinician will be objectively and subjectively assessing during the examination. Similarly, parental observations of other developmental areas relevant to particular concerns (such as hearing, language, motor skills, memory, intelligence, reading, social skills, etc.) can be encouraged. This process also enables the optometrist to explore parental expectations in relation to the child's problem and its remediation, and sets the stage for connecting parental observations with specific clinical findings following the optometric examination (Alpert & Wittenberg, 1986; Klein, 1982; Klein & Klein, 1987). By linking parental observations to clinical findings, the establishment of treatment priorities which are shared by the parents and optometrist is facilitated.

When treatment priorities require parental involvement with their child in a programme at home, the mutual participation or partnership model can prevent the optometrist from establishing unrealistic expectations which are likely to lead to non-compliance. For example, although a particular vision training programme may require that a parent and a child work together for thirty minutes a day, the optometrist can review how much time is actually available within the constraints of the demands of everyday family life and begin with smaller, more realistic increments of time. In this way, both parents and child can begin the process by feeling successful rather than feeling inadequate to the task. Gradually, the 'partners' can decide to increase the demands.

15.4   Written reports

Even under the best of circumstances, well-intentioned, intelligent parents are unlikely to remember everything communicated verbally by the optometrist (Alpert & Wittenberg, 1986). Encouraging parents to take notes or tape record meetings can be helpful. However, the most effective approach is to prepare a written report for parents, summarizing the discussion of the child's problems, clinical findings and recommendations in language understandable to lay persons.

Besides helping parents (and clinicians) remember the discussion and thereby prevent the ordinary distortions in memory that occur over time, such reports can often be more valuable than technical clinical reports for other professionals unfamiliar with eye-care jargon.

In conclusion, by utilizing the concepts of respecting the expertise of parents and encouraging them to be active participants in meeting the needs of their child and by integrating their own adaptations of the techniques described, optometrists can greatly increase the likelihood that a child's eye-care needs will be met and that the family will continue to perceive the optometrist as a valuable resource person.

15.5   References

Alpert, J.S. and Wittenberg, S.M. (1986) *A clinician's companion: a study guide for effective and human patient care.* Little Brown & Co., Boston.

Bernstein, L. and Bernstein, R.S. (1985) *Interviewing: a guide for health professionals,* 4th edn. Appleton-Century-Crofts, Norwalk.

Billings, J.A. and Stoeckle, J.D. (1989) *The clinical encounter: a guide to the medical interview and case presentation.* Year Book Medical Publishers Inc., Chicago.

Caplan, S. (1986) 'Blaming mother'. *Psychology Today,* **20,** No. 10, 20–25.

Kerns, R.D. and Turk, D.C. (1985) 'Behavioral medicine and the family: historical perspectives and future directions', in *Health, illness and families: A life-span perspective.* (D.C. Turk & R.D. Kerns, eds). John Wiley & Sons, New York.

Klein, S.D. (1979) 'Parent-school conferences: guidelines and objectives'. *Exceptional Parent,* **9,** E19–21.

Klein, S.D. (1982) 'The role of the family in helping the child with learning disabilities', in *The role of vision in multi-disciplinary approach to children with learning disabilities.* (M. Davis & J.C. Whitener, eds). Charles C. Thomas, Springfield.

Klein, S.D. and Klein, R.E. (1987) 'Delivering bad news: the most challenging task in patient education'. *J. Am. Optometric Assoc.,* **9,** 660–63.

Korsch, B. and Negrete, V. (1972) 'Doctor-patient communication'. *Sci. Amer.,* **66,** 227–30.

Mumford, E. (1985) 'The responses of patients to medical advice', in *Understanding human behavior in health and illness,* 3rd edn (R.C. Simons, ed). Williams & Wilkins, Baltimore.

Schopler, E. and Reichler, R. (1972) 'How well do parents understand their own psychotic child?'. *J. Autism and Child. Schizophrenia,* **2,** 387–400.

Selig, A.L. (1983) 'Common myths of family feedback conferences', *Dev. & Behav. Ped.,* **4,** 67–9.

Seligman, M. and Darling, J. (1989) *Ordinary families, special children.* Guilford Press, New York.

Seligman, M. and Seligman, P.A. (1980) 'The professional's dilemma: learning to work with parents'. *Exceptional Parent,* **10,** S11–13.

Szasz, T.S. and Hollender, M.H. (1956) 'A contribution to the philosophy of medicine: the basic models of the doctor-patient relationship'. *AMA. Arch. of Internal Med.,* **97,** 5585–92.

Vincent, L.J. (1988) 'What we have learned from families'. *OSERS News in Print,* **1,** 3.

Wolraich, M.L. and Reiter, S. (1979) 'Training physicians in communication skills'. *Dev. Med. and Child Neur.,* **21,** 773–8.

Zambone, A.M. (1990) 'Optometrists on the team: holistic care and the patient-parent-educator interface', in *Principles and Practice of Pediatric Optometry*. (A.A. Rosenbloom & M.W. Morgan, eds). J.B. Lippincott & Co., Philadelphia.

CHAPTER 16
The Management of Ametropia
David Edgar

Few decisions in optometry are more difficult than the question of what to prescribe to a child. With preschool children there are no subjective results to assist, and the precycloplegic retinoscopy data is often suspect, having been obtained from a child with unstable accommodation and fixation. Indeed, often the only reliable information available is a retinoscopy finding obtained under cycloplegia, and the practitioner must anticipate the likely modification required to this retinoscopy result when normal accommodation is restored. All prescribing decisions must take into account the likely effect of any new prescription on the patient's oculomotor balance. Other considerations include, for example, the decision to recommend contact lenses to an introverted young myope which may be motivated by the optometrist's assessment of the likely psychological impact of this form of correction, rather than by any major benefits to the patient's visual system. In infants particularly, there is the likely permanence of the refractive error to be considered. These and many other factors can influence the practitioner's prescribing decision.

The optometrists' approach to the refractive management of ametropia in children is considered in this chapter, which excludes pathological causes of ametropia such as keratoconus and pathological myopia. In other chapters of the book a chronological approach is used with four categories; birth to 18 months, 18 months to three years, three years to five years, and over five years. These are not always appropriate here, although when the term 'infant', which is not rigorously defined in the literature, is used in this chapter it refers to those in the age group from birth to approximately 18 months.

16.1   Myopia

A myopic eye is defined as an eye in which the optical system is too powerful for its axial length. Non-pathological myopia is increasingly regarded as a broad term embracing a number of distinct types, distinguishable by the age of onset of the error of focusing. Two of these types, congenital and juvenile onset myopia affect infants and children respectively, and are considered in detail here. A third type, early adult-onset myopia can begin in the mid to late teens.

Myopia is a relatively common disorder, with a prevalence in the western world estimated at around 25%, although there are marked racial variations. In those of Chinese origin, myopia is much more common – 70% of Hong Kong Chinese are myopic by the age of 17 years (Lam & Goh, 1991). Optometrists' concern with the management of myopia is closely related to the detrimental effect that relatively small amounts of myopia can have on distance acuity.

16.1.1   Congenital myopia

Congenital myopia has a high prevalence among premature infants (those of less than 35 gestational weeks), though by the age of 12 months their refractive errors are usually close to those found in full-term infants – unless retinopathy of prematurity (ROP) has occurred in which case they remain myopic (Kushner, 1982). In the absence of ROP, practitioners should be cautious when considering prescribing to premature infants under 12 months. Re-examination a few months after the initial assessment to establish the degree of permanence of the refractive error may be prudent.

Indeed, practitioners often do not prescribe to myopic infants, for several reasons. Infants' distance acuity is low, and contrast sensitivity poor, especially at high spatial frequencies. In any case myopia is little handicap, and may even be advantageous to infants, because their sphere of interest has a fairly short radius, related to the length of the mother's arms. Most myopic infants will experience vision of optimal clarity for periods when the object of interest is situated at, or closer to the eye than their far point, so there is no danger of them developing amblyopia. On the practical side, the difficulties of achieving successful spectacle wear in an infant should not be underestimated. When a myopic correction is eventually prescribed, the child will immediately achieve optimal acuity with the full correction. The decision when to prescribe is based on the infant's interest in, and need to interact with, their environment beyond the far point. Once this is impaired their development will suffer in the absence of the ability to see the world clearly, hence prescribing is indicated.

Exceptions to this non-prescribing approach are those infants with high degrees of myopia, and those with medium to high anisometropia, which is always a cause for concern. High myopia can be associated with a number of inherited diseases including Down's syndrome, Marfan's syndrome, albinism, and retinitis pigmentosa. Full correction of myopia is beneficial in most of these cases. Many patients suffering from inherited conditions are multihandicapped. In a multihandicapped group of patients, Orel-Bixler et al. (1989) found 73% to have a significant refractive error, but 63% of these were uncorrected. Deprived of optimal visual acuity such patients respond by further inhibition of their sensory, perceptual and cognitive development (Bader & Woodruff, 1980).

16.1.2 Juvenile (or youth) onset myopia

Juvenile onset myopia is not present at birth, but has its onset during the period of bodily growth. It develops when the axial elongation that occurs during childhood is not fully compensated by the reduction in the power of the cornea and the lens (Sorsby & Leary, 1960), resulting in a failure of the emmetropization process (see Chapter 3). Results from recent longitudinal studies that measured the optical components over a number of years in randomly selected children (Zadnik *et al.*, 1994), and in juvenile onset myopes (Grosvenor & Scott, 1993), show that corneal power does not change significantly with age. This suggests that it is changes in the crystalline lens, including flattening of its curvatures, and thinning, which are the chief contributors to the emmetropization process.

Both heredity, and a wide variety of environmental factors, have been suggested as possible causes for this lack of coordination between the eyes' ocular components. Heredity undoubtedly plays a part. Low refractive errors are multifactorial, while high refractive errors are usually autosomal recessive, as in pathological myopia, or occasionally autosomal dominant (see Chapter 1). Studies of uniovular twins lend support to the genetically determined nature of many refractive errors (Sorsby *et al.*, 1962; Knoblock *et al.*, 1985). However, there is also enough variation in refractive error between some sets of uniovular twins to demonstrate that it is not possible to give a comprehensive explanation of the development of myopia on the basis of hereditary factors alone.

On the environmental side, evidence is mounting to suggest a close relationship between prolonged close work and myopia. There is a high correlation between the amount of close work undertaken and the extent of myopic progression (Parsinnen *et al.*, 1989). One possible explanation for this relationship is that accommodation increases intraocular pressure, which may cause stretching of the relatively flexible coats of the child's eye, leading to an increase in axial length (Young, 1977). This suggestion of a possible link between accommodation and myopia is by no means new. Both Donders in the nineteenth century and Helmholtz, in the early twentieth century, believed excessive accommodation to be a possible cause of myopia. While accommodation is by far the most frequently cited environmental factor contributing to myopia, poor nutrition, and a variety of systemic diseases may also make a contribution.

Given this background it is hardly surprising that there have been numerous attempts to halt, or at least slow down, the progression of juvenile onset myopia by refractive management.

Undercorrection

By undercorrecting a myope for distance the need to accommodate for close work is reduced or eliminated. Undercorrection may be augmented by the prescribing of base in prisms, which reduce the convergence required for close work, which in turn reduces accommodative demand. The disadvantage of the undercorrection approach is the inevitable distance vision blur that may hinder the child for games and other activities requiring best acuity. For this reason there has been much more interest in the prescribing of bifocals, which achieve the same effect at near, but retain distance clarity. Nevertheless, if undercorrection at near is the aim, the prescription of single vision lenses is a cheap, cosmetically acceptable and 'easy-to-dispense' solution.

Bifocals

Several studies have claimed success in slowing myopia progression by the use of bifocals (Roberts & Banford; 1967, Oakley & Young, 1975; Goss, 1986). Others have found the bifocals to have no beneficial effect on the majority of patients (Grosvenor *et al.*, 1987; Parssinen *et al.*, 1989). There is no consensus view, but the balance of evidence, particularly from the more recent work, suggests that for most patients, the wearing of bifocals has no beneficial effect in slowing myopia progression.

However, bifocals may have a decelerating effect on the myopia of patients in that subgroup of juvenile myopes who are esophoric at near (Goss & Grosvenor, 1990). From the point of view of the patient, even if the ability of bifocals to slow myopia progression were proven, the argument in favour of prescribing them is not overwhelming. To illustrate this point, let us assume that bifocal therapy works, and can reduce a juvenile myope's final myopic state by 1 D. So a potential -6 D myope would emerge as a -5 D myope after bifocal therapy. Is this significant one dioptre reduction in myopia worth the expense, and the possible adverse psychological effects resulting from years of deliberate blurring in the distance, for a child who is still going to be a spectacle-dependent patient at the end of their bifocal experience? On the other hand it could be argued that another child who also emerged after bifocal therapy with a 1 D reduction in myopia, this time as a -1.25 D myope instead of -2.25 D, had benefited from bifocals. But once presbyopia had become well established, this patient might have found the higher degree of myopia to be advantageous. Clearly, in many cases, the estimation of relative benefit is complex and difficult to resolve.

Contact lenses

Conventionally-fitted contact lenses made from both rigid gas-permeable and PMMA materials have been shown to retard the development of juvenile myopia. In a longitudinal study over five years, Stone (1976) reported a mean increase in myopia of approximately 0.50 D for the PMMA contact lens wearing group, compared to 1.75 D for spectacle wearers. Similar findings emerge from the rigid gas-permeable contact lens study (Perrigin *et al.*, 1990). In both studies the deceleration in myopia progression is attributed to corneal flattening, with a possible contribution from a slight decrease in axial length. Grosvenor *et al.* (1991) demonstrated that the rate of progression of myopia increased markedly in a subgroup of their original sample, which discontinued contact lens wear for a period of 2.5 months after a 44-month period of wear. When contact lens wear resumed there was no additional progression of myopia over a period of six months. Not surprisingly, it is also possible to slow the rate of myopic progression with lenses designed to deliberately flatten the cornea, a procedure known as orthokeratology (Polse *et al.*, 1983).

Accommodation biofeedback

Biofeedback techniques are widely used in medicine to reduce stress, and thus ameliorate conditions such as cardiovascular disease and migraine. An application of biofeedback to myopia control has been proposed by Trachtman (1987), using the Accommotrac vision trainer, an infra-red optometer that measures the state of accommodation every 32 ms. A computer-controlled auditory signal is generated, the frequency of which varies according to the eye's accommodative state. When undergoing a training period, the patient wears headphones in darkness, and the task is to alter the auditory signal to a tone of higher pitch which indicates relaxation of accommodation. The method is claimed to promote greater accommodative control, which can reduce what Trachtman describes as 'functional' myopia. In their excellent review of the subject, Gilmartin *et al.* (1991) point out that Trachtman's functional myopia should properly be classified as pseudo-myopia because 'the mechanism by which myopia reduction occurs emanates in the initial stages of training from a relaxation of parasympathetically-induced spasm of accommodation'. It should be noted that those who are claimed to benefit from Trachtman's biofeedback technique are patients who developed myopia in their late teens and early twenties. However, since the method received extensive publicity when released commercially, optometrists involved in pediatric work may find themselves asked for advice by parents keen to know if the technique could benefit their child.

Clinical studies by Gallaway *et al.* (1987), and Koslowe *et al.* (1991) found no evidence to support any reduction in myopia using biofeedback. Gallaway found an improvement in visual acuity in several subjects, but this is attributable to an enhanced ability to interpret blurred letters on a chart. Despite the possible role of accommodation in the genesis of late-onset myopia, there seems little evidence to suggest that currently available biofeedback techniques have a role to play in its management.

Medical management

Atropine has a long and controversial history as an agent to reduce the progression of myopia by relaxing accommodation. Beneficial effects of long-term therapy have been claimed, but often in studies of poor design. Results from well-designed studies reveal the method to bring little benefit. Furthermore, subjects must wear bifocals, endure photophobia, and run the risk of systemic and local adverse reactions. Even the diagnostic use of atropine is in decline, and atropine management of myopia has few advocates today.

Visual hygiene

It has been suggested that the poor visual hygiene of many young myopes is a contributory factor to their myopia. In particular, the short working distances favoured by many myopes have been implicated as the likely culprit. Advocates of visual hygiene recommend that patients should adopt good posture while doing near work, use good lighting, and take frequent rests. All this is sound advice, but it has not been shown to have any benefit in terms of the development or progression of myopia.

Summary

Of the various methods of myopia control discussed above, only contact lens management can unequivocally claim to be effective. Further work in the area of contact lens management may improve current methods, and these improvements may eventually allow further deceleration of myopic progression. However, there seems little hope in the foreseeable future of contact lens wear halting, or reversing juvenile onset myopia. Evidence in favour of bifocals remains at best equivocal, although bifocal therapy may prove to be of benefit to subsets of the myopic population. In the long-term, the best prospect for myopia control may lie with laser refractive surgery, a treatment which offers the hope of a 'cure' for myopia. While the prospects for laser surgery in adults seem assured, such surgery on the growing myopic eye remains a distant hope. For the present, the author sees little alternative but to prescribe the full myopic correction to juvenile myopes.

16.1.3   Early adult-onset myopia

Before moving on from myopia, it is worth briefly considering early adult-onset myopia, since much of our current understanding of the etiology of myopia has come from recent work investigating early adult-onset myopia, and comparisons between the early adult-onset and juvenile forms. Early adult-onset myopia, also known as late myopia or late-onset myopia, is defined as myopia having its onset after the completion of bodily growth. It is usually considered to be due more to environmental influences rather than to hereditary. The increased prevalence of myopia in those in higher education, and in occupations demanding intensive close work is well known (Zadnik & Mutti, 1987; Adams & McBrien, 1992).

16.2 Spasm of accommodation (pseudo-myopia)

Hypermetropic and emmetropic patients can become myopic as a result of accommodative spasm, which can be brought on by prolonged close work, and may be associated with stress. Children who present with reduced distance acuity and are found to be myopic, can have signs which suggest that spasm of accommodation may be the cause. Good indicators of spasm are an amplitude of accommodation that is abnormally low for the patient's age, and marked esophoria. If cycloplegic refraction reveals the child to be emmetropic or hypermetropic, spasm is confirmed. In these circumstances prescribing the myopic correction merely invites further spasm, and is to be avoided. Improved visual hygiene can help, and the child should be given advice about posture when doing close work, to use good lighting, and to take frequent rests. If stress is the cause, the spasm usually resolves when the stressful period is over. Positive lenses for near, which aim to encourage accommodative relaxation, may help in stubborn cases.

16.3 Hypermetropia

The refractive management of hypermetropic patients with a manifest squint and other anomalies of binocular vision is covered in Chapter 19.

Moderate degrees of hypermetropia in infants cannot be treated so lightly as moderate degrees of myopia. Ingram & Walker (1979) found that the presence of two or more dioptres of spherical hypermetropia in both eyes was significantly associated with the child being identified two or more years later as having either squint, or amblyopia, or both. The value of prescribing at this level of hypermetropia was confirmed in young hypermetropes of greater than +2 D, who were much more likely to display below-average visual analysis skills than age-matched emmetropes and myopes (Rosner & Gruber, 1985). Those hypermetropes in this sample who obtained their first spectacles before the age of four years had a reduced incidence of visual analysis skills impairment than those first corrected after the age of four (Rosner & Rosner, 1986). However, it is difficult to apply a strict cut-off point at 2 D. Many practitioners would prefer to defer prescribing to an asymptomatic hypermetropic child, of more than 2 D, if he or she is doing well at school, has no binocular vision anomalies, no symptoms, and no family history of binocular vision anomalies. It is difficult to quarrel with this view, especially if the child is monitored regularly. On the other hand, prescribing should not be discounted for hypermetropes of less than 2 D if the child has symptoms or signs which suggest that they would benefit from spectacle correction.

In the case of previously uncorrected medium to high degrees of hyper-metropia (e.g. +5 D or +6 D), the question becomes one of how much positive power to prescribe. There are two distinct schools of thought here: those who prefer to give the full positive correction from the outset; and those who prefer to give a partial correction, say +3 D. The danger of giving the full prescription is that the patient may experience distance vision blur, because they are used to accommodating to see clearly in the distance. As a consequence, the child may refuse to wear the glasses, and both patient and parents may become antagonistic to the idea of the child wearing a spectacle correction. Those who favour the full-correction approach argue that the distance blurring is frequently very short-lived, and if the patient and parents are warned in advance to expect blurring, it rarely becomes a problem. One factor that could justify prescribing the full hypermetropic correction is the presence of marked esophoria. When prescribing the full correction for hypermetropia, some optometrists advocate the instillation of a cycloplegic, often 1% cyclopentolate, to aid the adaptation process.

Other practitioners advocate the partial correction approach, and they are content for this non-squinting child to exert a certain amount of accommodation for distance. Provided the child has a normal amplitude of accommodation, a 2 D or 3 D accommodative effort in the distance should be easily attained and maintained. The aim may be to increase the positive power over time, gradually building up to the full distance correction, in a manner which is likely to avoid any adaptation difficulties caused by distance blurring. Alternatively, in the continued absence of any signs or symptoms, it may be sufficient to leave the child with the partial correction. One advantage is that the child still has to accommodate for distance vision and, being used to accommodating in the distance, will not be so handicapped when removing the glasses for games and other activities.

The importance of taking into account the likely effect of any new prescripton on the patient's oculomotor balance is particularly relevant to hypermetropes. Most binocular anomalies have an accommodative element, and any significant alteration in the spherical component of the correction may alter the patient's binocular status. It is not always possible to predict with any certainty the effect of a new, or significantly altered, prescription on oculomotor balance. Where there is doubt, it is prudent for the practitioner to monitor the patient in the initial stages of wearing the new prescription.

16.4 Astigmatism

A feature of refractive development in infants is the high prevalence of astigmatism and its transient nature. Using near fixation retinoscopy Mohindra *et al.* (1978) found astigmatism over 1 D in 45% of infants in the first year of life. By the method of photorefraction, Howland *et al.* (1979) found a prevalence of 60% for astigmatism of 0.75 D or greater, in patients of similar age. No fewer than 12% of Mohindra *et al.*'s sample had astigmatism of greater than 3 D. They followed up a subgroup of 28 infants with more than 2 D of astigmatism when three to six months old. Re-examined at 50 weeks, 14 of these had zero astigmatism, and a further seven showed a marked reduction. Astigmatism continued to reduce in the second year, and no sign of astigmatic amblyopia was found until the end of the third year. Similar findings were reported by Atkinson *et al.* (1980), and have been confirmed subsequently in several other studies that have used various methods of determining the refractive error.

These research findings have important clinical applications for the optometric management of the astigmatic child. Prescribing for astigmatism in children is rarely indicated until after their second birthday, and many practitioners prefer to wait until around the child's third birthday before prescribing. Meridional amblyopia is unlikely before this age, and even if present it should rapidly disappear once a prescription is constantly worn. It is impossible to give hard and fast rules regarding most aspects of prescribing for infants, and prescribing for astigmatism is no exception. Each case must be judged on its own merits. In particular, the higher the astigmatism and the more stable it remains over time, the greater is the risk of meridional amblyopia, and the more likely is the practitioner to prescribe at an age closer to the second birthday than the third.

Children may present with medium to high degrees of uncorrected astigmatism. A typical example would be a child aged five years with 4 D of astigmatism, discovered during routine visual screening at school entry. At this age, meridional amblyopia is established and a prescription is required. In children of this age, most practitioners prefer to give the full correction in the first pair of glasses. This is a different approach from that taken when faced with a refractive error of 4 D of uncorrected astigmatism in an adult. Here, the optometrist is unlikely to prescribe the full cylindrical correction, since to do so would run the risk of intolerance as the patient struggles to cope with the distorted view of the world resulting from the now clear retinal image. With a child there is less danger of intolerance to the full prescription, presumably due to the lability of the visual system and adaptability of children to change.

16.5   Anisometropia

Trivial amounts of uncorrected anisometropia can be ignored, but there is general agreement that anisometropia of 1 D or greater can be significant, and correction should be considered. For ease of reference the term anisometropia will be used in the rest of this section to mean anisometropia of 1 D or greater.

Anisometropia is relatively common in newborns: Zonis & Miller (1974) reported a figure of 17.3%, and Thompson (1989) found a similar prevalence in her sample, but noted that only 3.4% of infants had a difference between the eyes of greater than 2 D. Anisometropia becomes less common during the first year of life, and there is convincing evidence that in infancy it can be transient. For example, in one group of children, the prevalence of anisometropia remained constant, at approximately 7%, when they were refracted at one year old, and refracted again at three-and-a-half years. However, only one-third of those initially anisometropic remained so, and they were joined at three-and-a-half years by a previously isometropic group (Ingram & Barr, 1979).

This labile nature of anisometropia in children of up to about three years of age makes prescribing difficult. Regular refraction is necessary to confirm that anisometropia is stable. Only once this has been established can an informed decision as to the need for correction be taken. Both amblyopia and squint are strongly associated with stable anisometropia. If both eyes are hypermetropic the risk of amblyopia, albeit of mild form, is real with even 1 D of anisometropia, and the benefits of prescribing are indisputable for children of any age. Ciuffreda *et al.* (1991) estimate the risk of amblyopia with 2 D of anisometropia in hypermetropes to be 50%. If both eyes are myopic the situation is not so clear-cut. A 1 D difference in an uncorrected myope is unlikely to produce amblyopia, because both eyes will receive a clear retinal image at times. Ciuffreda *et al.* estimate that in myopes a 5 D difference between the eyes is required to give a 50% chance of amblyopia. So the optometrist's non-interventionist approach to prescribing to infants with myopia can be extended to those with myopia plus a mild degree of anisometropia. However, the question of whether amblyopia is a likely occurrence if the child is left uncorrected becomes an academic one in most cases of juvenile myopia. Such children require a prescription for distance vision anyway, which itself will correct any anisometropia.

When prescribing following a cycloplegic examination, the practitioner should have access to both the pre- and post-cycloplegic findings. Where the degree of anisometropia differs between pre- and post-cycloplegia, it is advisable to pre-scribe the anisometropic difference found under cycloplegia. Accommodation can be unstable monocularly, leading to errors in the pre-cycloplegic estimates of the spherical power. With the benefit of accommodative relaxation under cycloplegia the difference in spherical power between the eyes is much more likely to be correct. If an incorrect anisometropic difference is prescribed to an amblyopic patient, their acuity is less likely to recover fully.

Sadly, the optometrist may be confronted all too often with an already amblyopic anisometropic child for whom little can be done to reduce the amblyopia. The average sensitive period for visual development lasts for about eight years (see Chapter 3), and while there are individual variations that allow some hope for improvement beyond this age, the author's experience suggests that if the child is older than ten years, a correction for anisometropia is unlikely to improve the acuity. A similarly gloomy prognosis is likely for those with anisometropic amblyopia which has reduced acuity to less than 6/60.

Contact lenses are often more successful than spectacles in the refractive management of anisometropia (see Chapter 18). Spectacles produce unequal prismatic effects between the right and left eyes, and require unequal amounts

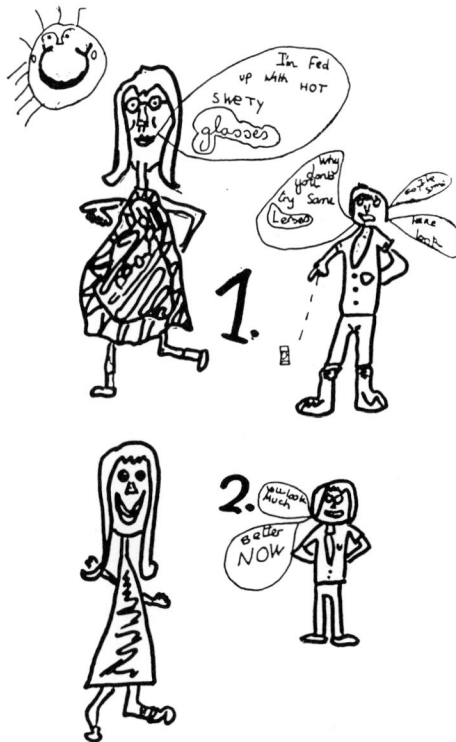

Fig. 16.1 A seven-year-old patient presented her optometrist with this artistic response to her recent switch from wearing glasses to her first pair of contact lenses.

of ocular accommodation. Both of these unwanted effects are absent in contact lens wear. Contact lenses may also reduce the aniseikonia produced by spectacle lenses (Bennett & Rabbetts, 1989).

16.6   Prescribing in general

Prescribing decisions are invariably made easier if made in the knowledge of previous measurements of refractive error. So, regular examinations, of at least every six months, are advised until the refractive state has stabilized. Infants, in particular, can undergo rapid changes in spherical error, in astigmatism, and in the extent of any anisometropia. It is often a mistake to prescribe too hastily, and it is good practice to bring a child back in a couple of months to establish the stability of the refractive state.

Apart from technical considerations, there are other significant, though less measurable factors in prescribing for children. When prescribing, a good practitioner should always consider the psychological effect his actions may produce in the patient. Few practitioners would quarrel with this statement when prescribing for adults. That it also applies to children is illustrated in the following case reported by Barnard (1990). The patient was a seven-year-old girl with 7 D of myopia who wore spectacles, but was keen to switch to contact lenses. Her dramatically improved self-image with contact lenses is joyfully illustrated in a drawing, shown here (Fig. 16.1), which she presented to the practitioner on the day after receiving her lenses.

16.7   References

Adams, D.W. and McBrien, N.A. (1992) 'Prevalence of myopia and myopic progression in a population of clinical microscopists'. *Optom. Vis. Sci.*, **69**, 467–73.

Atkinson, J., Braddick O. and French J. (1980) 'Infant astigmatism; its disappearance with age'. *Vis. Res.*, **20**, 891–3.

Bader, D. and Woodruff, M.E. (1980) 'The effects of corrective lenses on various behaviors of mentally retarded persons'. *Am. J. Optom. Physiol. Opt.*, **57**, 447–59.

Barnard, N.A.S. (1990) 'Case Report'. *Contact Lens Journal*, **18**, 282.

Bennett, A.G. and Rabbetts, R.B. (1989) *Clinical Visual Optics*, 2nd edn. Butterworth, London.

Ciuffreda, K.J., Levi, D.M. and Selenow, A. (1991) *Amblyopia. Basic and Clinical Aspects.* Butterworth-Heinemann, Oxford.

Gallaway, M., Scott, M.P., Winkelstein, A.A. and Scheiman, M. (1987) 'Biofeedback training of visual acuity and myopia: a pilot study'. *Am. J. Optom. Physiol., Opt.*, **64**, 62–71.

Gilmartin, B., Gray, L.S. and Winn, B. (1991) 'The amelioration of myopia using biofeedback of accommodation: a review'. *Ophthal. Physiol. Opt.*, **11**, 304–13.

Goss, D.A. (1986) 'Effect of bifocal lenses on the rate of childhood myopia progression'. *Am. J. Optom. Physiol. Opt.*, **63**, 135–41.

Goss, D. and Grosvenor, T. (1990) 'Rates of childhood myopia progression with bifocals as a function of nearpoint phorias: consistency of three studies'. *Optom. Vis. Sci.*, **67**, 637–40.

Grosvenor, T. and Scott, R. (1993) 'Three-year changes in refraction and its components in youth-onset and early adult-onset myopia'. *Optom. Vis. Sci.*, **70**, 677–83.

Grosvenor, T., Perrigin, D.M., Perrigin, J. and Maslovitz, B. (1987) 'Houston myopia control study: a randomized clinical trial. Part II, final report by the patient care team'. *Am. J. Optom. Physiol. Opt.*, **64**, 482–98.

Grosvenor, T., Perrigin, D.M., Perrigin, J. and Quintero, S. (1991) 'Rigid gas-permeable contact lenses for myopia control: effects of discontinuation of lens wear'. *Optom. Vis. Sci.*, **68**, 385–9.

Howland, H.C., Atkinson, J., Braddick, O. and French, J. (1978) 'Astigmatism measured by photorefraction'. *Science*, **202**, 331–3.

Ingram, R.M. and Barr, A. (1979) 'Changes in refraction between the ages of 1 and $3\frac{1}{2}$ years. *Brit. J. Ophthal.* **63**, 339–42.

Ingram, R.M. and Walker, C. (1979) 'Refraction as a means of predicting squint or amblyopia in preschool siblings of children known to have these defects'. *Brit. J. Ophthal.*, **63**, 238–42.

Knoblock, W.H., Leavenworth, N.H., Bouchard, T.J., and Eckert, E.D. (1985) 'Eye findings in twins reared apart'. *Ophthal. Ped. Genetics*, 5(1/2), 59–66.

Koslowe, K.C., Spierer, A., Rosner, M. and Belkin, M. (1991) 'Evaluation of Accommotrac biofeedback training for myopia control'. *Optom. Vis. Sci.*, **68**, 338–43.

Kushner, B.J. (1982) 'Strabismus and amblyopia associated with regressed retinopathy of prematurity. *Arch. Ophthalmol.* **100**, 256–61.

Lam, C.S.Y. and Goh, W.S.H. (1991) 'The incidence of refractive errors among school children in Hong Kong and its relationship with the optical components'. *Clin. Exp. Optom.*, **74**, 97–103.

Mohindra I., Held, R., Gwiazda, J. and Brill, S. (1978) 'Astigmatism in infants'. *Science*, **202**, 329–31.

Oakley, K.H. and Young, F.A. (1975) 'Bifocal control of myopia'. *Am. J. Optom. Physiol. Opt.*, **52**, 738–64.

Orel-Bixler, D., Haegerstrom-Portnoy, G. and Hall, A. (1989) 'Visual assessment of the multiply handicapped patient'. *Optom. Vis. Sci.*, **66**, 530–6.

Parsinnen, O., Hemminki, E. and Klemetti, A. (1989) 'Effect of spectacle use and accommodation on myopic progression: final results of a three-year randomised clinical trial among schoolchildren'. *Brit. J. Ophthalmol.*, **73**, 547–51.

Perrigin, J., Perrigin, D.M., Quintero, S. and Grosvenor, T. (1991) 'Silicone-acrylate contact lenses for myopia control: 3-year results'. *Optom. Vis. Sci.*, **67**, 764–9.

Polse, K.A., Brand, R.J., Schwalbe, J.S., Vartine, D.W. and Keener, R.J. (1983) 'The Berkeley orthokeratology study. Part II: Efficacy and duration'. *Am. J. Optom. Physiol. Opt.*, **60**, 187–98.

Roberts, W.L. and Banford, R.D. (1967) 'Evaluation of bifocal correction technique in juvenile myopia'. *Optom. Wkly* 58(38), 25–8; 58(40), 23–8; 58(41), 27–34; 58(43), 19.

Rosner, J. and Gruber, J. (1985) 'Differences in the perceptual skills development of young myopes and hyperopes'. *Am. J. Optom. Physiol. Opt.*, **62**, 501–4.

Rosner, J. and Rosner, J. (1986) 'The effects of early lens correction of hyperopia on visual perceptual skills development'. *Australian J. Clin. Exp. Optom.*, **69**, 166–71.

Sorsby, A. and Leary, G.A. (1970) 'A longitudinal study of refraction and its components during growth'. *Spec. Rep. Ser. Med. Res. Coun.*, No 309. HMSO, London.

Sorsby, A., Sheridan, M. and Leary, G.M. (1962) Refraction and its components in twins'.

London: Privy Council, *Med. Coun. Spec. Rep., No 303.*

Stone, J. (1976) 'The possible influences of contact lenses on myopia'. *Brit. J. Physiol. Opt.* **31**, 89–114.

Thompson, C.M. (1989) 'Infant refractive development during the first year: cross-sectional and longitudinal findings'. *Invest. Ophthalmol. Vis. Sci. Suppl.,* **30**, 517.

Trachtman J.N. (1987) 'Biofeedback of accommodation to reduce myopia: a review'. *Am. J. Optom. Physiol. Opt.,* **64**, 639–43.

Young F. (1977) 'The nature and control of myopia'. *Am. J. Optom. Physiol. Opt.,* **48** (4), 452–8.

Zadnik, K. and Mutti, D.O. (1987) 'Refractive error changes in law students'. *Am. J. Optom. Physiol. Opt.,* **64**, 558–61.

Zadnik, K., Mutti, D.O., Friedman, N.E. and Adams, A.J. (1993) 'Initial cross-sectional results from the Orinda longitudinal study of myopia'. *Optom. Vis. Sci.,* **70**, 750–58.

Zonis, S. and Miller, B. (1974) 'Refractions in Israeli newborns'. *J. Ped. Ophthalmol.,* **11**, 77–81.

CHAPTER 17
Spectacle Dispensing

Henri Obstfeld

17.1　Introduction

There are three aspects to the dispensing of spectacles, namely the choice of frame sizes, the fitting of the frames and the choice of lenses.

There have been complaints that children's spectacle frames are frequently scaled-down adult models (Sasieni, 1954; Veltmann, 1986). In fact, children's head and face dimensions depart in a number of aspects from those of adults. Very few manufacturers have paid attention to these differences and have made their interest public (Marks, 1961; Kasparek, 1981). A few others have done their own research into this matter, but have not published their findings. However, details are given in Kaye & Obstfeld's publication (1989). Dispensers will benefit from selecting purpose-designed children's spectacles because these will be easier to fit, and so will their patients.

Note that spectacle frame measurements are given according to British Standard BS 3199 (1991).

17.2　Facial and frame dimensions

Children's faces and their measurements change rapidly with growth. British Standard BS 6625: 1985 takes some account of this in specifying two grades based on performance. Grade B applies to metal spectacle frames for younger children where it is anticipated that the period of use will not exceed one year.

Facial measurements of two age-groups of Caucasian children, and adults can be found in Table 17.1. Most children have acquired adult facial measurements by the time that they have become teenagers.

There are considerable variations between individuals at a given age, and it is not possible to design a frame for, for example, 'a 4-year-old child'.

17.3　Frame fitting

When the frontal width of the frame matches the temple width of the head, the frame is usually cosmetically acceptable. One of the main features of a child's

Table 17.1 **Main variations in facial measurements of children and adults (compiled from Hantman, 1978; Kaye & Obstfeld, 1989).**

	Children		Adults
	<6 years	*6–12 years*	*Adults*
Interpupillary distance (mm)	45–54	54–58	56–72
Frontal angle (°)	30	22	22
Splay angle (°)	30	27	25
Height of crest (mm)	−2	+2	+5
Temple width (mm)	105–115		100–145

face is the flat nose. Hence, both the frontal and splay angles need to be large. Consequently, the vertex distance will be short, and since children's eyelashes are often long, they will smear the lenses with oily secretion (Lang, 1977). On the other hand, spectacle frames tend to slide down the nose thus increasing the vertex distance, and the eyelashes may clear the lenses. When a spectacle frame slips down the nose there is the risk that the child will look over the top of the frame. Because children live in an adults' world, much of which towers above them, even slight frame slippage can produce this effect. Frame slippage should be avoided, particularly with hypermetropic children. In very young children, this may be achieved by fitting loop-end sides to the front of the frame (Fig. 17.1). A ribbon is then passed through the two loops and tied at the back of the

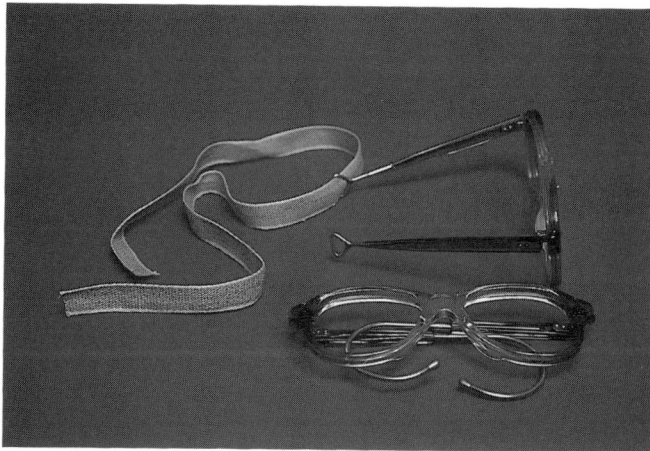

Fig. 17.1 A 'baby' size frame with curl sides, and one with loop-end sides, one loop threaded with tape: mode 1 PS 91 (courtesy of Pell Optical Co.).

child's head, or possibly in the form of a bow, on top of their head. An alternative to a tied knot, is an elastic band fitted with 'velcro'. This allows a certain measure of adjustment to the length of the band. A purpose designed frame with 'bridle' is shown in Fig. 17.2. For further reading see Albrecht (1985).

Slightly older children may be best fitted with curl sides. To avoid the possibility of the metal (nickel) of the wire binding of the curl producing an allergic response, it should be covered with a plastics sleeve. Many children of school age are fitted with drop-end (hockey-end) sides.

The splay angle of plastics pad frames is never made as large as required according to the facial measurements. If it were, one would not be able to insert the lens from the rear of the front into the eye of the frame. Hence, the dispenser must heat the pads and adjust them with the thumb to the required angle.

The shape of the pad should be such that its greatest width is situated towards the lower rim of the frame. Because of the large frontal angle the greater part of the bearing surface will then be nearer to the horizontal plane so that the weight of the frame is distributed over a larger bearing surface. This should increase comfort.

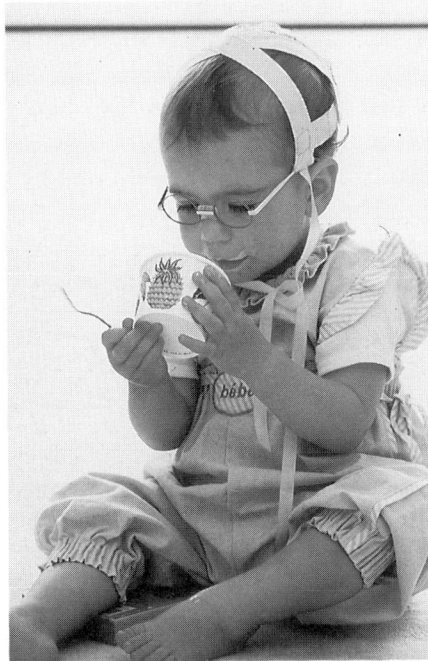

Fig. 17.2 A 'baby' size frame with silicone bridge and 'bridle': model 5935 (courtesy of Carl Zeiss Oberkochen).

Metal pad frames may be made into a frame with a regular or saddle bridge by replacing the two pads by twinned pads made of silicone rubber. This has the advantage of increasing the bearing surface on the nose, which reduces the pressure on any one spot thus increasing comfort.

Størseth *et al.* (1985) recommended that the eye shape of children's frames should be round or oval so that it would fit between eyebrow, nose and cheek. However, as long as the frame fits within this incomplete 'box' area, the actual lens shape seems to be less important provided it gives a large field of view. For cosmetic reasons, it is important that the eye and frame shape are compatible with the patient's facial features.

It has also been recommended (Størseth *et al.*, 1985) that the pantoscopic angle (between the visual axis of the eye when in the primary position, and the optical axis of the lens) should be 0° (for adults it is usually 7–10°). In view of the underdeveloped nasal bone of most children, the lower rim of the frame is likely to rest against the upper cheek if the pantoscopic angle were larger. In principle, the lower rim of any frame should stay clear of the skin. This may be achieved by adjusting the angle of side. However, some frame constructions (particularly metal), do not allow for any adjustment of this angle so that variations in the vertical position of the ear cannot be accommodated either.

Some children's frames are fitted with spring-loaded joints. These can be more robust than other types of joints, but may give the dispenser no opportunity to adjust the angles of side and control the angles of let-back and hence, the vertex distances (Harmer, 1994). Modern joints of the conventional type, are usually designed such that the angle of side can be adjusted easily, and by several degrees. Note that the angle of let-back may need to be adjusted, by filing out the joint. Adequate pressure can be exerted by the conventional types of side, at the ear point. The accurate shaping of the drop of the side so that it conforms to the shape of the mandibular bone, is also of great importance. This can increase the friction between side and skin which will help to retain the frame in the desired position.

For further discussion the reader is referred to Eakin (1964).

17.4   Plastics lenses

These days, glass spectacle lenses are seldom prescribed for children because their mass is about twice that of comparable plastics lenses, and their impact resistance, even when toughened, compares unfavourably with plastics lenses.

For the purpose of this text, children's spectacle frames have been divided into those for school-age children, with a horizontal boxed lens size of 48 mm, and those for preschool children, with a horizontal boxed lens size of 38 mm (Fig. 17.3).

Obstfeld (1991) weighed edged glass lenses for adult frames and showed that

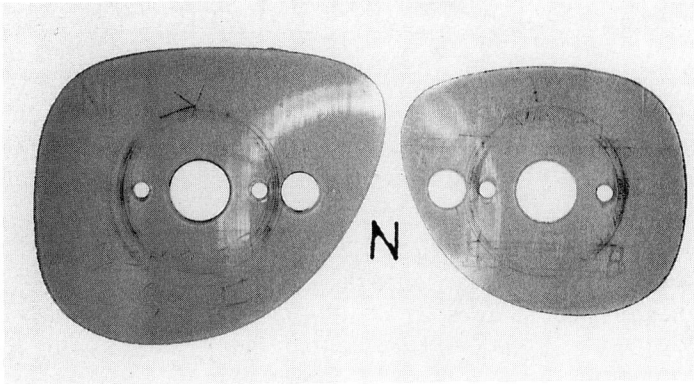

Fig. 17.3 The shapes of the edged 48 mm and 38 mm boxed lenses (N = nasal side).

the lens mass is little affected by the lens shape, with a difference of up to about 2 g, for the same edged boxed size. For plastics lenses, this difference will be less. In view of the smaller eye-size of children's frames, any differences will be smaller. The eye shapes used approximated to the pilot shape (BS 3521).

Table 17.2 shows the weight of edged plastics lenses, for back vertex powers from +9.00 DS to −9.00 DS. It shows:

(1) The higher the positive power and the larger the uncut diameter, the larger its centre thickness and edged mass (Fig. 17.4); the latter applies also to high index ($n = 1.6$) plastics lenses.

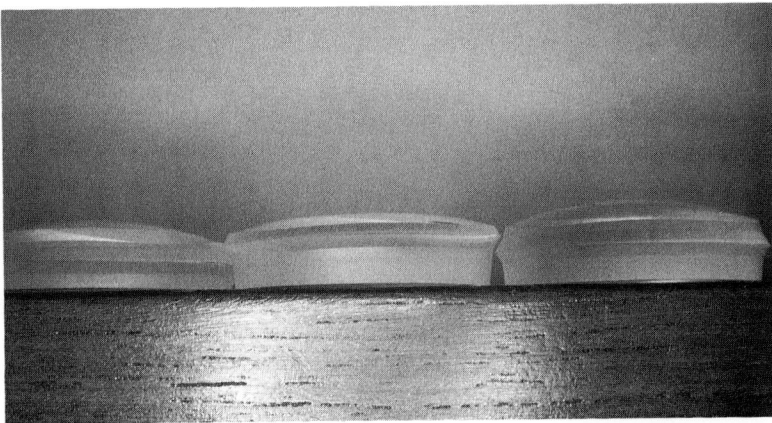

Fig. 17.4 The centre thickness differences of +9.00 DS edged 38 mm boxed lenses. Left to right (uncut diameter in mm): CR39 Hyperaspheric 58.5 mm; refractive index 1.6, 67.5 mm; CR39, 61.5 mm. Not shown: the smallest mass was recorded for the CR39 lens of uncut diameter 52.5 mm (compare with Table 17.2).

Table 17.2 Mass of edged plastics spectacle lenses in grams.

BVP (D)	Description	Uncut dia. (mm)	Thickness (mm) centre	Thickness (mm) edge	Mass 48 mm	Mass 38 mm
+9.00	index 1.6	67.5	9.2	K	15 M	11 M
	hyperaspheric	58.5	9.7	K	12 M	9 M
	CR 39	61.5	9.7	K	15 M	11 M
	CR 39	52.5	6.6	K	8 M	7 M
+5.00	CR 39	60	5.9	1.0	9 M	7 M
		52.5	4.5	0.6	6	5
+1.00	CR 39	60	2.6	1.7	5	3
		52.5	2.1	1.3	4	2
−1.00	CR 39	65	2.0	−	4	3
−5.00	CR 39	64	2.1	−	7 M	4
−9.00	CR 39	67	2.3	−	9 M	5

K = knife edge
M = mini-bevel

(2) Irrespective of power, edged negative lenses of 38 mm boxed size have a very similar mass (about 4 g).
(3) The mass of edged lenses of 48 mm boxed size, is 2–4 g more than that of the equivalent 38 mm boxed size lenses.
(4) Lenses worked to a knife-edge, and of a suitable uncut diameter, have the lowest mass.

Polycarbonate lenses have the highest impact resistance and should, therefore, be considered. Their unfavourable chromatic aberration is unlikely to bother a child.

Since there is little difference in density between the different plastics spectacle lens materials, the greatest reduction in mass can be effected by chosing or ordering the smallest uncut diameter, knife-edged lens commensurate with the eye size of the frame and any decentration required. Thus, when using plastics lenses the overriding aspect is their cosmesis.

Abrasion-resistant coatings should be applied by the dipping process, or be integral to *both* lens surfaces. Coatings applied by the vacuum process, are too thin to give extra protection to the lens surfaces (Wilkinson, 1984).

17.5 References

Albrecht, M. (1985) 'Spezialanfertigung und Anpassung von Kinderbrillen und Kleinst-kinderbrillen'. *Neues Optikerj.* **Part 3**, 21–5.

British Standard 3521: Part 2 (1991) *Glossary of terms relating to spectacle frames.* British Standards Institution, London.

British Standard 6625 (1985) *Specification for spectacle frames.* British Standards Institution, London.

Eakin, R.S. (1964) 'Designing and adjusting spectacles for children', in *Vision of Children.* (M.J. Hirsch & R.E. Wick, eds). Hammond, London, 271.

Hantman, D.P. (1978) *A comparison of facial measurements with age* (Final Year Project). City University, London.

Harmer, M.A. (1994) *Investigation of sprung-hinges in spectacle frames* (Final Year Project). City University, London.

Kaye, J. and Obstfeld, H. (1989) 'Anthropometry for children's spectacle frames'. *Ophthal. Physiol. Optics*, **9**, 293–8.

Kasparek, G. (1981) 'Anforderungskriterien an Kinderbrillen'. *Deutsche Optikerz.*, **Part 10**, 10–14.

Lang, J. (1977) 'Die Kinderbrille: Augenaertzliche und optische Probleme bei Kindern'. *Neues Optikerj.*, **19**, 575–8.

Marks, R. (1961) 'Some factors for consideration in the selection and fitting of children's eyewear'. *Am. J. Optom. Arch. Am. Acad. Optom.*, **38**, 185–93.

Obstfeld, H. (1991) "Weight of edged spectacle lenses'. *Ophthal. Physiol. Optics*, **11**, 248–51.

Sasieni, L.S. (1954) 'Considerations in the design of frames for children'. *Optician*, **128**, 481–2.

Størseth, G., Lundemo, T. and Lundemo, B. (1985) 'Barn og briller, 0–7 ar'. *Optikeren*, *Oslo*, **Part 4**, 15–16.

Veltmann, U. (1986) 'Stiefkind Kinderbrille'. *Augenspiegel*, **Part 10**, 46–55.

Wilkinson, P. (1984) 'Scratch resistance and optical properties of plastics lens coatings'. *Optician*, **188**, 18–21.

CHAPTER 18
Pediatric Contact Lens Practice
Judith Morris

18.1   Introduction

In addition to the therapeutic and prosthetic need for the use of contact lenses for some children, they may offer the child with a refractive error the same optical and mechanical advantages over spectacles that are afforded to the adult, but with certain additional attractions. The tolerance of spectacles by children below one year of age is usually low, often presenting the practitioner and parents with problems in keeping the appliance in place. In addition there may be difficulties in successfully fitting a pair of spectacles to the small face and nose of a very young child. The need for an adequate fit is exacerbated by the weight of higher powered prescriptions. These problems are discussed in Chapter 17.

In the presence of anisometropia, the aniseikonia that may be induced by spectacle correction can be an obstacle to the development of binocular vision and contact lenses may prove to be beneficial (Stone, 1979).

Owing to their advantages over spectacles, in recent years contact lenses have been used to treat children of all ages, including those as young as neonates. The fitting of scleral lenses to infants has been reported since the early 1960s (Lake, 1964) and child acceptance has been found to be good (Lewis, 1971). However, an analysis of cases from Moorfields Eye Hospital (Daniel, 1974) found that scleral lenses were disappointing from a visual and management point of view, and the main indication for these lenses is now considered to be for prosthetic purposes. Although corneal hard lenses have been fitted to infants for many years (Sato & Saito, 1959), the advent of soft lenses of various water contents has increased patient acceptance, giving rise to an increase in the use of contact lenses in pediatric practice.

18.2   Management of the patient

18.2.1   Parental relationship and management

The management of the pediatric patient cannot be discussed without consideration of the parents (see also Chapter 15).

Ocular conditions that manifest themselves in the first few weeks or months of life are usually psychologically traumatic to the parent, although, if the anomaly is familial the parents may be relatively prepared.

The most common of such anomalies is congenital cataract, and many parents have great difficulty in coming to terms with the need for surgery and subsequent optical correction. In these situations, the practitioner needs to spend time discussing with the parents the importance of contact lenses for their baby and to give them explanations and reassurance concerning the future management of their child. From the outset, the parents should always be present and included in such procedures as insertion and removal of a lens. In this way, they learn as much as possible about the handling of the lens and their responsibilities towards their child's contact lens treatment. The parent who is going to take the most responsibility for insertion, removal and disinfection of the lens should be encouraged to attend the clinic as much as possible so as to learn these techniques and to develop a relationship with the practitioner, thus aiding communication should any problems arise in the future.

The older child who, for example, may have developed myopia, may be brought to the practitioner by a parent who is unhappy with his or her child wearing spectacles for cosmetic reasons. If the child is happy with the spectacles and the clinical benefits are not obviously advantageous, then it may be in the child's best interest for the practitioner to persuade the parent against the idea of contact lenses.

18.2.2   Management of the child

Generally, babies are very easy to handle. Little communication is required other than pacification, which is best done by the mother. The babies attention may be gained by using lights and noise; such techniques are dealt with in Chapter 5.

Once infancy is attained, then the practitioner may use appropriate actions and speech to keep the attention of the young patient during such procedures as retinoscopy and lens evaluation. Insertion and removal of a contact lens can be a struggle at this age.

As the child gets older, he or she will learn to trust the practitioner, especially when shown care and patience over a period of time. Nevertheless, even after a few years of wear, insertion and removal of lenses may still be traumatic for child patients.

For the new patient who presents at the age of five or six years of age, fear of the unknown proves to be the most difficult problem for the child to overcome. Patience and kindness will eventually enable a lens to be inserted, and once this has been experienced the child will gain confidence, and managing the patient becomes progressively easier.

The use of the keratometer and slit lamp biomicroscope are essential in contact lens practice and the routine for carrying out these techniques on children will need adaption. Some infants can be examined on the slit lamp by the parent holding their child horizontally and positioning their head on to the headrest. The young child can often be made to kneel on a stool enabling keratometry and slit-lamp microscopy to be carried out. Continual verbal encouragement helps these procedures.

18.2.3   Insertion and removal

Insertion

Insertion of a contact lens with a baby is easily managed as there is a minimum of struggle. The practitioner should pull up the baby's upper lid and insert the lens under it (Fig. 18.1); then pull the lower lid over the lower edge of the lens.

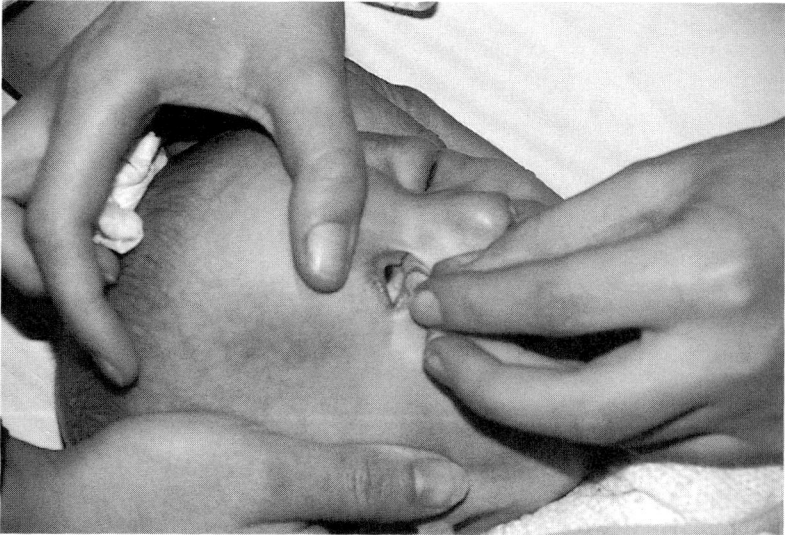

Fig. 18.1   Insertion of contact lens for an infant.

The contact lens should then be checked to ensure that it has not folded during insertion.

In the case of a two-year-old, a struggle might ensure. Insertion may be easier if the child is laid on a bed and his head held between the arms of a parent, whose hands are also holding down the child's shoulders and hands. It is often the father who learns to hold the child and the mother who learns to insert the lenses. With time, no holding is required and eventually the lenses can be inserted whilst the child is sitting in the consulting room chair.

From about the age of five years, it may be possible to encourage the child to begin to manage insertion and removal themselves. Insertion is not always so easily achieved and so initially help is required from a parent to hold the lids or guide the child's finger. Once the child has gained confidence and appreciates the advantages of being independent, his insertion technique improves, enabling him to handle the lenses without any assistance. Children then become remarkably responsible in looking after and handling their lenses, although some supervision of the cleaning regime is wise.

Children may find hard lenses easier to insert than soft because of the size, but then may need help with removal.

In the case of an older child, where there is a real difficulty and no progress is being made, hypnosis has been suggested to teach the child to insert their lenses (Barnard, 1989). A parent should always be present during such a procedure.

Removal

To remove a soft contact lens in a baby, the lids are pulled apart as much as possible and gentle pressure is put on the superior and inferior lens edges; this produces a break of the suction allowing the lens to be lifted out by the lids (Fig. 18.2).

As the infant grows, the same method may be employed, although in some cases it may be necessary to hold the infant's head. If there is struggling, the lids may be squeezed tightly shut and this may actually help ejection of the lens as the lids are pulled apart by the practitioner. Once the child is old enough the lens can be 'pinched' off in the conventional way.

From about the age of five years, children may 'pinch' soft contact lenses from their corneas without any prompting, and indeed the younger child may remove his lenses frequently in order to impress his mother, which can prove to be a nuisance.

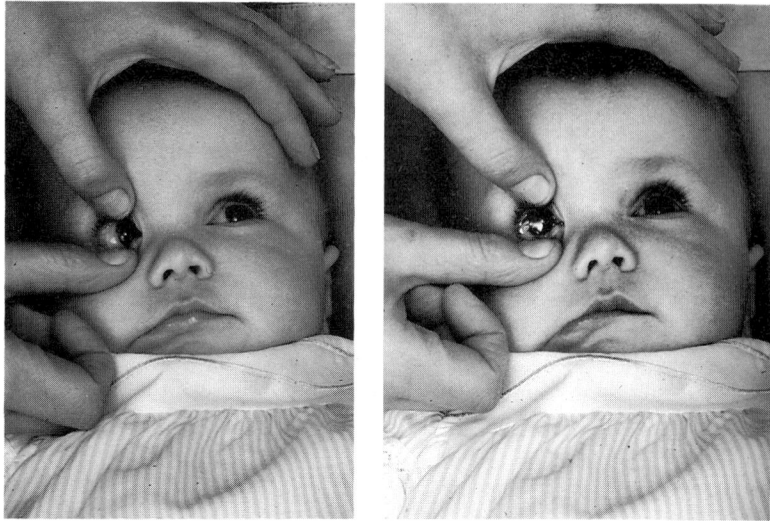

Fig. 18.2   Removal of contact lens for an infant.

18.3   Contact lens applications

18.3.1   Myopia

The correction of high myopia with contact lenses of all types may improve visual acuity and field of view, but if the risks of fitting and wear are to be justified then their superiority over spectacles must be demonstrated. The highly myopic child will usually develop normal monocular vision unaided, by holding objects close to their eyes. Therefore, the long-term effects of wearing contact lenses must be weighed up against the child's ability to cope firstly without, and then with spectacles.

With infants, the optometrist's first lens of choice is usually a soft lens. However, the complications that can arise due to the long-term wear of a large lens with a thick edge continually sitting on the limbus is of prime importance in the clinical judgement of this need. The parents must also be able to cope with eventual daily wear.

In extreme degrees of myopia, a child who will not wear their spectacles is in danger of becoming amblyopic. Sometimes, having tried wearing contact lenses but finding the experience too traumatic, they might have learnt to appreciate good vision and eventually take to their spectacles permanently.

The axially myopic eye is large and so infants of under one year may start with soft lenses of back optic radius (BOR) 8 mm and total diameter of between 13.5 and 14 mm (Speedewell, 1987). It may not be until they are four or five years old that they will accept a refitting with hard gas-permeable lenses that will obviously relieve the pressure on the limbus.

There have been a number of reports that hard lenses have a stabilizing or retarding effect on the progression of myopia (Morrison, 1956; Nolan, 1964; Baldwin, 1969; Kelly, 1975; Stone, 1976). The controlled clinical trial that Stone (1976) carried out over a five-year period involved a contact lens-wearing group fitted with PMMA lenses just steeper than the flattest keratometry reading, and a control group of spectacle wearers. The study showed a mean rate of increase in myopia of 0.1 D per year for the contact lens wearers as compared to 0.35 D per year for the spectacle wearers. Stone concluded that the effects of the contact lenses on the progression of myopia could not be accounted for entirely by corneal flattening, and suggested that the contact lenses might have a retarding effect on the axial elongation of the eye. We now know that PMMA is not good physiologically compared to hard gas-permeable (HGP) lenses; and fortunately hard gas-permeable lenses may give some degree of myopia control (Grosvenor *et al.*, 1989). Grosvenor's two-year study found an increase of 0.28 D in the contact lens wearers and 0.80 D in the control group. Corneal flattening, was also measured which was found to be 0.33 D in the contact lens wearers whilst only 0.13 D in the controls. Interestingly, they measured the axial length of the eyes and found an increase of only 0.1 mm in those wearing contact lenses but 0.6 mm in the spectacle wearers. This study, therefore, shows the importance of corneal flattening in the control of myopia. The follow-up study reported by the same team (Perrigan *et al.*, 1990) after three years of HGP lenses for myopia control showed that the mean increase in myopia was found to be 0.48 D for contact lens wearers as compared with 1.53 D for spectacle wearers. From other measurements they hypothesized that no more than one-half of the effect of contact lenses in controlling the progression of myopia could be accounted for by corneal flattening and that this flattening was accompanied by small amounts of elongation. These results concurred with those of Stone (1976) but they added the explanation of the change in keratometer readings by pointing out that the keratometer fails to measure the portion of the cornea that is crucial for determining the refractive error of the eye that has worn hard contact lenses.

18.3.2 Hypermetropia

Hypermetropes manage quite well with contact lenses. The cases which might benefit the most are the strabismic children, especially the group with accommodative esotropia (Calcutt, 1983). If soft lenses are chosen they must be of high water content from a physiological point of view, though in bilateral cases, hard gas-permeable lenses are often accepted.

18.3.3   Anisometropia

Unilateral myopes, or hypermetropes, are usually reluctant to wear their correction, as often the other eye is nearly emmetropic so they can see perfectly well without spectacles. Hence, contact lens wear, usually with a soft lens, may be the only method of attaining reasonable vision in the ametropic eye. This can also be helped by periods of occlusion of the good eye. The visual results obtained are better for the unilateral myopes than for the hypermetropic anisometropes (Geyer, 1974) although one would expect a problem from aniseikonia in the axial myope. It appears that the expected aniseikonia does not occur due to the perceived image size, depending not only on the retinal image size, but also on the distribution of the receptor units on the retina. These cases, therefore, seem to need the contact lens-induced larger image to cover the same number of receptors as the emmetropic eye (Stone, 1979). It has now been shown that aniseikonia with contact lens wear is less for axial and refractive anisometropia, therefore better stereopsis will develop the earlier contact lens treatment is employed (Winn *et al.*, 1986).

The results for unilateral aphakes are disappointing, even with contact lens wear and occlusion therapy from a few weeks of age (Moore, 1993). If elastoplast patching is not tolerated, then an occlusive contact lens can be tried or one of high power. With the occlusive lens, it is advisable to check the visual acuity through the lens as sometimes the good eye still sees better than the amblyopic one. In traumatic aphakia, dense amblyopia is common especially in children under nine, but a contact lens might help in reducing the amplitude of a secondary strabismus (Speedwell, 1989).

18.3.4   Aphakia

It is in bilateral aphakic children that the use of contact lenses in infancy has real long-term visual significance. Especially in bilateral congenital cataracts, the risks of continuous contact lens wear are fully justifiable by the results gained (Taylor *et al.*, 1979). Results show that early management of these patients, and of human amblyopes, enables essential early treatment and optical correction since the effects of visual deprivation start at about four months and continue with a cumulative, but decreasing degrees throughout the first decade of life. Contact lenses have been used in aphakic children for many years (Sato & Saito, 1959; Parkes & Hiles, 1967; Ruben, 1969; Levinson & Ticho, 1972; Morris *et al.*, 1979). Most of these authors achieved a high degree of tolerance in patients with hard lenses, but the advent of high water content soft lenses has provided even more potential for the full optical correction of aphakic infants and children.

Fitting under general anaesthesia does not seem to be an advantage, as the

Table 18.1   **Range of parameters of soft lenses in aphakic children.**

Age	Parameter	Value
Birth to 2 years	Back optic radius	7.00 to 7.60 mm
	Back vertex power	+34.00 to +22.00 D
	Total diameter	12.00 to 13.00 mm
2 years to 10 years	Back optic radius	7.80 to 8.10 mm
	Back vertex power	+24.00 to 16.00 D
	Total diameter	13.50 to 14.50 mm

cornea may be edematous, and also lens movement can not be assessed. Each eye is usually operated upon a week apart. The first eye is patched until the operation on the fellow eye to prevent the fellow eye becoming amblyopic. A week later the infant is fitted in the clinic. Keratometry has been found to be unnecessary as trial and error gives acceptable results (Morris *et al.*, 1979). The range of parameters for high water content soft lenses is shown in Table 18.1.

For infants the refraction is overcorrected, so that the anterior focal point of the eye/lens system is within arms'-reach, this being the sphere of interest in small children. The power is reduced as the child approaches school age and he or she is then prescribed bifocal spectacles for use at near. Initially, therefore, the retinoscopy will show a −2.00 D to −3.00 D over-refraction.

Silicone lenses are used for infantile aphakics. The lenses have either to be fitted under general anaesthesia, basing one's choice of parameters on a hard lens alignment fit done in the operating theatre (Clark, 1979), or basing it on a previous soft lens fitting. The lens is fitted about 0.2–0.4 mm flatter than a soft lens would be, for lenses of 10.80–11.70 mm in total diameter. Silicone lenses are often used on those infants who have lost a remarkable number of lenses and will not wear their spectacles.

The sustained wear of aphakic contact lenses has important connotations for the long-term visual prognosis in patients with congenital cataracts. The range of visual acuity achieved in those children attending the contact lens department of Moorfields Eye Hospital, London is from 6/60 to 6/12 in the better eye (Morris & Taylor, 1994). This allows many children to cope with normal education.

18.3.5   Cosmetic reasons

The reasons for fitting cosmetic lenses are much the same as for adults, and the variety of lens types available include sclerals, corneal hard lenses and cosmetic soft lenses.

Scleral lens-fitting can be done under general anaesthesia for the under three-year-olds if it is warranted in an unsightly blind eye. However, an impression can be taken in a young child sitting on their mothers lap with only the aid of a local anaesthetic. If the child will not sit quietly then he or she may be wrapped in a blanket and talked to by a parent whilst the practitioner carries out the necessary procedures (Kempster, 1983).

Soft lenses are most commonly fitted and often more acceptable to the child from a comfort point of view, as usually only one lens is needed. The use of hard corneal lenses is preferred in bilateral cases as they are physiologically better for the eye and are more readily accepted when both eyes are fitted.

Some of the conditions most commonly seen by the pediatric contact lens practitioner include the following.

Albinism

This is often associated with astigmatism and ametropia, as well as photophobia. In the infant, the correction of astigmatism provides little improvement subjectively, so a tinted spherical soft lens is much more beneficial. As the astigmatism in the older child is prone to be of a high degree, a tinted hard lens is probably better visually compared to a soft lens, but the optometrist should not be suprised if there may be no improvement over spectacles. The other factor worth nothing is that often the nystagmus present will increase from the agitation of adapting to wearing a hard lens.

Aniridia and iris coloboma

These cases need an opaque iris lens to occlude the light. These are available in soft lens materials but colour-matching with the normal fellow eye can be problematic. Scleral lenses can also be used, but involve more time for the fitting and are more occlusive to the ocular tissue.

Microphthalmos

These cases tend to have steep corneal radii and high hypermetropic prescriptions and so can be fitted in a similar way to an aphake. Those unilateral cases which only need cosmetic attention can be dealt with by fitting a tinted soft lens of plus power to help make the eye appear larger.

The use of a cosmetic lens for one disfigured eye is usually the parents' wish initially. However, once the child is aware of the cosmetic benefit they will often not go outside the home without their lens. The management of problems associated with contact lens wear then have to be thought through carefully.

18.3.6   Therapeutic reasons

Some corneal dystrophies call for a therapeutic soft lens (see Chapter 15). However, they are often fitted under general anaesthetic and eventual management in the clinic is very difficult because of the thinness of such lenses. They are not usually very successful.

18.4   Complications

In hospital practice, fitting high water content soft lenses for extended wear in infants initially shows a high rate of lens loss. In the pediatric contact lens clinic of Moorfields Eye Hospital, we found there to be an average loss of nine lenses in the first year and then 2.4 lenses a year thereafter. The major loss was by the one- to two-year-olds, but babies of a few months easily rub the lenses out during sleep. For continued optical correction, which is especially important for the bilateral aphakic babies, a spare set of lenses needs to be in store in the clinic, and with the parents. Once on daily wear, the problem decreases, and eventually lens deterioration is the major cause of lens replacement of about every six months.

Minor infections occur from time to time, especially if the child is on soft lens extended wear. The parents must always be carefully briefed on the removal of a lens if they see the slightest redness of the bulbar conjunctiva. If at this stage they are unable to handle the lens, then they must get local hospital or optometric help. If the infant is a bilateral aphake then removal of both lenses is advisable as amblyopia can quickly develop in the eye without a lens. The lens needs to be removed for a few days and a topical antibiotic instilled. Major infections have occurred in infants whose parents have been slow to deal with the redness, and all have had residual corneal effects.

Due to the risks incurred with extended wear of soft lenses, most infants and children are now fitted with daily wear lenses from the beginning. Neumann *et al.* (1993) concluded in their study of infantile aphakes that using daily-wear lenses avoids complications connected to extended wear use.

Vascularization of the cornea due to anoxia in various degrees has shown in about 25% of patients attending the pediatric contact lens clinic of Moorfields who were wearing soft lenses (Morris & Taylor, 1994). A child on extended wear must be refitted with a daily-wear lens, and if on daily-wear soft lenses, then hard gas-permeable lenses are needed. Otherwise, spectacles are often the preferred choice. This is also true for those children who develop contact lens-induced giant papillary conjunctivitis.

Studies of long-term polymethyl methacrylate (PMMA) wearers show many unacceptable changes in corneal structure and function (Holden & Sweeney,

1988). Lowering of sensitivity (Millodot, 1978) and endothelial polymegathism (Schoessler & Woloschak, 1981) have potential problems when the child is older, and so limiting the use of PMMA in children is advisable.

Children will present with all the common contact lens-related problems that one sees in adults, e.g. 3- and 9 'o'clock' staining. The main fact to bear in mind in pediatric practice is how much corneal compromise to accept clinically, remembering that the child is a potential long-term wearer of contact lenses. The importance of a backup pair of spectacles, and their use maybe once a week, cannot be put strongly enough to the child and their parents to minimize effects to corneal health.

18.5   Conclusion

In all young contact lens wearers, the demands of their social situation and medical associations of their ocular disease warrant close management by not only the contact lens practitioner, but also pediatricians, ophthalmologists, community nurses and educational officers. Good communication by all parties helps the child lead a full life.

As children are potential long-term wearers of contact lenses it is important to give them lens materials that are physiologically acceptable. Simple myopes and hypermetropes must be made to understand the importance of aftercare, as there is no ultimate material as yet. Only hard gas-permeable lenses and high water soft contact lenses allow adequate oxygen to reach the cornea but these are still fraught with problems.

18.6   References

Baldwin, W.R., West, D., Jolly, J. and Reid, W. (1969) 'Effects of contact lenses on refractive corneal and axial length changes in young myopes'. *Am. J. Optom. Arch. Am. Acad. Optom.*, **46**, 903–11.

Barnard, N.A.S. (1989) 'Hypnosis in contact lens practice'. *Con. Lens J.*, **17**, (5), 159–60.

Calcutt, C., Mathalone, B. and Holland, B. (1983) 'Contact lenses as an alternative to spectacles in accommodative esotropia'. *J. Brit. C.L. Assoc.*, **6**, (4), 137–40.

Clarke, A. (1979) 'Lectures by B.S Abrams: "Fitting Infants with Extended Wear Silicone Lenses"'. *Optician*, **41**.

Daniel, R. (1974) 'An evaluation of contact lenses in unilateral post traumatic aphakic children'. *Con. Lens J.*, **4**, 16.

Geyer, O. (1974) 'Contact lenses: the treatment of anisometropia in children'. *Con. Lens J.*, **4**, 6.

Grosvenor, T., Perrigin, J., Perrigin, D. and Quintero, S. (1989) 'Use of silicone-acrylate contact lenses for the control of myopia: results after two years' of lens wear'. *Optom. & Vis. Sci.*, **66**, (1), 41–7.

Holden, B.A. and Sweeney, D.F. (1988) 'Corneal exhaustion syndrome (CES) in long-term contact lens wearers: a consequence of contact lens-induced polymegethism'. *Am. J. Optom. Physiol. Opt.*, **65**, 95.

Kelly, T.S., Chatfield, C. and Canustin, G. (1975) 'Clinical assessment of the arrest of myopia'. *Brit. J. Ophthal.*, **59**, 529–38.

Kempster, A.J. (1983) 'Fitting cosmetic contact lenses in the Hospital Eye Service'. *J. Brit. C.L. Assoc.*, **6**, (2), 62–4.

Lake, L.H. (1964) 'Contact lenses in the treatment of infantile and juvenile aphakia'. *Brit. J. Physiol. Optics*, **21**, (4), 287–90.

Levinson, A. and Ticho, U. (1972) 'The use of contact lenses in children and infants'. *Am. J. Optom. & Arch. Am. Acad. Optom.*, **49**, (1), 59–64.

Lewis, T.E.M. (1971) 'Contact lenses for infants and children'. *Brit. J. Physiol. Optics*, **26**, (1), 61–8.

Millodot, M. (1978) 'Effect of long-term wear of hard contact lenses on corneal sensitivity'. *Arch. Ophthalmol.*, **96**, 1225–7.

Moore, B.D. (1993) 'Pediatric aphakic contact lens wear: rates of successful wear'. *J. Ped. Ophthalmol. Strabismus*, **30**, (4), 253–8.

Morris, J.A. and Taylor, D. (1994) '*Contact Lenses for Children. Contact Lens Practice*' (M. Ruben & M. Guillon eds). Chapman and Hall, London.

Morris, J.A., Taylor, D., Rogers, J., Vaegan and Warland, J. (1979) 'Contact lens treatment of aphakic infants and children'. *J. Brit. C.L. Assoc.*, **2**, (3), 22–30.

Morrison, R.J. (1956) 'Contact lenses and the progression of myopia'. *Optom. Wkly.*, **47**, 1487–8.

Neumann, D. Weismann, B.A., Isenberg, S.J., Rosenbaum, A.L. and Bateman, J.B. (1993) 'The effectiveness of daily wear contact lenses for the correction of infantile aphakia'. *Arch. Ophthalmol.*, **111**, (7), 927–30.

Nolan, J.A. (1964) 'Progress of myopia and contact lenses'. *Contacto*, **8**, (1), 25–6.

Parks, M.M. and Hiles, D.A. (1967) Management of infantile cataracts. *Am. J. Ophthal.*, **63**, (1), 10–19.

Perrigan, J., Perrigan, D., Quintero, S. and Grosvenor, T. (1990) 'Silicone-Acrylate Contact Lenses for myopia control: 3-year results'. *Optom. & Vis. Sci.*, **67**, (10), 764–9.

Ruben, M. (1969) 'Role of contact lenses in aphakia in infants and young children'. *Proc. Roy. Soc. Med.*, **62**, (7), 696–9.

Sato, T. and Saito, N. (1959) 'Contact lenses for babies and children'. *Contacto*, **3**, 12.

Schoessler, J.P. and Woloschak, M.J. (1981) 'Corneal endothelium in veteran PMMA contact lens wearers'. *Int. Contact Lens Clin.*, **8**, 19–25.

Speedwell, L. (1987) 'Contact lens fitting in infants and pre-school children'. *Optician*, 26–39.

Speedwell, L. (1989) '*Infants and pre-school children, Contact Lenses*' (A.J. Phillips & J. Stone, eds), 3rd edn. Butterworth, London.

Stone, J. (1976) 'The possible influence of contact lenses on myopia'. *Brit. J. Physiol. Optics*, **31**, 89–114.

Stone, J. (1979) 'Fitting children with contact lenses'. *Con. Lens J.*, **8**, (4), 22–6.

Taylor, D., Vaegan, Morris, J.A., Rodgers, J. and Warland, J. (1979) 'Amblyopia in bilateral infantile and juvenile cataract'. *Trans. Ophthal. Soc. UK.*, **99**, 170–76.

Winn, B., Ackerley, R.G., Brown, C.A., Murray, F.K., Prais, J. and St John, M.F. (1986) 'The superiority of contact lenses in the correction of all anisometropia'. *Transac. BCLA Annual Clin. Conf.*, 95–100.

CHAPTER 19

Management of Binocular Vision Anomalies

Ivan Wood

19.1 Introduction

Between 2% and 6% of the population express abnormal binocular vision in the form of a strabismus or amblyopia (Graham, 1974; Cuiffreda *et al.*, 1991). In many cases there is an inherited predisposition to these binocular deficits (Cantolino & von Noorden, 1969; Jay & Elston, 1987) which is reinforced by an environmental trigger in infancy.

The ideal goal of the treatment of these conditions is restoration of full binocular function. However, monocular restoration of visual acuity and cosmetic appearance is often achieved at the expense of binocularity, and in such cases the best that can probably be achieved is partial binocularity.

19.2 Management and treatment of infants below the age of 18 months

In this age group any eye investigation is principally concerned with diagnosing those infants who will suffer blindness through pathology or strabismus. The golden rule of 'no symptoms - no treatment' does *not* apply to the management of eyesight defects in infants. The clinician must rely upon an accurate history and objective observation of the infant when deciding on a diagnosis and treatment.

19.2.1 Management of disabling impairment in infants below the age of 12 months

The incidence of disabling impairment of vision is low in neonates, occurring in between two and four cases per 10 000 births (Hall, 1989). At birth, disabling impairments are principally caused through inherited congenital defects, retinopathy of prematurity (ROP) and gliomas. Neonates should be screened for various *risk factors* which might precipitate these disabling conditions, as shown in the following list giving risk factors for visual defects:

- Nystagmus
- Familial blindness
- Rubella
- Severe prematurity
- Mental subnormality
- Cerebral palsy
- Hydrocephalus
- Neonatal ophthalmia.

At birth pediatricians will detect any obvious ptosis, visible sign of cataract or nystagmus and refer for ophthalmological opinion (Illingworth, 1982). It is difficult at this stage to determine that an eye is blind, particularly cortically blind, because the behavioural responses of infants younger than two months may include apparent responses, including fixing and following faces, using a principally subcortical reflex. They may even produce a subcortical smile reflex. Even later, deciding whether a child is partially sighted or blind may be difficult.

Objective tests of flash and pattern electroretinogram (ERG) and visually evoked potential (VEP) may be used to investigate the patency and acuity potential of the macular area in suspicious cases. These tests may be complemented by electro-oculogram (EOG) eye movement analysis. Asymmetries in vestibular ocular reflex (VOR), optikinetic nystagmus (OKN), fixing and following eye movements can be used to check the patency of the visual and oculomotor pathways. For example, a sighted young infant will rapidly suppress post-rotational nystagmus following stimulation of the vestibular ocular reflex (VOR) by swinging the infant at arms' length (Mein & Trimble, 1991). Monocular asymmetries of OKN are observed in infants younger than three months of age. Temporal to nasal OKN is easily demonstrated, whereas nasal to temporal OKN shows little response. Infants of four to six months or older develop symmetrical OKN responses except in the presence of amblyopia. However, a positive OKN response may not necessarily indicate intact form vision (Marsh-Tootle, 1991).

Fixation preference is an oculomotor response which may be used to diagnose the presence of strabismic amblyopia. When the preferred eye is covered the clinician can grade the duration and 'quality' of fixation carried out by the non-preferred eye (Table 19.1). Strong fixation preferences may still remain despite increases in acuity following occlusion therapy (Birch *et al.*, 1990).

Table 19.1 Binocular fixation preference (after Rabinowitz, 1983; Garzia, 1990).

Grade	Description of fixation	Inferred acuity
0	Absolute preference for the fixing eye. The habitually fixing eye resumes fixation immediately the cover is removed. Unsteady eccentric fixation of the deviating eye.	6/60 or less
1	Strong fixation preference for the habitually fixing eye. The deviating eye can only hold central fixation fleetingly.	6/18–6/24
2	Moderate fixation preference for the habitually fixing eye. The deviating eye maintains steady central fixation until the next blink.	6/9–6/12
3	Slight fixation preference for the habitually fixing eye. The deviating eye is able to hold steady central fixation through the blink.	6/9
4	There is no fixation preference between the two eyes.	6/6 each eye

19.2.2 Management and treatment of amblyopia in infants less than 12 months old

Deprivation amblyopia

This severe type of amblyopia (amblyopia ex anopsia), also known as stimulation deprivation amblyopia, is most likely to occur in early infancy if there is any visual disruption due to, for example, lid lesions, congenital cataracts or persistent hypoplastic primary vitreous (PHPV). This type of amblyopia appears to affect the whole of the visual pathway (von Noorden & Maumenee, 1968).

To date, the reports of success of treatment for this type of amblyopia are mixed (Mein & Trimble, 1991). There is a risk of inducing occlusion amblyopia of the fellow eye if occlusion treatment of these young infants is not carefully monitored.

Refractive treatment of deprivation amblyopia with congenital cataract

Congenital cataract, which has a high prevalence in Down's syndrome, is generally screened for by pediatricians at birth, six weeks, six months, 10 months, 18 months and two years. Early detection should result in early referral to an ophthalmologist.

When diagnosed at birth, unilateral congenital cataract is usually aspirated within three weeks from birth (and certainly should have been aspirated by six weeks) to prevent deprivation amblyopia developing. Bilateral cataract extraction can be deferred for a few more weeks but should be carried out by eight to nine weeks after birth. Silicone (Gold *et al.*, 1988) or high water-content contact lenses (Morris & Gasson, 1992) may be fitted two weeks after surgery.

In order to select the parameters of the contact lens, keratometry readings may be obtained under general anaesthesia (Pratt Johnson, 1985) or by estimating the corneal contour. The specification of these lenses usually falls within the range 7.0–7.7 mm back optic zone radius (BOZR) and 13.0–13.5 mm total diameter (TD). The dioptric power of the lens required may be from about +6 D to up to +48 D and the lenses are ordered following a post-cataract refraction. These contact lenses may be deliberately overplussed by +1.50 DS to provide for intermediate vision.

Following insertion, lenses with a high oxygen permeability (Dk value) may be left in situ for a fortnight. These babies should be reviewed at four week intervals using preferential looking (PL) techniques to assess the visual acuity. Parents should be urged to visually stimulate the infant during waking hours with brightly coloured stimuli such as toys.

Extended-wear lenses are more likely to give rise to 'red eye'. Special prophylactic measures to reduce the risk of infection may include the parents instilling chloramphenicol 1% eyedrops morning and evening. If a 'red' or 'sticky' eye is noticed first thing in the morning then the lenses should be removed and medical advice sought.

The success of this type of treatment is dependent upon the cleanliness of the home environment, as well as the motivation of and the care provided by the parents. The expected resultant visual acuity from a bilateral extraction is approximately 6/12 Snellen at five years of age.

The success of treatment of infantile aphakia using intraocular lenses (IOLs) (Burke *et al.*, 1989) is difficult to assess due to the large power changes of the infant eye which occur during the first year of life. The refractive changes, if not properly compensated for, will affect the final level of acuity at five years of age.

19.2.3 Refractive treatment of amblyopia in strabismus

Strabismic amblyopia

Following cortical awakening at three months (Nelson, 1988) there is likely to be an increase in incidence of amblyopia with the onset of infantile esotropia (Costenbader, 1961; Dickey & Scott, 1987). One of the precipitating causes of this type of strabismus may be the excessive accommodative effort required by hypermetropes of about +3.00 DS or greater. However, for a number of reasons, there is a general reticence to prescribe spectacles before the age of twelve months. For example, there is no real consensus as to the direction and time course of refractive changes following birth (Thompson, 1987). However, in a preliminary study of refractive changes in infancy, Hodi & Wood (1991) suggested that the average spherical component rises from emmetropia at two weeks of age to +1.75 DS at six months and then decreases to +1.50 DS at twelve months. The large standard deviation of the average spherical component (~2.00 DS) measured in infants less than one year old may reflect the difficulty in obtaining a measurement.

Correcting the refractive error is critical to the success of amblyopia treatment (Kushner, 1988). In infants of twelve months with a previous family history of amblyopia and squint, the risk of amblyopia is significantly higher for refractions greater than +2.50 DS (Ingram *et al.*, 1979). For infants presenting infantile esotropia or a history of high hypermetropia there is a need to investigate and correct the refractive error because of the incidence of high degrees of hypermetropia (>+5 DS) associated with this condition. These patients should be refracted under cycloplegia and the resultant visual acuity checked, if possible, by an acuity card method and the deviation evaluated with the Hirschberg test and cover test.

In primary infantile esotropia, the full hypermetropic correction should be given. Additional positive correction up to a maximum of +1.00 DS may be given when this is demonstrated to change an intermittent deviation to a phoria.

In all cases the correction should be worn continuously and visual acuities, binocular assessment and cycloplegic refraction should be reassessed every three months.

19.2.4　Visual acuity assessment

For this age-group the method of choice for assessing visual acuity is by using the PL technique with acuity cards (McDonald *et al.*, 1988; Teller *et al.*, 1987). Improvement in the visual acuity of non-strabismic anisometropes or high hypermetropes is often spontaneous when the refractive error is corrected. However, the fine gratings employed with PL techniques do not produce crowding effects in strabismic amblyopes (Katz & Sireteanu, 1990). Indeed, aliasing of fine gratings may affect detection thresholds in the presence of optical blur (Thorn & Schwartz, 1990). At this age there are difficulties in maintaining compliance with respect to spectacle wear, and this may explain some of the differences in reported success in the treatment of amblyopia found in various studies using refractive treatment.

19.2.5　Assessment of stereovision

Although disparity detection has been *experimentally* observed in three-month-old infants, a *clinical* assessment of stereovision using the Lang test cannot be achieved until the age of six to nine months (see Fig. 19.1).

Where the full spectacle correction leaves a residual angle of squint, relieving

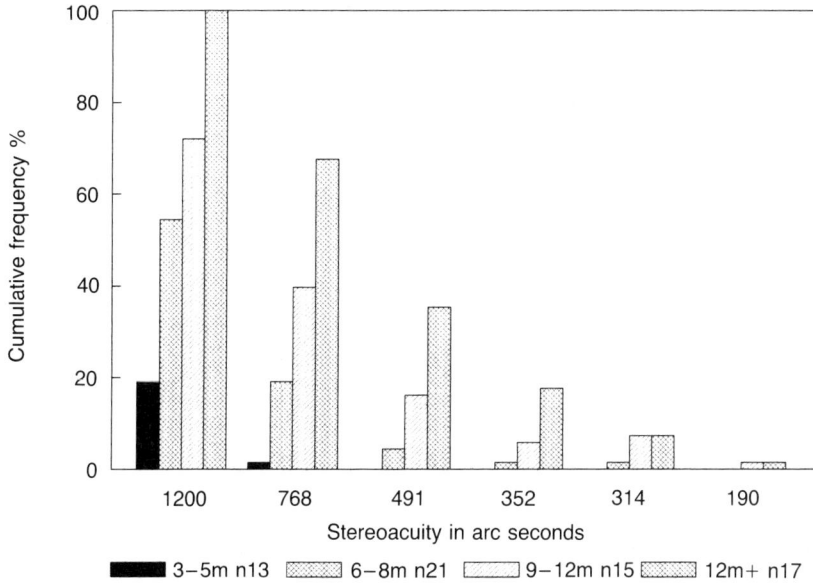

Fig. 19.1 Lang test for the assessment of stereopsis.

prisms may be incorporated into the prescription in an attempt to obtain bifoveal fixation. This may encourage full binocularity and equal stimulation of the cortex by each eye, with the result that visual acuity and stereopsis may develop normally. For angles of deviation of less than 45 Δ of misalignment, Fresnel prisms may be used prior to surgery. However, there are several disadvantages which may contra-indicate this type of prismatic treatment. With high powered prisms there is a reduction in visual acuity and overall spatial information. Moreover, prism adaptation (PA) may cause the angle of deviation to increase and subsequently return to its original magnitude after surgery (Bagolini, 1985). In those infants who lack fusion there is a possibility that an attempt at prismatic alignment may cause intractable diplopia.

19.2.6 Occlusion therapy for infants of less then 12 months old

With the correct spectacle correction in place, occlusion of the 'normal' eye is the usual way of improving visual acuity in an amblyopic (deviating) eye. The more profound the deviation and amblyopia, the longer the period of occlusion treatment required. However, continuous patching of young infants for more than three days may produce occlusion amblyopia and an esotropia in the occluded eye (Kushner, 1988). Therefore it is important to alternate occlusion to the fellow eye every fourth day. Fixation of each eye should be monitored by the parents who should be advised to remove the patch for half-an-hour per day and observe whether there is an esotropia of the 'normal' eye.

Fortunately, occlusion amblyopia and esotropia appear to be reversible. Weekly orthoptic assessment of visual acuity and fixation is required for this age-group. Once a plateau of acuity has been achieved the occlusion should be gradually reduced down to three hours per week. Such a regime of treatment appears to maintain the acuity gain in the amblyopic eye. For a more detailed discussion the reader is referred to von Noorden (1990).

Occlusion therapy using hypoallergenic patches is very successful, with the patch being stuck over the eye and not over the glasses. An opaque contact lens may be a viable alternative as an occluder.

In the presence of both nystagmus and strabismus, the visual acuity in the deviating eye often does not respond to occlusion therapy. Other therapies such as intermittent photic stimulation (Mallett, 1983) or biofeedback (Kirschen, 1983) may be considered when the child is older.

19.2.7 Management of strabismus in infants of less then 12 months old

About half of all neonates appear, by the Hirschberg test and the Bruckner light reflex test, to be orthotropic. The remaining neonates express an exodeviation because of their inability to fixate the target. Congenital exotropia presents in less than 0.05% of neonates (Moore & Cohen, 1985) and is uncommon in the absence of more profound neurological problems. A small percentage of divergent deviations may be associated with active pathology, particularly in the presence of incomitance and/or nystagmus. Therefore in any strabismus workup the presence of pathology must be excluded.

At birth, the presence of convergent strabismus is rare (0.1%) (von Noorden, 1988) or is quoted as begin non-existent.

Infantile esotropia syndrome, an acquired disorder of maturation of the visual system, is expressed from two months of age onwards. The syndrome can be subdivided into essential or true esotropia, nystagmus blocking syndrome and/or lateral rectus palsy. These squints are associated with large (>45° angles), good visual acuity in each eye and cross fixation. An ophthalmological opinion is recommended for surgery and to eliminate the possibility of active pathology such as, for example, retinoblastoma or cataract, which may be associated with convergent strabismus.

19.2.8 Surgical treatment for young infants

Infants with a sizeable and constant convergent strabismus are likely to develop a greater depth of amblyopia if their eyes are not surgically aligned. However, opinion is divided about the efficacy of surgery at an early age. Ing *et al.* (1966)

and Taylor (1962, 1967) claim that early intervention at six months is desirable for a functional cure. However, with surgery there are risks of under- or over-correction of the deviation. Schieman *et al.* (1989) have shown that late surgery for infantile convergent deviation is just as successful. Below the age of one year a conservative approach to surgery is applied to both constant and intermittent exodeviations and to intermittent esodeviations. A similar conservative approach is used with miotic and botulin drug therapy and the treatment of nystagmus in this young age-group.

19.3 Treatment and management of infants aged from 18 months to three years old

As infants mature, accommodative effort and visual acuity reaches near adult values and the incidence of accommodative convergent strabismus and amblyopia increases. Arousing the child's interest by playing games with matching tests for visual acuity, the cover test, ocular motility and stereotests helps make the assessment of the visual status in this age-group much easier. For example the infant may point to the various shapes displayed on a Lang test (Fig. 19.2).

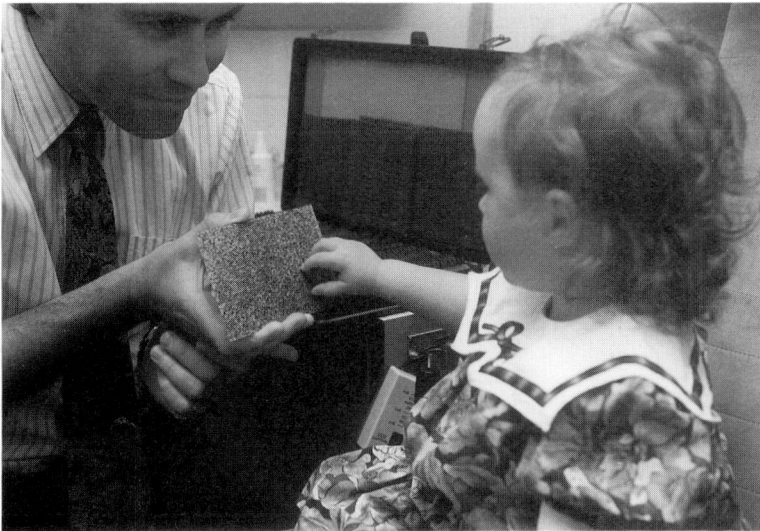

Fig. 19.2   20-month-old infant reaching for a shape on a Lang stereotest.

19.3.1   Refractive management of infants aged from 18 months to three years old

Testing acuity

From 18 months onwards a cooperative child may indicate differences in visual acuity through picture tests, as well as with the more sophisticated Sheridan– Gardiner test or crowded acuity cards. This enables the clinician to check the improvement of the acuity with the spectacle prescription in place. Single letters (angular acuity) will give an overestimate of visual acuity compared to a conventional Snellen test (morphoscopic acuity) because of the 'crowding phenomenon'.

Refractive management of convergent deviations

The refractive management of accommodative convergent deviations for this age-group is the same as discussed above for infants up to a one-year-old. Cycloplegic corrections greater than +1.50 DS and larger than 1.00 D cylinder may be prescribed. Over-correcting the dominant fixing eye by +0.50 DS causes insignificant blur and may encourage the non-dominant eye to fixate at distance.

In convergence excess cases, prescribing bifocals may be considered. The power of the addition may be determined by gradually increasing the plus power and for each spherical increase carrying out the cover test to determine the minimum lens power required to straighten the squint. An assessment of stereopsis can be carried with this correction in place. A straight top bifocal with a large reading segment (either an Executive bifocal or a large D segment bifocal with a segment diameter up to 45 mm) should be prescribed; the top of the segment should be placed 1 mm below the edge of the inferior edge of the pupil. This will make it difficult for the child to avoid looking through the addition when reading or viewing near tasks. A review of the effectivity of the addition should be made within three months at which time the cover test and an evaluation of stereovision should be carried out. The refraction should be reviewed every six months before and after instillation of a cycloplegic. After about one year of continuous wear the practitioner should aim to reduce the power of the addition by 0.50 DS decrements at regular intervals.

Refractive management of divergent deviations

For intermittent divergence excess cases a binocular minus addition of up to −5.00 DS may be used to control the exodeviation in order that bifoveal fixation is obtained, and at this age this may be confirmed with the cover test and, if available, a distance (6 m) stereotest.

19.3.2 Treatment of amblyopia in infants aged 18 months to three years old

Occlusion of the 'good' eye with the amblyopic eye refractively corrected for all waking hours, for three days per week is likely to produce the quickest gains in visual acuity. On the fourth day the occluder should be changed to the amblyopic eye (Burian & von Noorden, 1974).

As with infants of 18 months or less, follow up should be arranged at weekly intervals, over a five-week period, to check for improvements in visual acuity. The schedule of occlusion therapy should be gradually reduced as described above.

Fogging treatment (penalization)

This technique is used as an alternative or backup to conventional occlusion treatment. Table 19.2 outlines the different types of penalization therapy available.

Table 19.2 Types of penalization ranked from mildest to severest (D/V = distance vision; N/V = near vision)

Type	Indications	Aim	Method
Mild	To prevent amblyopia from reoccurring	Encourage D/V use of the amblyopic eye	Full distance correction with a +1.00 DS addition to non-amblyopic eye
Distance	In the presence of mild amblyopia or to prevent amblyopia developing	Encourage D/V use of amblyopic eye and near vision use of amblyopic eye	Full distance correction with a +3.00 DS addition to non-amblyopic eye
Near	In the presence of deep amblyopia with eccentric fixation	To encourage near vision use of amblyopic eye and distance vision use of non-amblyopic eye	Full correction with a +1.50 DS to +3.00 DS addition to amblyopic eye
Total	In the presence of high hypermetropia and moderate amblyopia	To encourage both D/V and N/V use of amblyopic eye	Full correction with a −4.00 DS addition to non-amblyopic eye
Total and cycloplegia	As above	As above	As above with cycloplegic

Mild and distance penalization without cycloplegia

The milder forms of penalization use a +1.50 DS to +3.00 DS lens over the non-amblyopic eye. This enables peripheral fusion to be maintained and helps to improve the acuity in the amblyopic eye.

Near vision penalization with cycloplegia

This fogging strategy is typically advocated in the case of a child with deep amblyopia who will not tolerate conventional occlusion (Rutstein, 1991). Several studies (McKenney & Byers, 1975; Timmerman, 1977; Willshaw & Johnson, 1979) have shown improvements in near visual acuity in a substantial number of patients, even in cases where conventional occlusion had failed.

This type of optical occlusion may be recommended in children with intermittent squint and nystagmus. A full correction for the non-amblyopic eye is prescribed for constant wear. To encourage the development of near visual acuity of the amblyopic eye, 1% atropine ointment can be applied once a week. In the presence of strabismus, a prism may be used to achieve ocular alignment. However, there is a risk that the preferred eye with the better acuity may fixate with a corresponding increase in the size of the deviation. The latter is due to the increase in the AC/A ratio caused by the atropine cycloplegia. A patient undergoing this type of treatment should be reviewed in a similar way as with occlusion therapy with the treatment also lasting for five weeks. Prolonged atropinization may not prevent the development of 'occlusion' amblyopia. Accordingly, the patient should be carefully monitored and the treatment interrupted if visual acuity in the normal eye deteriorates.

Total penalization using negative lenses and atropine

This type of treatment requires the dioptric blur, produced by a negative lens, to reduce the distance and near vision of the 'good' fixing eye below a 6/15 acuity threshold. Total penalization requires the vision in the non-amblyopic eye to be reduced for both distance and near vision (Deller, 1979). The treatment should last for two or three months until the amblyopic eye improves to within two lines of the 'good' eye. Although it has been claimed that this form of amblyopia treatment is less risky than conventional occlusion, in that it does not produce occlusion amblyopia, von Noorden (1990) does not take this view.

Like pleoptic treatment, penalization has not gained either practitioner or patient acceptance because the achievements in increased acuity are no better than those achieved by conventional occlusion (Rosner & Rosner, 1990). However, it may be considered as a treatment option if conventional occlusion fails.

19.3.3 Visual acuity improvements in the treatment of amblyopia

Unfortunately it is not possible to predict the acuity improvement for a given treatment regime. Most amblyopia treatment will last for four to six months and will involve that therapy every day for between 20 minutes to two hours. Levels of motivation must be kept high for these regular periods of treatment to produce successful results. Active therapy such as tracing exercises or computer training which help develop hand–eye coordination appear to enhance the efficacy of the treatment.

Further research into the change of monocular versus binocular abnormal interactions during treatment, the compliance of the patient, and the sensitivity of the acuity measures during the treatment is likely to provide more information about the prognosis using various treatment regimes.

19.3.4 Management of nystagmus

Nystagmus is a sign of an underlying pathological process affecting fixation and therefore although active pathology is rare in this age-group, every effort must be made to differentially diagnose the underlying cause of a nystagmus before initiating treatment. Significant loss of visual acuity is one of the main characteristics of nystagmus, the loss of acuity being related to the waveform of the eye movement and the duration of foveal fixation. To obtain a meaningful acuity threshold for those children suffering from subnormal acuity Grisham (1990) recommends the use of a Bailey–Lovie chart with its logarithmic progression of letters. If meridional amblyopia is suspected because of the presence of high astigmatism then tumbling E acuity thresholds may prove useful. In any event the goal of the treatment of a nystagmus is to dampen the amplitude and frequency of the oscillations which in turn may significantly improve the visual acuity. Fortunately the parameters of most types of congenital nystagmus naturally decrease with increasing age. However, the use of lenses, prisms and additions, vision therapy, medications and aligning surgery may help in this and subsequent age groups.

Optical management of congenital nystagmus

As a general guideline for infants and children over the age of one year with nystagmus the following refractive errors should be corrected: hypermetropia of >2 DS, astigmatism of >1 DC and anisometropia or myopia of >1.50 DS. However, subsequent three- and six-month checks may not reveal a significant improvement in acuity threshold.

Prismatic correction may be used alone or in conjunction with the correction of significant ametropia to dampen the nystagmus. A Fresnel base out prism ranging from 6 Δ to 20 Δ may be tried in the hope that increased convergence will help control the nystagmus. In some cases a head turn will move the eyes to a 'null position' where the nystagmus is minimal. Yoked prisms of 20–30 Δ may be used to move the image to the null position, thereby reducing the nystagmus and improving acuity without the need for the head turn. This latter type of prismatic treatment may assist in evaluating the likely success of a subsequent Kestenbaum operation to move the eyes to a null point.

Treatment of nystagmus with vision therapy and medication

Several 'amblyopia therapies' such as pleoptics and intermittent photic stimulation (Mallett, 1983) have been suggested to control and stabilize the fixation of the nystagmus patient. The use of an after-image in conjunction with the IPS treatment may provide the patient with feedback on fixation during the treatment

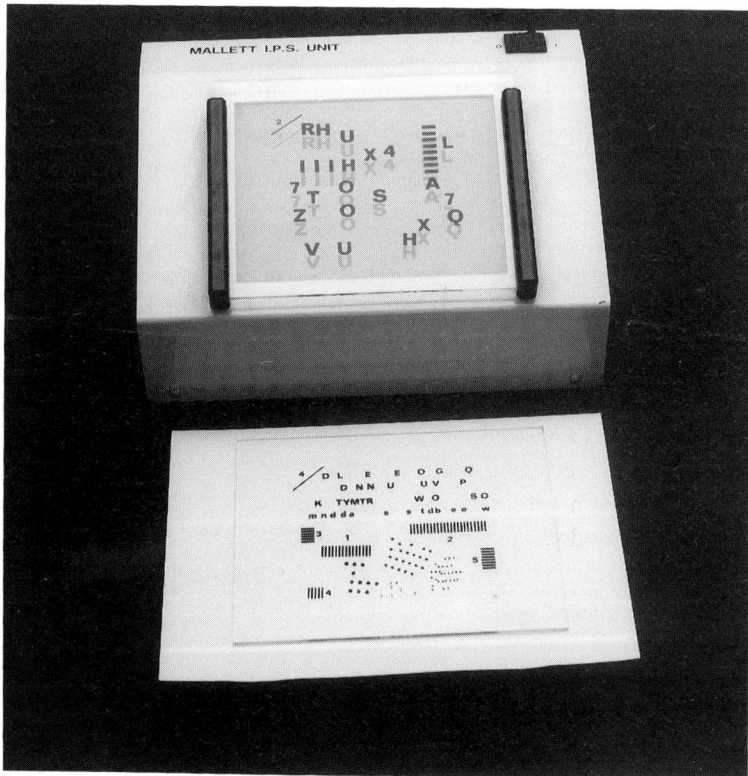

Fig. 19.3 Mallett IPS unit with slides for varying levels of acuity.

sessions. These treatment regimes are more suitable for school-age children than this age-group but require further studies on efficacy.

In the presence of oscillopsia, Baclofen, a glutamate inhibitor, has been reported to reduce nystagmus amplitude in congenital nystagmus (Yee *et al.*, 1982). However, these treatment regimes are expensive and not suitable for children.

19.3.5   Surgical treatment for infants aged 18 months to three years old

Surgery is indicated for cosmetically unacceptable deviations, usually greater than 10–15 Δ for divergent and 20–25 Δ for convergent deviations. Further attempts to align the eyes in infants suffering from infantile esotropia or non-accommodative esotropia may be attempted. Large (>25 Δ) intermittent deviations may require surgical intervention.

Surgical treatment for nystagmus

All types of surgery aim to rotate both eyes, whilst maintaining parallelism of the visual axes, into the null zone of the nystagmus. In the Kestenbaum procedure, the most successful technique, surgery is performed on all four horizontally acting muscles so that in the presence of, for example, a head turn to the right, each eyeball will be rotated left by resection of the right lateral rectus and the left medial rectus, and recession of the right medial rectus and left lateral rectus.

19.3.6   Miotic therapy in infants aged 18 months to three years old

Miotics, such as 0.5% ecothiophate or 1% pilocarpine, can be used as a useful diagnostic test and possible alternative treatment regime to decouple accommodation from accommodative convergence in accommodative squints of this age-group (London, 1990). The pharmacological action of a miotic will constrict the pupil and will act either directly or indirectly on the ciliary muscle to cause accommodative spasm. These peripheral neuromuscular actions reduce the amount of accommodation required for near vision, and hence reduce the amount of accommodative convergence expressed as an esotropia. The apparent reduction in excess convergence with this therapy increases the chance of sensory and motor fusion. However its use is usually reserved for hyperactive non-cooperative children who will not wear a spectacle correction (von Noorden & Attiah, 1986) and require correction of residual refractive errors following surgery (Kushner *et al.*, 1984). It should be noted that miotics are toxic and can cause side-effects (Folk, 1981).

19.3.7 Botulin toxin therapy

Injection of botulinum 'A' toxin into the appropriate extraocular muscle may be used to control both concomitant strabismus in infants and children (Scott, 1980), and inconcomitant strabismus in adults (Metz & Snell, 1985), instead of or as an adjunct to surgery. For example, a convergent deviation of the right eye may be corrected by injection of botulinum toxin into the medial rectus of the right eye. An exotropia may initially follow as a sequel. The subsequent alignment of the visual axes may allow fusion to build up and consolidate over the average two-month period that the botulinum toxin binds with the muscle. During this time antagonistic contracture may take place producing a long-lasting effect which may enhance the efficacy of subsequent surgical treatment of the strabismus. If intractable diplopia occurs instead of fusion following injection, then surgery to correct the deviation is contra-indicated.

19.4 Management and treatment of three- to five-year-old children

The onset of strabismus and its effects on the development of visual acuity and stereopsis become less of a threat in this age-group. The increasing span of attention of children of this age allows the clinician to refine the refractive correction by measuring acuity with tests to produce crowding. Subjective measures of stereopsis, suppression and abnormal retinal correspondence (ARC) may be obtained from a cooperative child. Observation of eccentric fixation with the ophthalmoscope may be achieved with this age-group. This additional information is useful in aiding the diagnosis and future management and treatment of these more subtle binocular anomalies. With increased cooperation it may also be easier to distinguish concomitant from incomitant deviations.

19.4.1 Refractive management of three- to five-year-old children

At this age glasses are more often tolerated once the initial trauma of wearing spectacles has been overcome. However, breakages of spectacles are frequent because of the normal rough and tumble of life at this age, and six-monthly optometric examinations are necessary even when a refractive error appears stable. Distance vision becomes increasingly important at this age, so that overplusing of any hypermetropic correction is not well tolerated. In the UK, the vision screening carried out at three years of age by community health doctors or orthoptists often reveals unilateral or bilateral reductions in visual acuity. This amblyopia is often associated with previously uncorrected anisometropia or astigmatism. In both cases the full amount of spherical and cylindrical correction should be prescribed from the cycloplegic examination.

Fortunately the visual system at this age of development is able, in most cases, to tolerate any induced aniseikonia.

19.4.2 Amblyopia treatment in three- to five-year-old children

A great deal of effort is required in monitoring occlusion therapy of strabismic, anisometropic and meridional amblyopic eyes at this age. Generally, the period of occlusion therapy needs to be longer. Up to four weeks between visits may be allowed as there is less susceptibility of the patched eye to develop occlusion amblyopia. The pattern of improvement of visual acuity varies tremendously from case to case. Unfortunately, many amblyopia treatment studies include any improvement in acuity as being a criteria of successful treatment. Most studies have small numbers of subjects and controls (Cuiffreda *et al.*, 1991). The clinical goal of obtaining 6/6 acuity in the treated amblyopic eye seems to be reached by very few at this age.

19.4.3 Management of abnormal retinal correspondence

It is possible to identify the presence of ARC using Bagolini-striated glasses in children of this age-group. However, treatment of ARC is contra-indicated because many patients have a useful, symptom-free pseudo-binocular vision with gross stereopsis which, if disturbed, may lead to intractable diplopia (Mein & Trimble, 1991). Of those treated for ARC, the 'cure' rate is only 5% (Wick & Cook, 1987).

19.4.4 Surgical treatment of three- to five-year-old children

Surgical intervention for all types of strabismus reaches a peak at this age primarily because of a desire for good cosmesis by the time the child starts school.

19.5 Management of children over five to seven years of age

Following any strabismus therapy that has been carried out at a younger age, a seven-year-old, or occasionally younger child, given sufficient practitioner and parental encouragement, may embark on a series of orthoptic exercises designed to further reduce any residual sensory deficits, such as suppression and amblyopia, and to improve motor fusion. The goal of all these orthoptic exercises is to improve both visual acuity and angle of deviation. For a good prognosis the manifest deviation will be ideally less than 10 Δ and the visual acuity of the deviating eye will be reasonably high.

19.5.1 Amblyopia treatment for older children

Conventional occlusion therapy may be used and has been described above. This may be supplemented by various active exercises such as tracing, drawing pictures with fine detail such as 'frog spawn', CAM treatment (Pickwell, 1989; Rosner & Rosner, 1990) and IPS. Whilst these exercises may be presented to the child as a form of game, he or she should be made to understand that the hard 'work' he or she will be expected to put in is designed to improve his or her vision. Many of these and similar exercises utilize hand/eye interaction and encourage foveal fixation and hand/eye coordination. Records of the patient's 'work', for example, the drawings and tracings, should be kept by the child to present to the practitioner who may wish to introduce a competitive structure to the exercises.

19.5.2 Pleoptic (after-image) treatment

Pleoptic treatment of functional amblyopia was championed in the 1950s and 1960s by Bangerter (1955) and Cüppers (1956). In this technique, an occluder is projected upon the fovea of the amblyopic eye and the remainder of the retina is briefly exposed to a bright flash of light. The patient is then encouraged to fixate on various targets using the unbleached fovea. The aim of this therapy is to encourage central fixation and instruments such as the pleoptophore were designed specifically for this purpose.

 After-image transfer treatment (AIT) was first suggested by Calorosa (1972) and has proved to be effective as both an in-practice and home treatment (Jenkins *et al.*, 1979) in older children with an amblyopic eye which has a VA of better than 6/36. To carry out AIT a photographic flash gun is modified by occluding the lamp with an opaque cardboard cover in which two narrow vertical slit apertures have been cut. A fixation target is positioned between the two apertures (Fig. 19.4).

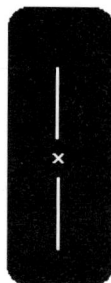

Fig. 19.4 Photographic flashgun, occluded apart from vertical apertures. The patient is asked to fixate the cross with the 'good' eye and the flash is fired.

The patient's amblyopic eye is occluded and he or she is directed to fixate the target with his or her 'good' eye. The flash gun is fired producing an after-image of the vertical aperture in line with the fovea. The 'good' eye is then occluded and the amblyopic uncovered. The after-image will be 'transferred' from the 'good' eye and is seen by the amblyopic eye in line with the fovea. Persistence of the after image can be assisted by arranging a lamp to flash in the treatment room at about 1 Hz. The patient is then directed to align the vertical after image markers seen through his or her amblyopic eye with various targets such as a letter on a Snellen chart. The working distance may also be varied. The after-image may be refreshed with the flash gun when it becomes faint, and the patient should be encouraged to cooperate and concentrate for as long as possible. With an enthusiastic parent, practitioner or clinical assistant, half-hour sessions should be obtainable by most patients and should be carried out two or three times a week if possible. Visual acuities should be recorded before each session, spontaneous improvements during the session should be noted, and finally the acuities should be checked at the end of each session.

The use of AIT in conjunction with Haidinger's brushes to detect ARC has been described by Cuiffreda *et al.* (1991). AIT therapy along with other active treatments of amblyopia such as the CAM apparatus may increase the percentage acuity improvement in those cases not responding to occlusion alone (Garzia, 1987).

Although many clinicians dismiss amblyopia treatment for children over the age of ten, there is ample evidence that therapy can be highly successful in older age groups (Kushner, 1988).

19.5.3 Orthoptic exercises

Orthoptic exercises may be used to treat amblyopia, and suppression and to increase fusional amplitudes. The ultimate goal of any orthoptic treatment is to increase motor fusional reserves and stereoacuity to 60″ of arc or better. The prognosis of such a full functional 'cure' for various types of binocular anomaly is shown in Table 19.3.

If the acuity response is adequate (i.e. 6/12 Snellen or better), orthoptic exercises may be used to treat suppression scotomata in the deviating eye initially, under static, and subsequently, under dynamic binocular viewing conditions. As motor fusional amplitudes are increased there may be an increase in stereoperception from peripheral coarse stereopsis through to fine stereoacuity.

There are many texts which discuss this topic in depth and the reader is referred to von Noorden (1990) and Pickwell (1989). However, the following discussion will provide the reader with some basic infomation on some of the training exercises currently used in practice.

Table 19.3 **Prognosis for a full functional 'cure' (modified from Rosner & Rosner, 1990).**

Prognosis	Indicator
Poor	None of the indicators shown below.
Guarded	Strabismus $>10\,\Delta$ with or without compensating prisms at distance or near.
Fair	Presence of microstrabismus with gross stereopsis (Wirt stereotest) or flat fusion with compensating prisms for the deviation.
Good	Presence of stereoacuity $<100''$. Recognizes presence of depth in random dot stereogram when tested through compensating prisms/spheres.
Excellent	Presence of high stereoacuity $<60''$ with random dot stereotests, and normal correspondence when tested at far and/or near through compensatory prism/spheres.

19.5.4 Anti-suppression exercises

Firstly, static therapy is carried out at the distance of binocular fixation, with or without compensating lenses/prisms. A traditional antisuppression training exercise utilizes the synoptophore and two brightly imaged targets, one presented to each eye, such as a lion and a cage. The patient is encouraged to see both slides simultaneously and superimposed. It is necessary to check for bifoveal fixation by carrying out a 'cover test' by switching off alternate synoptophore tubes whilst observing the eyes. Nowadays, simpler 'free space' exercises, such as the use of physiological diplopia, are commonly used.

Physiological diplopia techniques are primarily used in the treatment of suppression associated with the latent deviation of a heterophoria or the manifest deviation of a strabismus. These techniques utilize the binocular perception of non-corresponding points of the retina and cortex outside of Panum's fusional space. The symmetry of these diplopic points about the fixation target assures that normal correspondence occurs within Panum's fusional space. Once the suppression mechanisms of either uncompensated heterophoria or manifest strabismus are overcome, fusional amplitudes which oppose the heterophoria or heterotropia can be exercised and increased. To make certain that physiological and not pathological diplopia is being observed in the presence of strabismus (Capobianco, 1985), a cover test must be applied at the beginning of the exercise with the patient fixing the test target which is positioned in the primary position. The distance at which the target is set, the working distance, is determined by the lack of movement during cover testing. The physiological test target is then introduced, usually behind the fixation target, so that it can be seen in uncrossed diplopia. The patient is then given the tasks of controlling the fixation on the first target whilst observing the introduced target in physiological diplopia over an increasing viewing range. Having obtained a reasonable range of physiological diplopia, the patient's fusion range is then increased by diverging the eyes for convergent deviations and converging the eyes for divergent deviations by changing the position of the fixation targets. Physiological diplopia exercises can be supplemented using vectographic fusion slides (e.g. Vodnoy or Optomatters slides). These flat fusion and stereoslides are used to maximize the uncrossed (divergent) and crossed (convergent) fusion ranges (Fig. 19.5).

Convergence insufficiency

Physiological diplopia exercises can be used in the treatment of convergence insufficiency where the suppression of the non-dominant/deviating eye is accompanied by poor convergence and accommodation. By stimulating uncrossed disparate points on the retina/cortex, the patient is made aware of uncrossed physiological diplopia of a target while concentrating on a non-diplopic near fixation target placed at the limit of the reduced near point of convergence. Once the patient is aware of the physiological diplopia, the separation distance between the fixation target and the physiological diplopia target is slowly reduced until the patient is still aware of physiological diplopia with both fixation targets almost touching. By this time the binocular suppression mechanism which inhibits disparity vergence will have started to respond to the treatment and therefore the near target can be brought closer to the patient's nose and the anti-

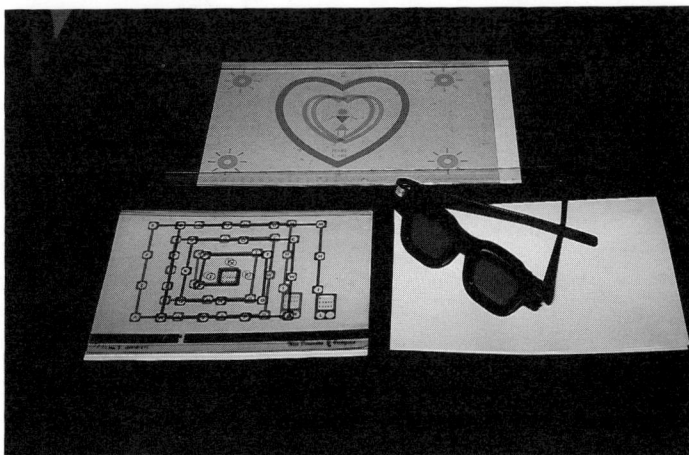

Fig. 19.5 Photograph showing examples of flat fusion slides (top) Optomatters (red/green) and (bottom) Vodnoy vectogram spirangle (polarized), both of which can be used to exercise fusional reserves in free space, and are ideal for both home or in-practice therapy.

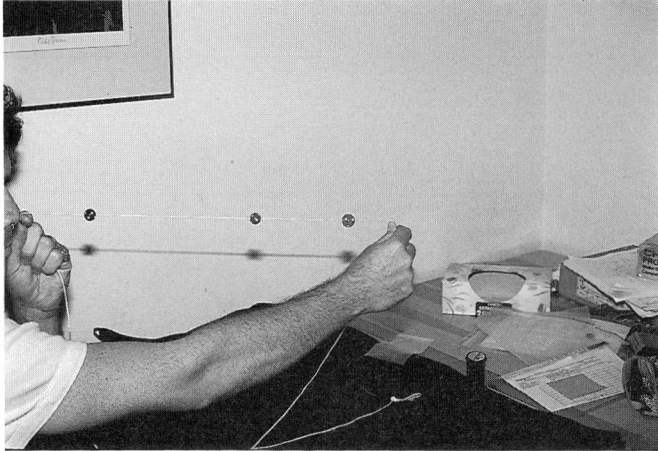

Fig. 19.6 The 'beads and string' shown may be used to exercise vergence whilst utilizing awareness of physiological diplopia. Red/green glasses may additionally be worn to aid awareness of suppression.

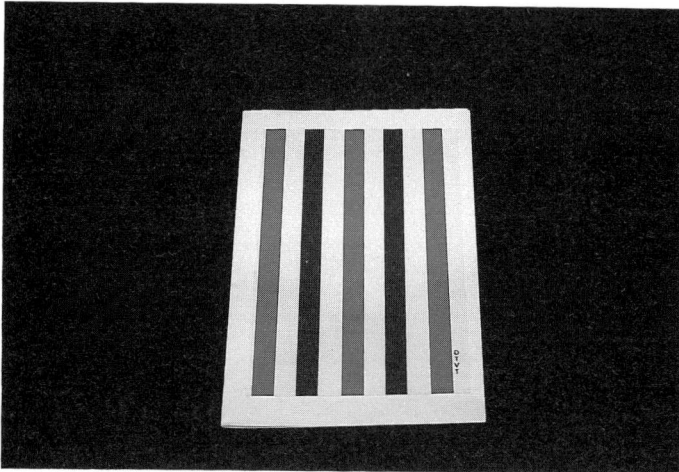

Fig. 19.7 The physiological 'bar reader' illustrated here is available with either red/green or polarized bars. The patient wears red/green or polarized spectacles and the 'bar reader' is placed over a page while the patient reads. This technique is used as a treatment for suppression.

suppression exercise repeated. This condition is quite rare in children below the age of seven years and is usually associated with an intermittent distance exodeviation. After 10 years of age the incidence of convergence insufficiency increases.

19.5.5 Biofeedback

From an uncertain start in the 1960s, biofeedback is now accepted as a valid treatment and has been advocated for problems which range from stress relief to refractive error. Halperin & Youlton (1986) reviewed the ophthalmic applications of biofeedback, including the correction of refractive error and treatment of nystagmus, strabismus and amblyopia. For each of these clinical entities, the review presented evidence to suggest that biofeedback might have a positive effect. The authors state that the precise mechanisms by which biofeedback treatment may work are not explained.

Hypnosis

Treatment of various ophthalmic problems by hypnosis probably falls into the same category of treatment as biofeedback. Although practised in the UK, there is very little written about the efficacy of this form of therapy. The technique can be most useful in teaching a patient to suppress an image when other methods of management have failed or are unacceptable.

19.6   References

Bagolini, B. (1985) 'Objective evaluation of sensorial and sensorimotor status in esotropia: their importance in surgical prognosis'. *Br. J. Ophthalmol.*, **69**, 725–8.

Bangerter, A. (1955) *Amblyiopiebehandlung*, 2nd edn. S Karger AG, Basel.

Birch, E.E., Stager, D.R., Berry, P. and Everret, M.E. (1990) 'Prospective assessment of acuity and stereopsis in amblyopic esotropes following early surgery'. *Invest. Ophthalmol. Vis. Sci.*, **31**, 758–65.

Burian, H.M. and von Noorden, G.K. (1974) 'Principles of nonsurgical treatment', in *Binocular Vision and Ocular Motility*, CV Mosby, St Louis, 424.

Burke, J.P., Willshaw, H.E. and Young, J.D.H. (1989) 'Intraocular lens implants for unilateral cataracts in childhood'. *Br. J. Ophthalmol.*, **73**, 860–63.

Calorosa, E. (1972) 'After image transfer: therapeutic procedure for amblyopia'. *Amer. J. Optom. & Arch. Amer. Acad. Optom.*, **51**, 862–71.

Cantolino, S.J. and von Noorden, G.K. (1969) 'Heredity in microtropia'. *Arch. Ophthalmol.*, **81**, 753–7.

Capobianco, N. (1985) 'Physiological diplopia in binocular vision (Normal and Anomalous)'. *Am. Orthopt. J.*, **35**, 30–41.

Costenbader, F.D. (1961) 'Infantile esotropia'. *Trans. Am. Acad. Ophthalm. Soc.*, **59**, 397–429.

Cuiffreda, K.J., Levi, D. and Selenow, A. (1991) 'History, definitions, classifications and prevalence', in *Amblyopia, basic and clinical aspects*. Butterworth-Heinemann, Boston.

Cüppers, C. (1956) 'Moderne Schielbehandlung'. *Klin. Monastbl. Augenheilkd.*, **129**, 579–604.

Deller, M. (1979) 'Are Amblyopic Man and Ape related'. *Trends in Neuroscience*, **20**, 216–18.

Dickey, C.F. and Scott, W.E. (1987) 'Amblyopia–the prevalence in congenital esotropia versus partially accommodative esotropia: results of treatment', in *Orthoptic Horizons*, *11–14*, (M. Lenk-Schafer, ed.). Mm. Trans. 6th Int. Orthopt. Cong., Harrogate.

Folk, E. (1981) 'Strabismus', in *Principles and Practice of Ophthalmology*. (G.A. Payman,

D.R. Sanders & M.F. Goldberg, eds). Saunders, Philadelphia/London, 1827.

Garzia, R. (1990) 'Management of amblyopia in infants, toddlers and pre-school children', in *Pediatric Optometry, Problems of Optometry*. (M. Scheiman, ed.). Lippincott, Philadelphia.

Garzia, R.P. (1987) 'Efficacy of vision therapy in amblyopia: a literature review'. *Am. J. Optom. & Phys. Opt.*, **64**, 3393–404.

Gold, R., Simon, J. and Sax, R.D. (1988) 'Contact lens fitting in the aphakic infant', in *Ophthalmol. Annual Review*. (Reinecke ed.). Raven Press, New York, 79–80.

Graham, P.A. (1974) 'Epidemiology of strabismus'. *Brit. J. Ophthalmol.*, **58**, 224–31.

Grisham, D. (1990) 'Management of Nystagmus in young children', in *Pediatric Optometry, Problems of Optometry, Vol 2.*, (M. Scheiman, ed.). Lippincott, Philadelphia.

Hall, D.M.B. (1989) 'Screening for vision defects', in *Health for all Children*. Oxford University Press, Oxford.

Halperin, E. and Youlton, R.L. (1986) 'Ophthalmic applications of biofeedback'. *Am. J. Optom.*, **63**, 985–98.

Hodi, S. and Wood, I.C.J. (1991) 'Refractive findings of a longitudinal study of infants from birth to one year of age'. *Invest. Ophthalmol.*, **33** (**S**), 971.

Illingworth, R.S. (1982) 'Vision', in *Basic developmental screening 0–4 years*. Blackwell Scientific Publications. Oxford, 59.

Ing, M., Costenbader, F.D., Parks, M.M. and Albert, D.G. (1966) 'Early surgery for congenital esotropia'. *Am. J. Ophthalmol.*, **61**, 1419–21.

Ingram, R.M., Traynar, M.J., Walker, C. and Wilson, J.M. (1979) 'Screening for refractive errors at 1 year of age: a pilot study'. *Brit. J. Ophthalmol.*, **63**, 243–50.

Jay, B. and Elston, J. (1987) 'Genetic aspects of strabismus. Orthoptic horizons 11–14'. (M. Lenk-Schafer ed.). Trans 6th Int. Orthopt. Cong. Harrogate, UK.

Jenkins, T.C.A., Pickwell, D.I. and Sheridan, M. (1979) 'After image transfer–evaluation of short-term treatment'. *Brit. J. Phys. Opt.*, **33**, 33–7.

London, R. (1990) 'Passive treatments for early onset strabismus'. in *Problems of Optometry*. (M. Scheiman, ed.). Lippincott, Philadelphia.

Katz, B. and Sireteanu, R. (1990) 'The Teller Card Test: a useful method for clinical routine'. *Clin. Vis. Sci.*, **5**, 307–23.

Kirschen, D.G. (1983) 'Auditory feedback in the control of congenital nystagmus'. *Am. J. Optom. & Phys. Opt.*, **60**, 364–8.

Kushner, B. (1988) 'Functional amblyopia', in *Ophthalmology Annual 1988*. (R.D. Reinecke, ed.). Raven Press, New York.

Kushner, B., Morton, G.V. and Wood, S. (1984) 'Use of miotics in post-operative esotropia'. *Am. Orthopt. J.*, **35**, 18–23.

McDonald, M., Sebris, S.L., Mohn, G., Teller, D. and Dobson, V. (1986) 'Monocular acuity in normal infants: the acuity card procedure'. *Am. J. Optom. Physiol. Opt.*, **63**, 127–34.

McKenney, S. and Byers, M. (1975) Aspects and results of penalisation treatment. *Am. Orthopt. J.*, **25**, 85–9.

Mallett, R.F.J. (1983) 'The treatment of idiopathic nystagmus by photic stimulation'. *Ophthal. Physiol. Opt.*, **3**, 341–56.

Marsh-Tootle, W. (1991) 'Clinical methods of testing visual acuity in amblyopia', in *Problems of Optometry*. Lippincott, Philadelphia, **2**, 219.

Mein, J. and Trimble, R. (1991) 'Ocular movements', in *Diagnosis and Management of Ocular Motility Disorders*. Blackwell Scientific Publications, London.

Metz, H. and Snell, L. (1985) 'Botulin toxin for the treatment of strabismus'. *Am. Orthopt. J.*, **35**, 42–7.

Moore, S. and Cohen, R.L. (1985) 'Congenital exotropia'. *Am. Orthopt. J.*, **35**, 68–70.

Morris, J. and Gasson, A. (1992) *Contact Lens Manual: A Practical Fitting Guide.* Butterworth-Heinemann, Oxford.

Nelson, J. (1988) 'Amblyopia: the cortical basis of binocularity and vision loss in strabismus', in *Optometry.* (Edwards & Llewllyn, eds). Butterworth, London, 189.

Pratt-Johnson, J.A. and Tillson, G. (1985) 'Hard contact lenses in the management of congential cataracts'. *J. Paed. Ophthalmol. Strabismus*, **22**, 94–6.

Rabinowitz, I.M. (1983) *Amblyopia* (Ch. 11, vol. 1) in *Pediatric Ophthalmology.* (R.D. Harley ed.), W.B. Saunders Philadelphia.

Rosner, J. and Rosner, J. (1990) *Pediatric Optometry.* Butterworth, Boston.

Rutstein (1991) 'Alternative treatment for amblyopia', in *Problems of Optometry Amblyopia.* (Rutstein ed.). Lippincott, Philadelphia.

Scott, A.B. (1980) 'Botulinum toxin injection as an alternative to strabismus surgery'. Ophthalmology, **87**, 1044–9.

Scheiman, M., Ciner, E. and Gallaway, M. (1989) 'Surgical success rates in infantile esotropia'. *J. Am. Optom. Assoc.*, **17**, 100–102.

Schmidt, P.P., Wood, I., Lewin, S. and David, H. (1992) 'Stereoacuity changes in infancy measured by preferential-looking'. *Optom. Vis. Sci.*, **69**, (12 Suppl.), 106.

Taylor, D.M. (1963) 'How early is early surgery in strabismus?'. *Am. J. Ophthalmol.*, **70**, 152–3.

Taylor, D.M. (1967) 'Congenital strabismus, a common sense approach'. *Am. J. Ophthalmol.*, **7**, 478.

Teller, D.Y., McDonald, M., Preston, K., Sebris, S.L. and Dobson, V. (1987) 'Assessment of visual acuity in infants and children: the acuity card procedure'. *Dev. Med. Child Neurol.*, **28**, 779.

Timmerman, G.J. (1977) 'The results of penalisation'. *Doc. Ophthalmol.*, **42**, 385–90.

Thompson, C. (1987) *Objective and psychophysical studies of visual development.* PhD thesis, University of Aston, Birmingham.

Thorn, F. and Schwartz, F. (1990) 'Effects of dioptric blur on Snellen and grating acuity'. *Optom. Vis. Sci.*, **67**, 3–7.

Von Noorden, G.K. (1988) 'Current concepts of infantile esotropia'. *Eye*, **2**, 343–57.

Von Noorden, G.K. (1990) *Binocular Vision and Motility.* C.V. Mosby, St Louis.

Von Noorden, G.K. and Attiah, F. (1986) 'Alternating penalisation in the prevention of amblyopia reoccurrence'. *Am. J. Ophthalmol.*, **102**, 473–5.

Von Noorden, G.K. and Maumenee, I.H. (1968) 'Clinical observations on stimulus deprivation'. *Am. J. Ophthalmol.*, **65**, 220–24.

Wick, B. and Cook, D. (1987) 'Management of anomalous correspondence: Efficacy of therapy'. *Am. J. Optom. Physiol. Opt.*, **64**, 405–10.

Willshaw, H.E. and Johnson, F. (1979) 'Penalisation as primary treatment of strabismic amblyopia'. *Brit. Orthoptic J.*, **36**, 57–62.

Yee, R.D., Baloh, R.W. and Honrubia, V. (1982) 'The effect of baclofen on congenital nystagmus', in *Functional basis of ocular motility disorder.* (G. Lennerstrad, D.S. Zee & E.L. Keller, eds). Pergamon Press, Oxford.

CHAPTER 20

Psychosomatic Visual Anomalies (Visual conversion reactions)

Simon Barnard

20.1   Introduction

Psychosomatic disorders are physical conditions in which emotional factors play an important part. The term 'psychosomatic' comes from 'psyche' and 'soma' meaning 'mind and body'. Emotional factors play an important part in most, if not all, disease processes but in predominantly 'physical' conditions their part is relatively small. Even in such clearly organic disorders as pneumonia or appendicitis, the individual's emotional state and attitude towards treatment and recovery affect progress. But these are not psychosomatic disorders as usually defined. Functional disorders of a psychosomatic nature may be described as those in which disordered psychopathology and physiology are so closely associated that both components actively and concurrently contribute to the natural course of the disorder (Barker, 1979).

20.2   Etiology

Freud (1910) suggested that oedipal-genital conflicts lead to unconscious 'conversion' of psychic energy into physical symptoms, thus giving rise to the term 'conversion hysteria'. It has also been argued that oedipal-genital conflicts are not the only factors involved in such a process (Kathol *et al.*, 1983a) and it can be seen from Table 20.1 that hysteria is by no means the only possible cause of visual psychosomatically-induced anomalies.

Because of the differing theories of etiology of this anomaly there has been much discussion concerning nomenclature (Table 20.2). Freeman (1983) believed that the term 'hysteria' should be abandoned because of frequent misuse and confusion. He believed, for example, that many practitioners with no psychiatric training wrongly associate 'hysteria' with malingering. Although he suggested the term 'conversion reaction' even this term is open to discussion because of its Freudian connotations. However, for the eye-care practitioner, a descriptive label is useful and the term 'visual conversion reaction' (VCR) is used in the discussions in this text and it is suggested that the term 'hysteria' be avoided unless a specific diagnosis has been made.

Table 20.1 Etiologies of VCR described in literature.

Etiology	Comments
Conversion (hysteria) (Freud, 1910)	Oedipal-genital conflicts.
Anxiety, depression, psychoneurosis or hysteria (Rada *et al.*, 1969)	
Neurosis (Van Balen & Slijper, 1978)	Neurotic conflict on basis of wish to express feelings of hostility and wish not to lose love of parents.
Stress (Mantyjarvi, 1981)	Stress at time of prepuberty and puberty.
'Complex family problems' (Leaverton *et al.*, 1977)	Conflicts centred around relationship between the 11 year-old patient and her father and stepfather.
Anxiety (Lincoff & Ennis, 1956)	10 year-old boy suffering from feelings of rejection and inadequacy in relationships with family and friends.
(Yasuna, 1963)	Pattern of school and home adjustment difficulties (26 children).
Abuse (Barnard, 1989)	Psychiatric trauma of sexual abuse producing amblyopia.
(Wolpe, 1953)	Amaurosis in 2 year-old girl due to rigid feeding and toilet training.
(Schlaegel, 1957)	Blindness in 3 year-old after being reprimanded by mother.

Table 20.2 Various terms used to describe visual dysfunction without organic cause.

Psychogenic visual disturbance (Freud, 1910)
Hysterical blindness (Wolff & Lachman, 1938)
Hysterical amblyopia (Yasuna, 1963)
Ocular conversion reaction (Krill & Newell, 1968)
Visual conversion reaction (Rada *et al.*, 1969)
Psychogenic amblyopia (Van Balen & Slÿper, 1978)
Amblyopic schoolgirl syndrome (Mantyjarvi, 1981)
Functional visual difficulty (Shute, 1991)

20.3 Epidemiology

Although not common, VCR will be seen fairly frequently by the practitioner who has a busy pediatric practice.

Eames (1947) found that 9% of 193 unselected schoolchildren exhibited tubular fields, with hysteria being positively diagnosed in 33% of the 9%. Yasuna (1963) reported having seen 26 children with hysterical amblyopia over a

16-year period representing an average of 1.6 cases per year. Van Balen and Slijper (1978) reported a total of 43 children between the ages of 8 and 16 years of age who were referred over a five-year period and were diagnosed as having functional vision anomalies. Mantyjarvi (1981) found an incidence of 1.4 cases per thousand children per year from a large population of 7 to 18 year olds.

The author has observed a higher frequency of mild VCR cases amongst large orthodox religious families where it is likely that stresses such as sibling rivalry may be greater.

20.4   Age and sex

Friesen & Mann (1966) cite Wolpe (1953) who reported a case of a four-and-a-half year girl with bilateral 'hysterical amblyopia' who had a well-established amaurosis at the age of two years. She was a poor eater who was rigidly fed and toilet trained. Therapy of a less rigid nature 'cured' her in seven months. Schlaegel (1957) reported a case of a three year-old girl who complained of sudden blindness after having been reprimanded by her mother. It would appear that the condition occurs most commonly at a mean age of about 10 or 11 years, although modal peaks have been found in the 13 to 14-year-old age-groups (Yasuna, 1963; Mantyjarvi, 1981; Rada *et al.*, 1969). This may suggest a possible pubertal association.

Analysis of the literature suggests that VCR is four times more common amongst girls (Barnard, 1989). Mantyjarvi (1981) even named the condition 'Amblyopic Schoolgirl Syndrome'.

20.5   Signs and symptoms of visual conversion reactions

20.5.1   Vision

These include:

- Monocular blindness (Leaverton *et al.*, 1977; Clarke & Clarke, 1987);
- Binocular blindness (rare) (Smith *et al.*, 1983);
- Amblyopia (light perception to 6/9) (Yasuna, 1963);
- Variable acuity between examinations or with suggestion (Rada *et al.*, 1978).

20.5.2   Visual fields

These include:

- Monocular hemianopia (Kathol *et al.*, 1983b);
- Bitemporal defects (Smith *et al.*, 1983);

- Binasal defects (Smith *et al.*, 1983);
- Central and ring scotomas (Lincoff *et al.*, 1956);
- Tubular fields in which the field is reduced in size and remains constant in size irrespective of the testing distance (Rada *et al.*, 1978);
- Spiral fields (Smith *et al.*, 1983);
- Oscillatory and star-shaped fields (Krill & Newell, 1968);
- Static quantitative anomalies (Barnard, 1989).

20.5.3 Colour vision

These signs include:

- Total colour blindness (Pickford, 1972);
- Non-recognition of Ishihara demonstration plate (Barnard, 1989);
- Non-consistent test results (Krill & Newell, 1968; Barnard *et al.*, 1990).

20.5.4 Accommodation

These signs include:

- Paralysis (Parinaud, 1900);
- Spasm (Souders, 1982).

20.5.5 Dark adaptation

These signs include:

- Elevated absolute thresholds ('exhaustion phenomenon') (Krill, 1967).

20.5.6 Diplopia

Includes:

- Monocular diplopia (Records, 1980).

20.5.7 Extraocular muscle palsy

Includes:

- Sixth nerve palsy (Meloff *et al.*, 1980).

20.5.8   Other anomalies

These signs include:

- Disturbances of reading and writing (Corboz & Felder, 1982; Barnard, 1989);
- Frequent blinking;
- Blepharospasm (Corboz & Felder, 1982);
- Pains in the eyes (Corboz & Felder, 1982).

20.6   Investigation and diagnosis of VCR

20.6.1   VCR versus organic disease

The possibility of an ocular, neuro-ophthalmic defect or organic disease MUST be ruled out. Misdiagnosis of VCR has been reported (Stroudmire *et al.*, 1982) and it should be remembered that conversion reaction can occur concurrently with organic disease (Kathol *et al.*, 1983b). VCR must therefore not even be tentatively diagnosed until the optometrist has carried out investigations to preclude the presence of an organic disease as far as is possible. Even then a referral for further investigations should be made when no improvement in the anomaly can be produced.

20.6.2   VCR versus malingering

Malingering may be defined as the 'wilful, deliberate and fraudulent feigning or exaggeration of symptoms of illness or injury done for the purpose of a consciously desired end' (Kramer *et al.*, 1979). In contrast, conversion reaction is a subconscious process. Whilst the malingerer is conscious of his deceit and is actually refusing, for example, to read something that is visible to him, the patient with VCR cannot see any more than he is reading at the moment and has a definite 'illness'. Theoretically then, the differential diagnosis of VCR and malingering is clear cut. It is the difference between simulation in malingering and unconscious determination in conversion. In practice, however, the delineation is not always so sharply and easily made, since there are varying degrees of awareness of the secondary gains that might follow in a conversion reaction (Kramer *et al.*, 1979). Conversion reaction and malingering can co-exist (Lincoff & Ennis, 1956; Barnard *et al.*, 1990). To confuse matters, the tests that may be used to diagnose VCR are often the same as those used to expose a malingerer.

It is likely that malingering is uncommon in children (Freeman, 1983; Van Balen & Slijper, 1978) as, at least initially, there is an absence of conscious gain although secondary gain may be recognized subsequently by the child. Shute

(1991) suggests that distinguishing between VCR and malingering does not serve any useful purpose and is potentially damaging. Shute rightly argues that a malingerer should not necessarily be condemned as 'bad' or 'wilful'. However in practice there will invariably be these connotations. Shute proposes the use of the term 'functional visual disability'. Whatever the term a practitioner decides to use, it is important that the parent does not see the problem as being malingering.

To tentatively diagnose visual conversion reaction, a high degree of suspicion is required (Kramer *et al.*, 1979). If, for example, a child claims a reduced visual acuity and examination of the eyes and visual system appear normal then suspicion may be aroused. This suspicion is enhanced if the visual acuity fluctuates or if the child exhibits visual field anomalies that disobey normal physical or physiological laws. Once suspicion has been aroused a number of tests may be employed in the consulting room to facilitate the diagnosis of conversion reaction. It is important that the optometrist thoroughly knows the tests to be employed so that they can be conducted rapidly and without hesitation so that the child is not disturbed by the tests.

The following tests and techniques are useful in the examination of children suspected of VCR.

20.6.3   Improvement of vision with plano lens and suggestion

The child is told in an optimistic tone that the practitioner has discovered what will make him see better. A plano lens is then placed before the amblyopic eye and the child is encouraged to read the 6/6 line on the test chart.

20.6.4   Size constancy

If a child is only able to read the same or similar size line on the Snellen chart when the testing distance has been reduced to 2 m or 3 m, then this is suspicious.

20.6.5   Tests for stereopsis

Assessment of stereoscopic vision of the patient with monocular functional visual loss may show normal or near normal stereopsis, an impossibility with true monocular vision. Levy & Glick (1974) found a close correlation between stereoacuity on the Titmus test and Snellen angular separation with perception of the target representing 40 seconds establishing the VAs to be better than 6/9 in each eye. Certainly if the child was able to read only 6/18 on Snellen then a correct response to 40″ gives a strong indication of the prescence of VCR.

20.6.6   Binocularity tests

A variety of tests of binocularity/suppression are employed in practice and these can give useful information with respect to suspected VCR. For example the Mallett near unit incorporates a useful test for suppression. For aiding the diagnosis of conversion reaction the test may be used in two ways: first, as a test for suppression; and second, as a polarized binocular test for near visual acuity. If a child exhibiting unilateral amblyopia of a significant degree is still able to read all the letters on the 5′ of arc line (CLOVEN), then this should arouse suspicion. If, however, he is able to read only half of the word at any level or reports seeing the other half as illegible dots then this is evidence against VCR. Care must be taken to ensure that the patient has not ascertained which eye is seeing which half of the target.

20.6.7   The mirror test

For the patient with severe amblyopia or blindness in one, or both, eye(s) a large mirrior ($\simeq$ 33 × 67 cm) is held close to the patient's face, with the practitioner looking over the top of the mirror to observe the patient's eyes. The mirror is either rocked from side to side, or up and down. In a patient with vision of a truly better level than manifested, the eye will move in correspondence to the mirror. According to Kramer *et al.* (1979) the mirror test is more reliable than opticokinetic tests.

20.6.8   Visual field testing

VCR in children appears to occur most commonly in children from the age of about seven years (Mantyjarvi, 1981) and at this age visual field investigation is usually possible in cooperative children.

The presence of tubular, spiral or other non-physiological fields may add to the index of suspicion.

20.6.9   Colour vision test

The author finds that children with VCR may misread or be unable to read the demonstration plate on Ishihara colour vision test, a figure that should be recognizable regardless of the type of colour vision defect present.

Rada *et al.* (1978) used any one of the following criteria as a basis for diagnosing VCR: (1) fluctuating VA, (2) tubular visual fields, an upward shift of dark adaptation thresholds after prolonged testing.

20.7 Optometric management of the child

Once the practitioner has been alerted to the possibility of VCR then techniques such as those outlined above may be added to the routine. Some of the procedures, such as the use of a plano lens, will involve a degree of suggestion which may immediately produce an apparent improvement in visual function. This improvement will confirm the diagnosis. However, the practitioner must not forget that VCR can occur concurrently with other anomalies.

20.7.1 Discussion with parents

Having confirmed the diagnosis the management should be dealt with in the following manner.

(1) Do not confront the child (that is, do not say anything that the child may conceive as you disbelieving him or her). Politely ask the child to sit in the waiting room while you have a chat with the parent(s) alone.

(2) Explain the anomaly to the parents in terms of the visual defect being akin to the very real feeling of 'butterflies in your tummy' when nervous or the real pain of a headache when under stress.

(3) Explain that the symptoms are real and the child is not malingering. (Occasionally, a child will conciously be pretending, but such cases are rare in children and the term should therefore be avoided.)

(4) Ask the parents if the child is under any particular stress that they might be aware of (examples of this might include sibling rivalry, academic pressures, bullying at school, parental marital problems). If nothing is forthcoming, do not push the parents.

(5) Explain that you wish to write a routine report (or a referral letter) to the family doctor and discuss your own proposed management, if applicable.

20.7.2 Discussion with child

(6) Ask the parents to leave the consulting room and invite the child back in for a 'chat'. Be very friendly and positive. Explain to the child how pleased you are to report that his or her eyes are very healthy.

(7) If the visual anomaly resolved with suggestion during the routine, reassure the child that the problem has now disappeared and will not trouble him or her again. The practitioner may wish to prescribe some simple home orthoptic exercises, such as 'pencil-to-nose', to further reinforce the 'improvement'. The author is of the opinion that placebo spectacles should only very rarely be prescribed, if at all.

(8) If the VCR was intractable during the routine, a question may be cau-

tiously directed towards the child as to whether they have any 'other problems'. The practitioner should be reminded not to confront the child and to remember that the determination of the underlying cause may need the skills of a counsellor or psychotherapist. Only in rare instances will referral for a psychiatrist's opinion be necessary.

For most patients, a report should be written to the family doctor, who may have information appertaining to previous non-visual psychosomatic disturbances suffered by the child. In some cases the optometrist may wish to suggest that counselling assistance may be required after other investigations to rule out possible organic causes of the visual anomaly have been carried out.

The practitioner should always be aware that, although suggestion may alleviate the VCR, the underlying cause, unless it was primarily a worry about vision or eyes, will not usually have been directly helped and may resurface in another manner.

20.8   Case history

The following case history has been included to illustrate the possible etiological complexity of psychosomatic visual anomalies. The name of the patient has been changed.

Miss Ella P. (aged seven years) was brought for an annual routine eye examination. Her mother requested that she speak with the optometrist alone and reported that Ella had recently been seen at an eye hospital because of her 'low vision'. This had been diagnosed as being psychological in origin, probably due to her mother having recently been hospitalized. The mother also said that Ella had 'made up' symptoms following a 'bump on the head.'

Examination of Ella showed unaided vision of 6/18 with each eye. This did not improve with correction of the low degree of hypermetropia, nor with suggestion. Stereopsis was poor and she misread the demonstration plate on the Ishihara test. Oculomotor balance, convergence, ocular media and fundi all appeared normal.

Throughout the examination, Ella continually sought the attention and reassurance of her mother, seeking cuddles and making eye contact with her each time she underwent a test or task.

In view of the lack of improvement in vision it was suggested to the mother that she take her family doctor's previous advice, which had up to now been ignored, that Ella be assessed by a child psychiatrist.

The whole family were subsequently seen by a consultant child psychiatrist who described Ella's presenting problems as that of 'complaining of symptoms in an attention-seeking way which produces sympathy from school or her parents, difficulty in making friends (she has no close friend and is rarely invited to parties), generalized attention-seeking behaviour, such as shouting or speaking in a loud voice in public and generally getting out of control'.

20.8.1   The consultant's report

Family composition

Ella's father was a businessman who worked long hours and who had a history of attending child-guidance type sessions when his parents sought help for his sister. He felt a 'scapegoat' at these meetings and was defensive about 'psychiatric type' interventions. He lost his father in the year of his marriage and became quite tearful when talking of his father's death.

Ella's mother was a part-time scientist who suffered puerperal psychosis at the time of Ella's birth. In addition, the mother described herself as having been diagnosed as allergic to her baby *in utero*. It was a most traumatic pregnancy with forceps delivery followed by a puerperal psychotic episode which lasted at least one year before recovery.

Ella has one sister aged four years. In addition the family have a series of live-in helps who undertake much of the child-care.

Early history

Ella's early history was very troubled, particularly in her relationship with her mother, including her mother's psychotic episode and the mother's need to return to work early and involving herself in local government three evenings a week.

Ella was said to have reached her milestones normally but she did have to cope with her mother's psychotic illness and approximately ten caregivers in the form of temporary nannies.

On meeting with her alone the psychiatrist found her to be a very frightened little girl struggling with a sense of loss and isolation and aggressive feelings.

During the family session, both little girls became wildly out of control and the parents struggled relatively ineffectually to control them with sundry threats. The younger sister tended to wind Ella up but was absolved by the father. Ella tended to be in the scapegoat position with her sister seen as the baby who could not help herself.

Formulation

The psychiatrist described a complex family history involving the father's unresolved bereavement and his leftover feelings about his wife's psychosis, which was extremely shocking for him. The mother is a very caring woman but desperation and sadness are very near the surface and she feels herself to have lost touch with Ella, and perhaps has never really been in touch with her.

Ella found herself to be out of control, with a sense of deprivation and she would do almost anything to attract attention to herself, even if this involved negative attention. At the same time, she got stirred up to a pitch of fear and excitement by being able to provoke out-of-control behaviour and threats from her parents (for example, that she would be sent to boarding school or adopted).

Advice

The psychiatrist advised the parents to seek individual psychotherapy for Ella and at the same time have sessions themselves in behaviour management advice in order to help Ella. The parents rejected the idea of individual therapy and opted for behaviour management.

Psychotherapeutic follow-up

Two months later the consultant reported a great improvement in Ella's difficulties. The mother had given up some of her extra work and was spending more time at home. Both parents had worked hard to intervene neutrally in sibling disputes. Therapy was continuing.

Optometric follow-up

A subsequent optometric follow-up two months later showed a complete resolution of all the initially reported visual anomalies.

20.9   References

Barker, P. (1979) *Basic Child Psychiatry*, 3rd edn. Granada, London, 157.

Barnard, N.A.S. (1989) 'Visual conversion reaction in children'. *Ophthal. Physiol. Opt.*, **9**, 371–8.

Barnard, N.A.S., Birch, J. and Wildey, H. (1990) 'Concurrent visual conversion reaction and simulated colour vision defects in a 12-year-old child'. *Ophthal. Physiol. Opt.*, **10**, 391–3.

Clarke, J.R. and Clarke, D.J. (1987) 'Hysterical blindness during dental anaesthesia'. *Brit. Dent. J.* **162**, 267.

Corboz, R.J. and Felder, W. (1982) 'Psychomatische wechselbeziehungen in der paediatrischen ophthalmologie'. *Klin. Mbl. Augenheilk*, **181**, 266–9.

Eames, T.H. (1947) 'A study of tubular and spiral fields in hysteria'. *Am. J. Ophthalmol.*, **30**, 610–11.

Freeman, R.D. (1983) 'Emotional components in paediatric ophthalmology', in *Paediatric Ophthalmology*, vol II. (R.D. Harley, ed). W.B. Saunders, Philadelphia, 1396–7.

Freud, S. (1910) 'Psychogenic visual disturbance according to psychoanalytic conceptions', in *Collected Papers, Vol. 2*. Basic Books, New York, 105–112.

Friesen, H. and Mann, W.A. (1966) 'Follow-up study of hysterical amblyopia'. *Am. J. Ophthalmol.*, **62**, 1106–15.

Kathol, R.G., Cox, T.A., Corbett, J.J., Thompson, H.S. and Clancy, J. (1983a) 'Functional visual loss: I. A true psychiatric disorder?'. *Psychol. Med.*, **13**, 307–14.

Kathol, R.G., Cox, T.A., Corbett, J.J., Thompson, H.S. and Clancy J. (1983b) 'Functional visual loss: II. Psychiatric aspects of 42 patients followed for 4 years'. *Psychol. Med.*, **13**, 315–24.

Kramer, K.K., La Piana F.G. and Appleton, B. (1979) Ocular malingering and hysteria: diagnosis and management. *Surv. Ophthalmol.*, **24**, 89–96.

Krill, A.E. (1967) 'Retinal function studies in hysterical amblyopia. A unique abnormality of dark adaption'. *Am. J. Ophthalmol.*, **63**, 230–7.

Krill, A.E. and Newell, F.W. (1968) 'The diagnosis of ocular conversion reaction involving visual function'. *Arch. Ophthalmol.*, **79**, 254–61.

Leaverton, D.R., Rupp, J.W. and Poff, M.G. (1977) 'Brief therapy, for monocular hysterical blindness in childhood'. *Child Psych. Hum. Devel.*, **7**, 254–63.

Levy, N.S. and Glick, E.B. (1974) 'Stereoscopic perception and Snellen visual acuity'. *Am. J. Ophthalmol.*, **78**, 722–4.

Lincoff, H.A. and Ennis, J. (1956) 'Differential diagnosis of hysteria and malingering'. *Am. J. Ophthalmol.*, **42**, 415–21.

Mantyjarvi, M.I. (1981) 'The Amblyopic Schoolgirl Syndrome'. *J. Paed. Ophthalmol. Strabismus*, **18**, 30–33.

Meloff, K.L., De Meuron G. and Buncic, J.R. (1980) 'Conversion sixth nerve palsy in a child'. *Psychosomatics*, **21**, 769–70.

Parinaud, M. (1900) 'The ocular manifestations of hysteria', in *System of Diseases of the Eye*, vol. 4. (W.F. Norris & C.A. Oliver, eds). Lippincott, Philadelphia.

Pickford, R.W. (1972) 'A case of hysterical colour blindness reconsidered'. *Mod. Prob. Ophthalmol.*, **11**, 165–7.

Rada, R.R., Meyer, G.G. and Krill, A.E. (1969) 'Visual conversion reaction in children. I. Diagnosis'. *Psychosomatics*, **10**, 23–8.

Rada, R.R., Meyer, G.G. and Kellner, R. (1978) 'Visual conversion reaction in children and adults'. *J. Nerv. Mental. Dis.*, **166**, 580–7.

Records, R.E. (1980) 'Monocular diplopia'. *Surv. Ophthalmol.*, **24**, 303–306.

Schlaegel, T.F. (1957) *Psychosomatic Ophthalmology*. Williams & Wilkins, Baltimore, 370.

Shute, R.H. (1991) *Psychology in Vision Care*. Butterworth-Heinemann, Oxford, 72.

Smith, C.H., Beck, R.W. and Mills, R.P. (1983) 'Functional disease in neuro-ophthalmology'. *Neurol. Clin.*, **1**, 955–71.

Souders, B.F. (1982) 'Hysterical convergence spasm'. *Arch. Ophthalmol.*, **27**, 361–5.

Stroudmire, A., Stork, M., Simel, D. and Houpt, J. (1982) 'Neuro-ophthalmic system lupus erythematosis misdiagnosed as hysterical blindness'. *Am. J. Psychiat.*, **139**, 1194–7.

Van Balen, A.Th.M. and Slijper, F.E.M. (1978) 'Psychogenic Amblyopia in Children'. *J. Paed. Ophthalmol. Strabismus*, **15**, 164–7.

Wolff, E. and Lachman, G.S. (1938) 'Hysterical blindness in children'. *Am. J. Dis. Child.*, **55**, 743–9.

Wolpe, Z.S. (1953) 'Psychogenic visual disturbance in a four year old child'. *Nervous Dis. Child.*, **10**, 314.

Yasuna, E.R. (1963) 'Hysterical amblyopia in children'. *Am. J. Dis. Child.*, **106**, 68–73.

CHAPTER 21
Children with Low Vision

Janet Silver & Elizabeth Gould

The practitioner in pediatric optometry occasionally comes across the problem of children with visual impairment; they present a very considerable challenge. Most often such children are already under the care of the appropriate medical and ophthalmological services. Occasionally they are not and, if discovered, must be referred on immediately.

In 1992 a World Health Organization (WHO) working group developed a definition of low vision as follows:

> A person with low vision is one who has impairment of visual functioning even after treatment and/or standard refractive correction and has a visual acuity of less than 6/18 to light perception, or a visual field of less than 10° from the point of fixation, but who uses, or is potentially able to use, vision for the planning and/or execution of a task.
>
> (WHO 1993)

It should be noted that this includes many children who are registerable as 'blind'.

Other important WHO-defined terms used in this chapter include:

Impairment: is any reduction of function.
Disability: is when that impairment makes *any* task difficult or impossible.
Handicap: is when that [difficult or impossible task] is a *desired* task.

Thus an uncorrected myope needing −1.00 has an *impairment* (his distant vision acuity is likely to be 6/18); his *disability* is that he is unable to see the blackboard from the back of the classroom; and his *handicap* is removed if he sits right at the front of the class, or obtains spectacles.

In the developed countries children represent less than 5% of the recognized visually disabled. But, although small in number (since most visual disability is due to degenerative processes and occurs among the elderly), children represent a lot of 'patient years'. The aim of low vision practice is to develop the child's visual abilities to his absolute limit and allow him to use normal materials in a normal environment, so far as it is possible.

360

21.1   Etiology

Although much visual disability is unrecognized and unreported, on the whole children are a well-served group, though the occasional child remains unrecognized until a fairly late stage. Disorders may be congenital, or acquired, with a further group with genetically determined disease becoming manifest during education. Typical of the latter group are some of the pigmentary degenerations.

Although accurate statistics are hard to obtain, the largest group of visually disabled children have *optic atrophy*. This may be due to some perinatal event or be inherited as dominant or recessive or be associated with another disorder.

Cataracts

These are the next largest group and are managed optically in various ways. From the point of view of the optometrist, much depends on the optical correction. If there has been early surgical intervention in both eyes there is a chance of binocular function. The low vision practitioner must bear in mind that, along with the lens, the child has lost accommodation although the near and distance acuities are often anomalous. At present, few children are pseudophakic, with contact lenses probably providing the best correction and spectacles the alternative. For some children with low vision, the 30% larger image size produced by spectacles has advantages.

Albinism

Tyrosinase negative albinos are instantly recognizable, but the tyrosinase positive and the rarer syndromes, such as rufous albinos, are easily missed. Although many albinos do have strabismus, in others crude binocular function can be demonstrated, and nearly all prefer to have both eyes open. Indeed, better acuity can be demonstrated with both eyes than with one occluded. The refractive error should be fully corrected. Very often full hypermetropic correction can reduce, or even eliminate, the need for near aids, because nearly all albino children have N8 or better with simple refractive connection if they are encouraged to select the best near vision position.

Pigmentary degenerations

Of the other congenital disorders, the pigmentary degenerations, rubella retinopathy, buphthalmos, aniridia and high myopia all make significant contributions. Despite current knowledge, retrolental fibroplasia is still seen. Even sadder are the cases of trauma particularly when the other eye is amblyopic. The optometrist will need some good reference books for the rare syndromes which do occasionally occur, often associated with skeletal or metabolic abnormalities. Furthermore, multiple disability is increasing.

21.2 Diagnosis and referral

Although in a few cases the optometrist may be the first person to recognize a visual disability in a child, most congenital disability is picked up very early in life, usually by the parents. Pediatricians will probably have been involved and the child is likely to be under the care of an ophthalmologist. The doctors should have made the parents aware of many of the problems that the child might have – the diagnosis, prognosis, and so on. Some parents report having explored the literature and are very knowledgeable about the child's disorder. Yet others will even be ignorant of what the diagnosis is and it frequently falls to the optometrist to explain the visual effects of the disorder and what the child can and cannot do.

It is common to find parents who are determined that the child will do everything that his fully-sighted peers can do. Others over-protect the child so that his or her impairment turns the child, in effect, into an invalid, and there is every variation in between.

Referral to an optometrist may originate from the parents. It is often at the suggestion of a well-informed teacher; but usually the referral comes from an ophthalmologist. In the UK, handicapped children have usually been put through the battery of tests needed for a statement of educational needs, and a referral is often a consequence of this.

If the child is in special education or is receiving help from a peripatetic teacher of the visually handicapped he or she may have been supplied with a magnifier. These are usually large magnifiers which will help with large print, but will be inappropriate to small print. He or she may have been given special enlarged materials, use the blackboard very little and may even have closed-circuit television available. Children with very low vision may be learning Braille which is learned easily young and may well be useful for some purposes in the presence of very low acuity, even if the prognosis is stable.

21.3 The consulting room

Any practitioner intending to see low vision patients needs a basic set-up, i.e. normal refraction equipment, plus some extra dedicated equipment, including:

(1) simple magnifiers with and without illumination, both hand-held and stand-mounted;
(2) spectacle magnifiers, etc;

(3) distant vision telescopes, monocular and binocular, hand-held for auxiliary use;
(4) spectacle and other head-mounted telescope, monocular and binocular;
(5) special frames suitable for the above;
(6) electronic reading machines;
(7) masks, etc;
(8) appropriate test material.

Most practitioners will adopt one of the large kits available from major manufacturers. Keeler produce an excellent range, so do Zeiss (from Germany) as do Designs for Vision (in the USA). For reasons that are not clear, some patients will do very well with one device and reject a technically very similar device from another manufacturer. Therefore, the practitioner will need alternatives available at every level. For young children, a closed-circuit colour television is very useful for looking at picture books, even though colour perception is usually seriously impaired. Although each practitioner will develop his or her own preferences, and much depends on local supply conditions, he or she will nonetheless need to be fully aware of everything that is available, and develop a good system for accessing information on devices that he or she does not hold. The British Standards Institution (BSI) has developed standards for optical low vision aids, and international standards are close to publication.

Manufacturers are inconsistent in their terminology when describing magnifiers, especially when referring to the magnification of the device. The optometrist needs to familiarize himself with the characteristics of the equipment he uses. Two calculations of magnification for hand/stand magnifiers and simple spectacles are commonly found:

$$\text{(Eq. 1)} \quad M = \frac{F}{4} \qquad\qquad \text{(Eq. 2)} \quad M = \frac{F}{4} + 1$$

(when F is the equivalent power of the lens in dioptres.)

The problem of magnification is probably easiest to tackle if one thinks in terms of angular subtense at the retina – which is how many telescope are described, the others using straightforward linear multiplication.

In addition to the optical and electronic devices, it is necessary to have some special assessment material. We consider that young children can give an accurate acuity by matching from the age of about $2\frac{1}{2}$ years. Single-letter optotypes are not a good predictor of reading acuity, therefore modern tests have been developed that allow measurement for both near and distant vision. With optotypes close enough for the possibility of confusion at every level, the Sonksen–Silver acuity system is preferred by the writers, but the Lea test, using simple symbols, is very comprehensive and includes simple to use colour vision and contrast sensitivity tests, and the Cardiff test also has advantages. The McClure reading chart ensures that the child's vision is measured rather than his reading ability.

With a limited amount of time available because of the normal child's short attention span, it is important to prioritize the tests that we do so that, although contrast sensitivity is becoming more and more important, it probably cannot be justified as part of low vision assessment in every case at this time.

It is helpful if materials that are known to be problematic are available too. For example, a comic, picture material or photographs, an atlas, an Ordnance Survey map, a compact disc, a dictionary and so on.

Ideally, the child should leave the first assessment visit with a device that will help. Therefore, the practitioner needs to hold an adequate stock of the most frequently-used appliances. Prescription devices invariably cause a delay and the child will need to come back to have the use of the aid taught, the parents instructed, and the acuities confirmed.

In the UK, low vision aids are loaned to the patient and no charges are made. This system has a number of merits. No patient is barred from appropriate help by financial restrictions; aids can be given on trial and improved; rejected or outgrown devices can be recycled.

21.4   Low vision assessment

Any patient attending a low vision clinic needs to make preparations in advance. The child should bring to the examination any visual material that is causing problems as perceived both by the child and also the carers, plus examples of visual material that can be managed, and any devices in current use. We try to agree early on the problems that we expect to resolve, as things should not be left open-ended. For example, 'we agree that you would like to see the scoreboard at the cricket ground and read your comics as well as your school books'. At later visits, these aims can be expanded or renegotiated. It is very important to establish a good rapport with the child. To this end the practitioner is often wise to abandon his white coat and be rather less formal. We emphasize that it is not only school tasks that cause problems, as far more time is spent at home. The child should be enabled to join in family activities on terms that are as equal as possible.

Present spectacles must be checked and acuity for distance and near measured carefully. Six metres is often too great a distance over which to communicate with a small child, mirrors are confusing and the error introduced by a closer distance is usually irrelevant. Any prescription can be adjusted, if need be, to compensate for such introduced errors. If the child is uncooperative about having one eye covered, a binocular acuity is far better than no acuity at all. We tend to allow the child to sit on mother's lap or even the floor if he prefers. Many children, though, like to show how grown up they can be.

Accurate objective refraction is crucial. Subjective results are not terribly helpful in young children but a competent refractionist will expect to be accurate to half a dioptre, which does not make a crucial difference when vision is low. Refraction under cycloplegia would have to be done at another visit since near vision is going to use any available accommodation. Alternatively, a cycloplegic refraction can be done at the end of the session. Using any of the visual acuity tests described above, it is possible to predict the level of magnification required, since they all have an arithmetic relationship between the optotype sizes. The distance at which any acuity is measured either for distant or near vision must be recorded.

If the child is aphakic, or for any other reason has no accommodation, a near addition will be needed; in either case, plus lenses are added, and the working distance reduced to achieve the level of vision required in the original contract. We prefer not to jump straight to a 20-dioptre reading add from a classic +4.00, but rather to move closer in two or three steps.

We recommend that spectacle magnifiers are described in terms of dioptric power, but regrettably they are often described in terms of magnification. It is important to remember that the magnification will be modified by the child's refractive error. For example, from Equation 2 above, for an aphakic child a $6 \times (+20\,\text{D})$ spectacle magnifier may well give only $3\times$ magnification with a working distance of 12 cm rather than the stated $6\times$ at the expected 5 cm.

Once the practitioner has established how much magnification is required then alternatives can be demonstrated to the child and parent. The young child may not be able to assess every suitable device in the place, and choices will have to be made. It may be necessary to limit this process at the first visit. Loan a 'good enough' device and continue at a subsequent visit. If the child goes away able to perform one of his required tasks then the visit will be adjudged a success.

It is important for the parents and the child to realize the possibilities of the device but also its limitations. Children will adapt very quickly, the parents less so; and the parents often have to be shown the limitations of the device. School is not the only place where acute vision is required. We have watched the delight on the face of a small boy looking at an ant under a magnifier, and a small girl who told us that with her distance vision telescope she had been able to see 'a real bird on a real tree' is always quoted.

The congenitally visually handicapped child is literally not aware of what he or she is missing. They may not have any visual material that is causing problems, or indeed not be aware that there is a problem at all. Bright children gain a lot of information from context and parents can be very confused, having been told that the child is registerable as blind but then see him or her rushing about and kicking a football as competently as their peer group. It is important to explain to the parents how the child does perceive the world, what he or she can and cannot do. Research has demonstrated that preschool children develop at a better rate if encouraged to use low vision aids. If it becomes normal for them to use a magnifier to acquire information, then the skills will be available later.

21.5　Prescribing

We tend to have a fairly relaxed attitude about the choice of devices at any given visit. If the child feels that pressure is being put on him to use a device, depending on his temperament he may conform but he may rebel. We stress to child and parent that the device is an available option to be used only when appropriate so, while he may use a telescope at a cricket match, for watching cricket on TV it usually makes more sense to have a cushion on the floor much closer to the set. We are concerned about cosmesis; any low vision aid announces the problem and, while some children seem to have no difficulty being different, others hate it. The device is more likely to be accepted if the practitioner does not pressurize and says that it can be used at home only if that is preferred; the device is then less likely to be rejected altogether. Sometimes the child appears to be put in a position where there is a conflict of loyalties. He or she may feel that abandoning a device loaned by a teacher involves rejection of the teacher, and will need to be reassured on this.

In some countries, training of low vision patients to use low vision aids is offered as a service. This has not been supported by properly structured research and there is no proof that training, as distinct from instruction, is of benefit. Here an exception must be made for low vision children who have been educated as 'blind'. Such children certainly do need considerable input to encourage them to use vision, and this is best structured by specialists who are usually orthoptists or teachers who themselves have been trained for this task.

21.6　Light sensitivity

Glare can be defined as 'unwanted light' and certain groups of patients do have this problem. The children with lamellar cataracts need shielding rather than tinted lenses. Albinos may well need protection outdoors, but need the best possible contrast indoors and for reading. Patients with RP certainly need fairly heavy shielding when they go out, ultra-violet must be cut out, and there is evidence that short wavelength visible light should be reduced, i.e. the lenses should be red or brown in colour. Perhaps 25% luminous transmission factor is optimal in the UK. Anything darker is for use on snow or the beach, and it is important to shield side vision in order to prevent the back surface of the lens acting as a mirror.

In the presence of cone dysfunction or achromatopsia, it is well worth seeing the response to very dark filters: somewhere between 2% and 5% luminous transmission factor should be tried. This should, under most circumstances, reduce the light to rod level with resulting improvement in performance. Such patients can be picked up quite easily. They are truly photophobic and find the chart easier to read without back illumination.

All children should be given plastic lenses, to prevent accidental damage and also because CR39 reduces UV transmission to a negligible level.

21.7 Follow-up

Very rigorous follow-up is necessary for small children. The first follow-up vision should never be more than three months after the appliances are collected. It is our view that devices should be supplied one or perhaps two at a time at the most. This way they become absorbed into the child's personal equipment and it is easy to add more at a second visit to solve other defined problems. If an attempt is made to solve all the problems at the first visit, it is often found that nothing is used. At follow-up visits there should be a certain amount of general chatter, talk of activities, holidays, hobbies, etc., involving both parent and child. This should elicit remarks about the use of the devices and the environment and occasions on which they were found to be of benefit and perhaps, more importantly, those when they were not useful. Many children express some distress at a follow-up visit if a device has been broken, scratched, etc. It is, of course, an excellent sign that the device has been well used, and can be quite useful to ask how long a pair of shoes should last and reassure the child appropriately. Acuities with and without the devices must be checked. Often a dramatic increase in acuity with the appliance can be shown. This demonstrates both that the appliance has been used a lot and that the child's skills have developed. It may be appropriate to reduce magnification. If a simple device such as a hand or stand magnifier has been well used, the merits of a face-mounted appliance will now be obvious and they can be added. It is worth remarking that children seem to respond better being given slightly more than minimal magnification. It can be reduced later, but the mechanism appears to be that, if the task is visually easy then the child will develop the other skills, and if the task is difficult the project gets abandoned.

Children should be reviewed frequently until their personal aids kit is stabilized, probably annual review is then sufficient as long as parents and child feel they can return to the clinic if problems arise sooner and for repairs.

21.8 Psychology

Visual disability invariably affects the psychological process of the individual concerned. When the individual is a child the parents share this burden. Parents may refuse to accept that the child has a problem and repeatedly request spectacles for the child that do not include telescopic lenses. Other parents can be terribly over-protective and restrict the child's development by doing too much for him or her. The optometrist is not an appropriate person to deal with these behaviours but he must recognize them and try to enlist the cooperation of the parents in a constructive manner. Some children seem to be quite happy and function well within their limits, preferring to swim than play table tennis; others seem very angry and try unsuccessfully to keep up with the peer group.

The advent of computers and the use of screens has made a big difference to visually handicapped children. We are concerned that the child should be equipped rather than the place and that, if a CCTV is provided ahead of an optical device, the child may become limited to one place. For the older academic child a CCTV is an excellent extra device. Adolescence is always painful and we have seen many children who use low vision aids happily at 12 years old refuse to use them at 14 years. We prefer not to be confrontational about this, knowing that the child is likely to return to the aid later, or perhaps to continue to use it in private.

Not every practitioner is suited to work with children. The qualities required are difficult to identify, but perhaps the most important is simply to be happy with children and to be able to communicate easily with them. With children, speed is essential, and therefore only practitioners very experienced in low vision work should attempt to work in this field.

21.9   References

Collins, B. and Silver, J.H. (1989) 'Recent Experience on the Management of Visual Impairment in Albinism'. *Ophthalm. Paed. Gen. In press.*
World Health Organization. *Management of Low Vision in Children. WHO/PBL* **93**, 27.

Index